Medically Accurate Illustrations

Concepts come to life with vibrant, clear, consistent, and scientifically precise images.

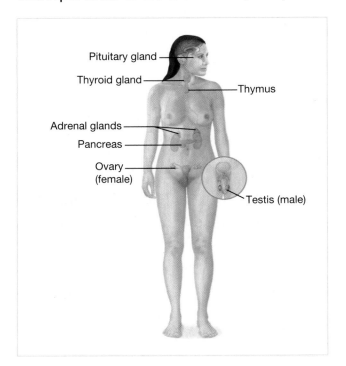

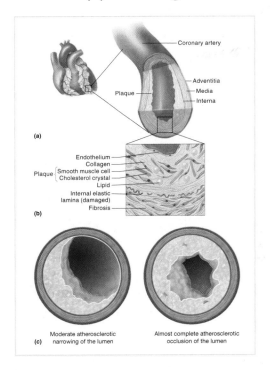

Image Labeling Frames

These frames provide you with opportunities to actively engage
with the illustrations, helping to reinforce your knowledge of anatomy.

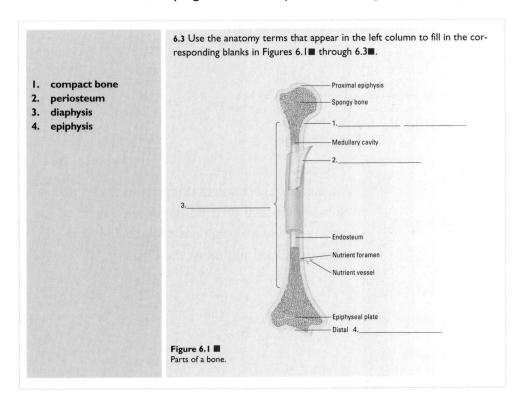

1. **compact bone**
2. **periosteum**
3. **diaphysis**
4. **epiphysis**

6.3 Use the anatomy terms that appear in the left column to fill in the corresponding blanks in Figures 6.1■ through 6.3■.

Figure 6.1 ■
Parts of a bone.

Word Building, Step by Step

At-a-glance tables provide a preview of the word parts and definitions you'll learn in each framed section that follows. Then, in the frame for each constructed term, word part reminders show how the individual word part meanings combine to form the constructed term. Word part breakdowns show, by using slash marks, how the constructed term is broken down. Word parts are colored here, too, for further word building reinforcement.

polycythemia pall ee sigh THEE mee ah	**7.18** The prefix *poly-* means "many." When combined with the word root that means "cell" (*cyt*) and the suffix that means "condition of blood" (*-emia*), the term _____ is formed. This constructed term is written poly/cyt/hem/ia. Polycythemia, which is an abnormal increase in the number of red blood cells in the blood, may also be called **erythrocytosis** (eh RITH roh sigh TOH siss). This is also a constructed term, written erythr/o/cyt/osis, that literally means "condition of red cell."

Did You Know?

These special frames reveal fascinating facts about the Latin or Greek origins of a medical term and provide interesting, relevant facts and figures.

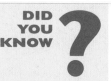

Inflammation

The Latin word *inflammatio* is the origin of this term, which literally means "to ignite or set ablaze." Because the symptoms of inflammation are heat, swelling, redness, and pain, this term is aptly named!

Words to Watch Out For!

These special frames provide tips about commonly misspelled or error-prone terms and word parts.

-ectomy or -tomy?

These two suffixes look very similar, but how do you tell them apart? One easy way is to remember that *-ectomy* means "excision" (see how they both start with an "e"?). The suffix *-tomy* means "incision" or "to cut," and this meaning does not start with an "e."

PRACTICE: Signs and Symptoms of the Skeletal and Muscular Systems

Break the Chain

Analyze these medical terms:

a) Separate each term into its word parts; each word part is labeled for you (**p** = prefix, **r** = root, **cf** = combining form, and **s** = suffix).

b) For the Bonus Question, write the requested definition in the blank that follows.

The first set has been completed for you as an example.

1. a) arthralgia   *arthr / algia*
                              r   s

    b) *Bonus Question:* What is the definition of the suffix? *condition of pain*

2. a) ataxia   ____/____/____
                          p   r   s

    b) *Bonus Question:* What is the definition of the word root? _____

3. a) atrophy   ____/____/____
                          p   r   s

    b) *Bonus Question:* What is the definition of the word root? _____

4. a) bradykinesia   ____/____/____
                              p   r   s

    b) *Bonus Question:* What is the definition of the prefix? _____

Practice Exercises

These are exercises that follow each chapter sub-section and provide opportunities to pause and review with practices such as *The Right Match, Linkup,* and *Break the Chain.*

Reinforcement Activities Conclude Each Chapter

Word Building Exercises
Practice opportunities to hone your understanding
of assembling word parts to form medical terms.

▶▶▶▶ **Chapter Review**

Word Building

Construct medical terms from the following meanings. (Some are built from word parts, some are not.) The first
question has been completed as an example.

1.	reduced ability of blood to deliver oxygen	an*emia*
2.	presence of red blood cells of unequal size	_____cytosis
3.	any abnormal condition of the blood	dys_____
4.	a serious protozoan infection of red blood cells	_____ia
5.	abnormal reduction of red blood cells	erythro_____
6.	inherited defect in blood coagulation	_____philia
7.	cancer originating in red bone marrow	_____emia
8.	abnormally large red blood cells	macro_____
9.	a condition of staphylococci in the blood	staphylococc_____
10.	disease caused by immune reaction against own tissues	_____ disease
11.	abnormal increase in number of red blood cells	_____emia
12.	red blood cells that are tear-shaped	_____cytosis
13.	presence of bacteria and toxins in the blood	septic _____
14.	a drug that reduces blood clotting	anti_____
15.	transfusion of blood donated by another person	_____logous transfusion
16.	measures percentage of red blood cells in a sample	hemato_____
17.	stoppage of bleeding	_____stasis
18.	calculation of the number of platelets in blood	_____ count
19.	cancer of lymphatic tissue	_____ disease
20.	inflammation of the lymph nodes	_____itis
21.	bacterial disease that causes a membrane in the throat to form	_____ia

Clinical Application Exercises
Scenarios that use critical thinking questions to help you
develop a firmer understanding of the terminology in
real-world context.

Medical Report

Read the following medical report, then answer the questions that follow.

Metropolis County Hospital

5500 University Avenue Phone: (211) 594-4000
Metropolis, TX Fax: (211) 594-4001

Medical Consultation: Dermatology

Date: 7/07/2007

Patient: Sally Garcia

Patient Complaint: Redness, swelling, pruritus, and pain reported on the skin of the right
upper arm, with skin elevations that open with scratching that is producing scars

History: 22-year-old Hispanic female has complained of occasional skin elevations that
cause discomfort from pruritus. No treatments have been provided previously. Patient reports that she works in an environment that is unusually humid and dusty.

Family History: Father, age 72, with melanoma; older brother with seborrheic dermatitis
spreading to the scalp to contribute to alopecia.

Allergies: None

Evidences: Generalized inflammation of right upper arm spreading to shoulder and thorax
with vesicle formation. Open vesicles are forming cicatrices and keloids.

Treatment: Debridement of damaged tissue and administration of oral antibiotic therapy.
Future surgery with autograft may be advised for keloid removal.

Jane K. Hernandez, M.D.

1. What is the actual cause of the cicatrices on the skin? _____

2. If the symptom of pruritus returns after the initial treatment, how might the formation of new scar tissue be

   prevented? _____

3. Why do you think antibiotic therapy is included in the treatment? _____

Key Terms Double-Check
Provides an alphabetical checklist exercise for each term, that allows
you to test yourself and confirm your knowledge before moving on.
Frame numbers are provided so you can go back and review any
needed content.

▶▶▶▶ **Key Terms Double-Check**

Remember that the chapter's key terms appeared alphabetically within each section of this chapter. This exercise
helps you to check your knowledge AND review for tests.

1. First, fill in the missing word in the definitions for the chapter's key terms.
2. Then, check your answers using Appendix F.
3. If you got the answer right, put a check mark in the right column.
4. If your answer was incorrect, go back to the frame number provided and review the content.

Use the checklist to study the terms you don't know until you're confident you know them all.

Key Term	Frame	Definition	Know It?
1. abrasion	5.7	a _____ scraping injury to the skin	☐
2. abscess	5.8	localized skin inflammation that may be accompanied by _____	☐
3. acne	5.36	bacterial infection of sebaceous glands and ducts resulting in numerous _____	☐
4. actinic keratosis	5.37	precancerous condition of the skin caused by exposure to _____	☐
5. albinism	5.38	genetic condition characterized by reduction of the skin pigment _____	☐
6. alopecia	5.39	baldness; may be a sign of an _____ of the scalp, high fevers, or emotional stress	☐
7. biopsy	5.64	minor surgery involving the removal of tissue for evaluation; abbreviated _____	☐
8. burn	5.40	caused by excessive exposure to fire, chemicals, or sunlight, and measured by _____ _____, and depth of the damage	☐
9. carbuncle	5.41	a skin infection composed of a cluster of _____	☐
10. carcinoma	5.42	skin cancer; varieties include _____ cell carcinoma and squamous cell carcinoma	☐
11. cellulite	5.9	a local uneven surface of the skin caused by _____	☐
12. cellulitis	5.43	inflammation of the _____ tissue in the dermis caused by an infection	☐

Multimedia Preview
Page that concludes each chapter and directs readers to the
wealth of features on the student DVD-ROM and website.
This is a gateway to deeper understanding.

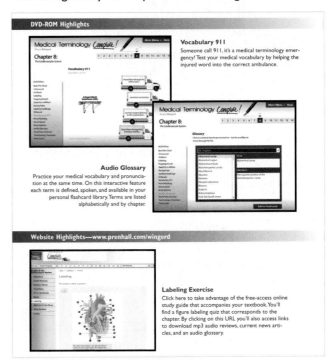

DVD-ROM Highlights

Vocabulary 911
Someone call 911, it's a medical terminology emergency! Test your medical vocabulary by helping the
injured word into the correct ambulance.

Audio Glossary
Practice your medical vocabulary and pronunciation at the same time. On this interactive feature
each term is defined, spoken, and available in your
personal flashcard library. Terms are listed
alphabetically and by chapter.

Website Highlights—www.prenhall.com/wingerd

Labeling Exercise
Click here to take advantage of the free-access online
study guide that accompanies your textbook. You'll
find a figure labeling quiz that corresponds to the
chapter. By clicking on this URL you'll also access links
to download mp3 audio reviews, current news articles, and an audio glossary.

The Complete Teaching and Learning Package ▶▶▶▶▶

We are committed to providing students and instructors with exactly the tools they need to be successful in the classroom and beyond. To this end, *Medical Terminology Complete!* is supported by the most complete and dynamic set of resources available today.

Student DVD-ROM

A bonus DVD-ROM is included with every text, and provides 12 different interactive game modules, animations, videos, an audio glossary, and more. Here are some highlights:

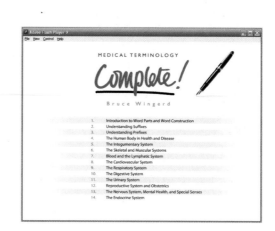

- **Custom Flashcard Generator**—allows students to create and print their own flashcards by selecting glossary terms on which to focus.

- **Audio Glossary**—provides definitions and audio pronunciations of each of the key terms presented in the text.

- **Terminology Translator**—contains the Spanish translations and audio pronunciations of over 5,000 medical terms.

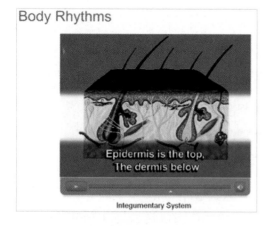

Body Rhythms

Integumentary System

- **Body Rhythms**—a collection of music videos featuring originally written songs that describe each body system. Thousands of students have found these videos to be fun yet educational study breaks.

- **12 different game modules**—provide students with a diverse and fun array of study tools.

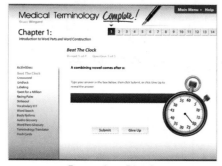

Beat the Clock

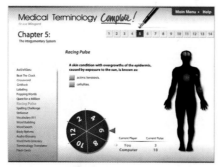

Racing Pulse

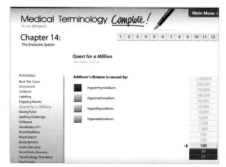

Quest for a Million

Online Learning ▶▶▶▶▶

No medical terminology textbook has as extensive a selection of web-based resources as **Medical Terminology Complete!** Whether you are looking for a basic Internet study experience, a robust, self-paced online course delivery system, or anything in between we offer the solution that suits your needs.

Medical Language Link

The most complete, dynamic, online medical terminology course available today! Compatible with any learning management system, this revolutionary, self-paced program engages students with activities, assessments, and rich media that is unmatched in the market. Features include:

■ **Integrated e-book**—provides a one-to-one match with the text and allows readers to access videos and animations straight from the "page."

■ **Interactive modules**—designed for readers to step through a self-paced tutorial program screen by screen.

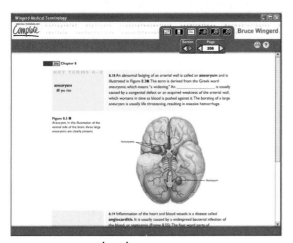

e-book

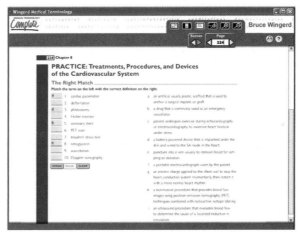

Interactive Modules

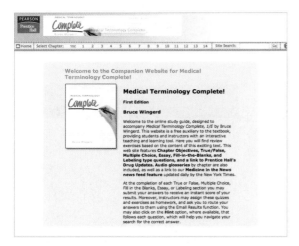

Companion Website

Our most basic online option, this is a free-access online study guide located at www.prenhall.com/wingerd. It contains:

■ Quizzes in multiple-choice, true/false, labelling, fill-in, and essay formats. Instant feedback and explanations are provided and results can be emailed to instructors.

■ An audio glossary in which key terms are pronounced.

Tools for the Instructor

Medical Terminology Complete! offers a rich array of ancillary materials to benefit instructors and help infuse a spark in the classroom. The full complement of supplemental teaching materials is available to all qualified instructors from your Pearson Health sales representative.

Instructor's Resource Manual

This manual contains a wealth of material to help faculty plan and manage the medical terminology course. It includes:

- A complete test bank of over 1,300 questions.
- Comprehensive lecture notes that contain abstracts, factoids, teaching strategies, and concept maps.
- A wealth of worksheets and handouts.
- *Medical Terminology Pearls of Wisdom,* a collection of best teaching practices shared by a national panel of master medical terminology educators.

Instructor's Media Library

A DVD contains all the electronic resources necessary for an instructor to manage a course.

- The complete test bank of over 1,300 questions that allows instructors to generate customized exams and quizzes.
- A comprehensive, turn-key lecture package in PowerPoint format containing discussion points, with embedded color images from the textbook, as well as bonus animations and videos to help infuse an extra spark into the classroom experience.
- PowerPoint content to support instructors who wish to use Classroom Response Systems ("clickers"). For more information, visit www.prenhall.com/crs.
- A complete image library that includes every photograph and illustration contained in the textbook, provided three ways: with labels, with leader lines only, and unlabeled.

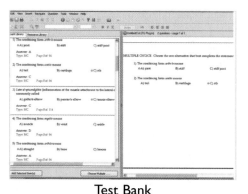

Test Bank

The Gastrointestinal System

Videos

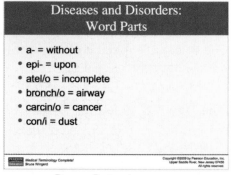

PowerPoint Lectures

Preface ▶▶▶▶▶

Medical Terminology Complete! is an introductory text presenting the most current and accepted language of health care in a programmed learning approach. Its goal is to prepare students for careers in the healthcare professions by providing them with a self-guided tool for learning medical terminology. The book may be used as a text to support lectures, or as an independent student workbook. The flexibility of its application is made possible by the book's text-like format combined with its self-guided learning program, self-assessment questions, and reinforcement exercises. In order to provide an optimum learning format, the text discussions are basic, clear, and concise. The programmed learning modules are simple and easy to follow, and the self-assessment questions and exercises provide reviews and clinical applications of the information at frequent intervals.

Pedagogy

Medical Terminology Complete! is a total pedagogical program that is centered on the programmed learning approach, combining narrative, visual, self-quiz, and clinical insert features. Each chapter is written at a level targeting introductory students. The programmed learning frames contain brief, clear, and concise statements, usually describing a single medical term. The advantage of this is to allow the student to focus on one term at a time. Each frame includes at least one blank space, which can be completed based on clues within the frame. The answer to the blank is provided in the left column of the page. Students can either cover the answer column, or can leave it uncovered. Either way, the kinesthetic component of filling in the blank provides another level of learning that ensures student retention.

Our format assists students in focusing on the most important terms. Following the first four introductory chapters, the body systems chapters present the most important terms (or "Key Terms") in the answer column with color-coded word parts, where applicable. Prefixes appear in **blue**; word roots and combining vowels are **red**; and suffixes are **purple**. An added benefit of this Key Terms answer column is that the terms are presented in alphabetical order, which provides a way for students to quickly review the priority terms. Each term is accompanied by its phonetic pronunciation.

Other terms that are related to the Key Terms in the answer column, yet are not as vital for the student to understand, are presented in the main frame section in boldface type.

The visual program provides an important supplement to learning medical terminology. Full-color diagrams and photographs complement nearly every page of the book, illustrating both the normal structures of the body and the various features of many diseases.

The self-program features enable students to learn the material with a minimum of instructor guidance. In addition to the programmed learning frames, other self-study features include blocks of review questions (**Practice**) that are placed at frequent intervals throughout each chapter. In these **Practice** sections, students are given the opportunity to self-test their new understanding by answering questions in **The Right Match, Linkup,** and **Break the Chain** activities. Answers to these activities, along with those for the end-of-chapter review questions, appear in Appendix F.

The book also includes inserted boxes intended to promote additional interest in medical terminology. They include **Did You Know?**, which reveal fascinating facts about the Latin or Greek origins of a medical term and provide interesting and relevant facts and figures that draw a connection between a particular term and its clinical point of interest and **Words to Watch Out For!**, which provide tips about commonly misspelled or error-prone terms and word parts.

Chapter Format

Each chapter begins with a brief list of **Learning Objectives**, informing the reader of the tasks ahead. In each chapter beginning with Chapter 5, a brief review of the structure and function of the particular body system discussed in the chapter follows the objectives. The section is titled **Anatomy and Physiology Terms**, which begins with an at-a-glance table with the major combining forms and definitions for that body system. The Anatomy and Physiology section then presents only two or three programmed learning frames—enough to give students an opportunity to review essential anatomy and physiology, without overwhelming them or providing redundancy to students who have already taken an anatomy course as a prerequisite. The illustrations accompanying this section provide additional fill-in-the-blank activities.

The primary text of each chapter consists of a brief narrative introduction discussing the pathophysiology of the body system, followed by numerous programmed learning frames that are divided into three sections:

- **Signs and Symptoms**
- **Diseases and Disorders**
- **Treatments, Procedures, and Devices**

Supportive features such as **Did You Know?** and **Words to Watch Out For!** boxes are interspersed throughout. Each programmed section concludes with **Practice** exercises, including a matching exercise called **The Right Match** and word part construction exercises called **Linkup** and **Break the Chain.**

The next section of the chapter presents the **Abbreviations** for the terms that are in common use. Each abbreviation is listed and defined, and a **Practice** activity follows to reinforce this new information.

A concluding **Chapter Review** section provides several review exercises, including **Word Building** and **Clinical Application Exercises** with a medical report and case study. Then, the chapter concludes with a unique review exercise called **Key Terms Double-Check,** which provides an alphabetical listing of all priority terms ("Key Terms"), a fill-in-the-blank exercise for each term, and a reference to the original frame number should the student need to go back to review the content. Once students are certain that they know the term, they place a check in the **Know It?** box.

Organization of the Book

The organization of this text is unique in that it provides a slow, building approach to teaching medical terminology. Students can often be overwhelmed by this new language, so here's what we've done to address this and make the learning experience more comfortable for students:

- The text begins with three chapters devoted exclusively to word building and word parts. We then present a chapter that introduces anatomy and physiology word roots and combining forms, both of which create the foundation for the majority of medical terms. This chapter also introduces other foundational terms, such as anatomical and directional terms. This allows the student to take a slow, logical approach to learning word parts and word building.

- Then, the student can put that knowledge to work and learn about medical terms as they apply to each body system. The body system chapters progress from the least complex body system (integumentary) to the most complex body system (endocrine). This approach enhances learning by allowing the student to build confidence as they work their way through the chapters.

A complete description of the contents of each chapter follows.

Introductory Chapters (1–4): Chapter 1 provides an introduction to medical terminology and to the programmed learning approach. Basic definitions of terminology and word construction are first described here. Also, the importance of learning the most common Latin and Greek word parts is emphasized as a starting point. Chapter 2 provides an opportunity for students to learn the common prefixes that are in frequent use in building medical terms. Chapter 3 covers suffixes and their common uses in medical terms. Chapter 4 provides an overview of anatomy and physiology as an effort to introduce the primary terms and concepts of these two important fields. The chapter begins with the introductory concepts of anatomy and physiology, such as directional terms, body organization, regional terms, and the importance of homeostasis as a unifying body function.

Body Systems Chapters (5–14): Chapter 5 covers the medical terminology of the most external system, the integumentary system. Chapter 6 follows the format of the previous chapter, but describes the terminology of the skeletal and muscular systems. The medical terminology of the two systems is combined in this chapter due to their close association with the function of body movement. Chapter 7 covers the lymphatic system, but also includes the medical terms associated with blood because of the close functional connection between blood and lymph. It includes the most common terms associated with infectious diseases. Chapter 8 describes the medical terms of the cardiovascular system. It is followed by the respiratory system in Chapter 9, the digestive system in Chapter 10, and the urinary system in Chapter 11. In Chapter 12, the male and female reproductive systems are combined, but discussed separately. The field of obstetrics is also included in the chapter. In addition, sexually transmitted infections are described here. Chapter 13 provides a study of the nervous system, and includes the eyes and ears. Additionally, it includes the most common forms of mental disease. It is followed by the medical terms of the endocrine system in Chapter 14, which concludes the major part of book.

Appendices: Appendix A provides a complete glossary of all word parts that are presented in the text, along with their definitions. Appendix B lists abbreviations commonly used in the health care professions. In Appendix C, common terms used in pharmacology are included for your reference. Appendix D provides common color terms, and Appendix E provides common numerical terms. Appendix F provides the answers to the Practice exercises and to the end-of-chapter Chapter Review questions.

About the Author

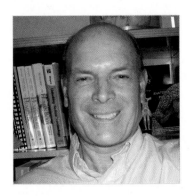

Bruce Wingerd is Associate Dean of Biology at Broward College in Florida and previously taught at San Diego State University for 25 years. His degrees are in the fields of Zoology and Physiology. While at SDSU, he taught medical terminology, human anatomy, advanced human anatomy, and anatomy and physiology. He has written numerous textbooks, lab manuals, and multimedia learning resources in medical terminology, human anatomy, anatomy and physiology, histology, and comparative mammalian anatomy. His goal in teaching and writing is to provide students with learning tools that will help them unlock their minds and release their potential through education. As a college administrator/professor, he enjoys counseling students in the Allied Health fields, developing novel approaches to teaching and learning, and leading faculty in the drive for excellence in education.

About the Illustrators

Marcelo Oliver is president and founder of Body Scientific International, Llc. He holds an MFA degree in Medical and Biological Illustration from the University of Michigan. For the past 15 years, his passion has been to condense complex anatomical information into visual education tools for students, patients, and medical professionals.

Body Scientific's lead artists in this publication were medical illustrators Liana Bauman, Carol Gudanowski, and Katie Burgess. They each hold Master of Science degrees in Biomedical Visualization from the University of Illinois at Chicago. Their contribution in the publication was key in the creation and editing of artwork throughout.

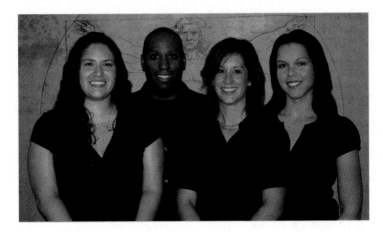

Acknowledgments

This book is a product of listening carefully to reviewer's comments on the best possible method of teaching and learning medical terminology. Rather than being the result of one author's vision, as the title page suggests, it is a compilation of work driven by a talented team with the goal of putting together a valuable learning tool that is unique in its simple, student-friendly approach and logical flow of information using the popular programmed learning methodology.

Our team received direction from Mark Cohen, who spearheaded the project from start to finish as the Executive Editor by providing the resources needed to attract a large body of peer reviewers and contributing his experience in identifying and applying effective ways of learning. Elena Mauceri of Dynamic WordWorks, Inc., provided expert daily management of the project, made important contributions to the content of each chapter, and established most of the compositional details of every page to maximize the learning benefits of the book. Elena's talented contributions to the final product are enormous. Sara Wilson provided many solutions to the technical problems associated with the creation of the text, relying upon her substantial skills in technical writing while simultaneously experiencing the development, birth, and infancy of her second child. Janine Nameny drew upon her experience with *Unlocking Medical Terminology* to contribute much of the content in the first several chapters and assist in the editorial details of each page. To each of these individuals, I express my sincere appreciation for their contributions.

There are many other talented people who worked hard to make this book a valuable teaching and learning resource. I extend to each of them my warmest gratitude:

Melissa Kerian, Managing Development Editor, who coordinated the development of a world-class teaching and learning package that you can read about on page viii.

Nicole Ragonese, Assistant Editor, who executed the complex process of managing our peer review program.

Marcelo Oliver and his team of medical illustrators at Body Scientific International, Inc., who created a dynamic, clear, and precise art program.

Mary Siener, Design Director, who coordinated the development of a beautiful, yet highly functional book design.

Christina Zingone, Production Liaison, who directed the flow of textual and visual content throughout the production of the book and ancillary materials.

Jessica Balch, Production Editor for Pine Tree Composition, who oversaw the copyediting and page composition processes.

I invite and welcome your reactions, comments, and suggestions to be sent to me directly so that subsequent editions may reflect your educational needs even better.

Bruce Wingerd
Biological Sciences
Broward College
Davie, Florida 33314
bwingerd@broward.edu

Our Development Team

The fresh, unique vision, format, and content contained within the pages of *Medical Terminology Complete!* comes as a result of an incredible collaboration of expert educators from around the United States. This book represents the collective insights, experience, and thousands of hours of work performed by members of this development team. Their influence will continue to have an impact for decades to come. Let us introduce the members of our team.

Manuscript Reviewers

Lynn Alexander, MEd, SBB(ASCP)
Assistant Professor, Clinical Laboratory
  Science
Winston-Salem State University
Winston-Salem, North Carolina

Martha Arnson, RN
Instructor, Allied Health Sciences
Gwinnett Technical College
Lawrenceville, Georgia

Cindy Ault, MS, MT(ASCP)
Assistant Professor, Biology
Jamestown College
Jamestown, North Dakota

Mary Jo Belenski, EdD
Coordinator, Undergraduate Health
  Programs
Montclair State University
Montclair, New Jersey

Linda A. Bell, BS, MEd
Professor & Chair, Business Division
Reading Area Community College
Reading, Pennsylvania

Bradley S. Bowden, PhD
Professor of Biology
Alfred University
Alfred, New York

Amy Bowersock, PhD
Assistant Professor, Exercise Science
Coordinator, Pre-Professional Allied Health
The University of Tampa
Tampa, Florida

Vera Brock, RN.C, DSN
Assistant Director, Nursing
Georgia Highlands College
Rome, Georgia

Mary Elizabeth Browder, BA, AAS, CMA
Assistant Professor, Medical Assisting
Raymond Walters College/UC|Blue Ash
Cincinnati, Ohio

Barbara Burri, MBA, BS, CVT, LVT
Instructor, Allied Health
New Hampshire Community Technical
  College
Stratham, New Hampshire

Christina Campbell, PhD, RD
Associate Professor, Nutrition
Montana State University
Bozeman, Montana

Sandra Carlson, RN, BSN, CNOR
Chair, Allied Health
Director, Surgical Technology
New Hampshire Community Technical
  College
Stratham, New Hampshire

Phyllis Clements, MA, OTR
Coordinator, Occupational Therapy
  Assistant Program
Macomb Community College
Clinton Township, Michigan

Pam deCalesta, OD
Online Instructor, Business Technology
Linn-Benton Community College
Albany, Oregon

Litta Dennis, BSN, MS
Adjunct Faculty, Health Careers
Illinois Central College
Peoria, Illinois

Rosemary DeSiervi, MEd
Part-time Instructor, Healthcare
  Technologies
West Valley College
Saratoga, California

Sherry Gamble, RN, MSN
Director & Assistant Professor, Surgical
  Technology
The University of Akron
Akron, Ohio

Steven B. Goldschmidt, DC, CCFC
Professor, Biology
North Hennepin Community College
Brooklyn Park, Minnesota
Professor, Health Care Management
Inverhills Community College
Inver Grove Heights, Minnesota

Karen R. Hardney, MS Ed
Assistant Professor, Health Studies
Chicago State University
Chicago, Illinois

Pamela Harmon, RT (R)
Clinical Coordinator, Radiology
Triton College
River Grove, Illinois

Kathy Harward, RN, BSN
Professor, Practical Nursing
Florida Community College at Jacksonville
Jacksonville, Florida

Rachel M. P. Hopp, PhD
Associate Professor, Biology
Houston Baptist University
Houston, Texas

Diana Houston, AAS
Director, Medical Assisting
San Jacinto College North
Houston, Texas

James E. Hudacek, MSEd
Adjunct Faculty, Allied Health/Nursing
Lorain County Community College
Elyria, Ohio

Marcie Jones, BS, CMA
Program Director, Medical Assisting
Gwinnett Technical College
Lawrenceville, Georgia

Marie L. Kotter, PhD
Professor & Chair, Health Sciences
Weber State University
Ogden, Utah

Paul Lucas, CMA, CPbt, PN, AS
Program Director, Medical Assisting
Brown Mackie College
Fort Wayne, Indiana

Mandy Mann, CMA
Program Coordinator, Medical Assisting
Big Bend Community College
Moses Lake, Washington

Cheryl Meyer, RN MSN
Professor, Allied Health & Nursing
Delaware County Community College
Media, Pennsylvania

Sandra Mullins, EdD
Associate Academic Dean
Bluegrass Community and Technical College
Lexington, Kentucky

Lisa Nagle, BSed, CMA
Program Director, Medical Assisting
Augusta Technical College
Augusta, Georgia

Anne Nez, RN, MSN
Assistant Professor, Nursing
Central Wyoming College
Riverton, Wyoming

Arthur J. Ortiz, MA, LPN, LRCP
Instructor, Medical Assisting
Southeast Community College
Lincoln, Nebraska

Elizabeth Pagenkopf, RN, BSN, MA
Coordinator, Health Science
Harper College
Palatine, Illinois

Felicity F. Penner, BSc, MSPH
Online Adjunct Professor, School of
   Business and Information Systems
Southwestern Community College
Chula Vista, California

Carol Reid, MS, RN
Instructor, Nursing
Century College
White Bear Lake, MN

Lawrence Rosenquist, MS, RN
Assistant Professor, Nursing
Wilkes University
Wilkes-Barre, Pennsylvania

Lorraine M. Smith, MBA
Instructor, Business and Technology
Fresno City College
Fresno, California

Steven C. Stoner, PharmD, BCPP
Clinical Professor, Division of Pharmacy
   Practice
UMKC School of Pharmacy
Kansas City, Missouri

Roger Thompson, BS, RRT
Associate Professor, Respiratory Therapy
Mountain Empire Community College
Big Stone Gap, Virginia

Judy Traynor, MS, FNP, RN, CASAC
Assistant Professor, Nursing
Jefferson Community College
Watertown, New York

Twila Wallace, MEd
Instructor, Office Technology
Central Community College
Columbus, Nebraska

Margaret T. Warren, PhD, RN
Professor, Emergency Medical Services
Rockland Community College
Suffern, New York

Lynn C. Wimett, RN, ANP, EdD
Chair, Post Licensure Programs In Nursing
Regis University
Denver, Colorado

Kathy Whitley, MSN, FNP
Associate Professor, Nursing
Patrick Henry Community College
Martinsville, Virginia

Kathy Zabel, BS, AAS
Instructor, Medical Assisting
Southeast Community College
Lincoln, Nebraska

Companion Website Author

Pamela A. Eugene, BAS, RT, (R)
Associate Professor, Allied Health
Delgado Community College
New Orleans, Louisiana

Classroom Response System Authors

Trisha LaPointe, PharmD, BCPS
Assistant Professor, Pharmacy Practice
Massachusetts College of Pharmacy
   and Health Sciences
Boston, Massachusetts

Kathy Zaiken, PharmD
Assistant Professor, Pharmacy Practice
Director, MCPHS/Harvard Vanguard Medical
   Associates Pharmacy Practice Residency
Massachusetts College of Pharmacy
   and Health Sciences
Boston, Massachusetts

Test Bank Authors

Jennifer Esch, BS, PA-C
Instructor, Medical Assisting
Bryant and Stratton College
Milwaukee, Wisconsin

Jean M. Krueger-Watson, PhD
Faculty, Health Occupations
Clark College
Vancouver, Washington

Instructor's Resource Manual Author

Donna Jeanne Pugh, BSN, RN
Chair, Medical Programs
Florida Metropolitan University
Jacksonville, Florida

PowerPoint Lecture Author

Linda C. Campbell, CMT, FAAMT
Medical Transcription Instructor
The Andrews School
Oklahoma City, Oklahoma

A Commitment to Accuracy ▶▶▶▶

As a student embarking on a career in health care you probably already know how critically important it is to be precise in your work. Patients and co-workers will be counting on you to avoid errors on a daily basis. Likewise, we owe it to you—the reader—to ensure accuracy in this book. We have gone to great lengths to verify that the information provided in *Medical Terminology Complete!* is complete and correct. To this end, here are the steps we have taken:

1. **Editorial Review**—We have assembled a large team of developmental consultants (listed on the preceding pages) to critique every word and every image in this book. No fewer than 12 content experts have read each chapter for accuracy. In addition, some members of our developmental team were specifically assigned to focus on the precision of each illustration that appears in the book.

2. **Medical Illustrations**—A team of medically-trained illustrators was hired to prepare each piece of art that graces the pages of this book. These illustrators have a higher level of scientific education than the artists for most textbooks, and they worked directly with the author and members of our development team to make sure that their work was clear, correct, and consistent with what is described in the text.

3. **Accurate Ancillaries**—The teaching and learning ancillaries are often as important to instruction as the textbook itself. Therefore, we took steps to ensure accuracy and consistency of these components by reviewing every ancillary component. The author and editorial team studied every PowerPoint slide and online course frame to ensure the context was correct and relevant to each lesson.

While our intent and actions have been directed at creating an error-free text, we have established a process for correcting any mistakes that may have slipped past our editors. Pearson takes this issue seriously and therefore welcomes any and all feedback that you can provide along the lines of helping us enhance the accuracy of this text. If you identify any errors that need to be corrected in a subsequent printing, please send them to:

> Pearson Health Editorial
> Medical Terminology Corrections
> One Lake Street
> Upper Saddle River, NJ 07458

Thank you for helping Pearson reach its goal of providing the most accurate medical terminology textbooks available.

Contents ▶▶▶▶▶

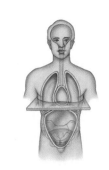

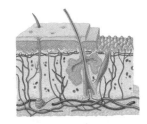

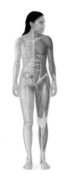

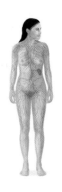

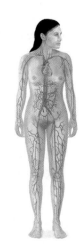

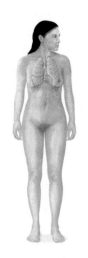

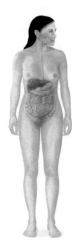

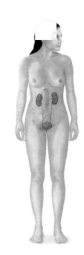

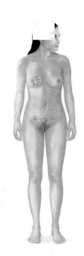

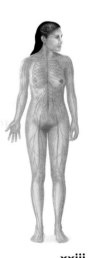

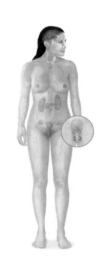

Introduction to Word Parts and Word Construction ▶▶▶▶▶

Learning Objectives

After completing this chapter, you will be able to:

- Use the technique of programmed learning and frames.

- Apply the phonetic pronunciation guides that are used in frames.

- Recognize that medical terminology has both constructed and nonconstructed terms.

- Identify each of the three word parts (word roots, prefixes, and suffixes) used to construct medical terms.

- Identify the function of a combining vowel that is added to a word root to form a combining form.

- Recognize that many medical terms are constructed from word parts and can be deconstructed into their word parts.

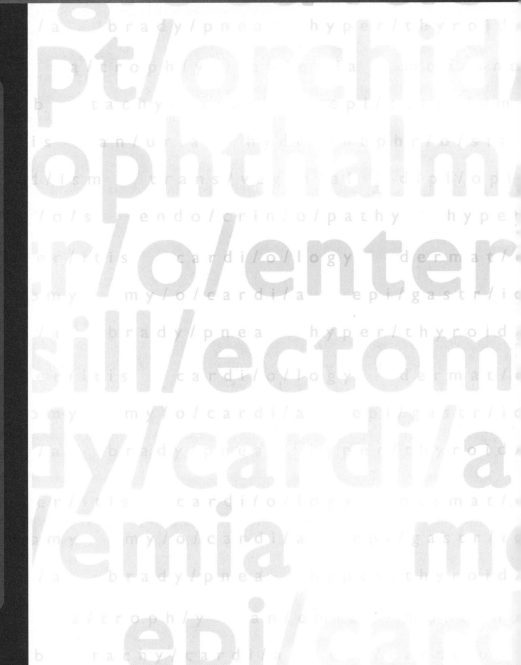

The Programmed Learning Approach ▶▶▶▶▶

frame

1.1 This textbook teaches you medical terminology by using the friendly technique of **programmed learning**. This technique has been used for many years to teach many subjects, such as math, world languages, and of course, medical terminology. It consists of blocks of information, known as frames, which contain one or more blanks. The blanks are provided for you to write in the missing word. In some cases, the missing word is easy to determine, and in other cases it becomes more of a challenge. In either case, the missing word is provided in the left margin of the _____, so you don't have to feel frustrated if you have trouble identifying or spelling the missing word correctly.

number

1.2 As you can see, each frame consists of a block of information with the blank in the box on the right side of the page. Note the frame _____. This number enables you to locate and flip back to a previous frame with ease if needed.

blank

1.3 The far left box in each frame contains the missing word. As you proceed from frame to frame, you should write the missing word into the _____. Try to work without looking at the answer first to make each frame a challenge. By doing so, the activity will engage your mind and help you to learn the meanings of the words.

spelling

1.4 Spelling is very important when learning medical terminology. By writing the missing word in the blank and then comparing your answer with the one provided in the far left margin, you will be practicing the _____ of the word. Always check your answer before moving to the next frame. Pay special attention to the "Did You Know?" and "Words to Watch Out For" boxes in this text. These will alert you to tricky spelling issues or terms that might easily be confused.

phonetic
phoh NET ik

1.5 In addition to spelling, correct pronunciation of medical terms is also important. To help you with pronunciation, the phonetic ("sounds like") form of the word is provided in parentheses whenever a new term is introduced, for example, _____ and pronunciation (proh NUN see AYE shun). You should say the new word aloud whenever possible, using the phonetic guide to assist you.

guides

pronunciation

1.6 In the phonetic _____ that appear in this text, note that the syllable with the most spoken emphasis is shown in all capital letters. Here are some examples:

- The term *cardiology* is pronounced kar dee ALL oh jee. Note that the middle syllable *ALL* carries the most emphasis.
- The term *gastrohepatic* is pronounced GAS troh heh PAT ik. Note that the long *o* sound in the second syllable is demonstrated when spelled phonetically as *oh*, and the short *e* sound is demonstrated when spelled *eh*.
- The term *osteopathic* is pronounced oss tee oh PATH ik. Note that the long *e* sound in the second syllable is shown as *tee*.

You can also refer to the CD for audio samples of the pronunciation of each medical term presented in this text. Spend time listening to the _____ of each term presented in each chapter. Doing so will help you complete the pronunciation exercise in this chapter, "Talking Shop."

PRACTICE: The Programmed Learning Approach

The Right Match

Match the term on the left with the correct definition on the right.

_____ 1. pronunciations

_____ 2. spelling

_____ 3. blank

_____ 4. programmed learning

_____ 5. Words to Watch Out For boxes

a. alert you to terms that might easily be confused

b. learning technique that consists of blocks of information, known as frames, which contain one or more blanks for the student to fill in

c. by comparing your filled-in answer with the one provided in the far left margin, you will be practicing this

d. as you proceed from frame to frame, you should write the missing word into this

e. you can also refer to the CD for audio samples of these

Talking Shop

In the blank, write the letter of the pronunciation that matches the term. The first one is completed for you as an example. Visit the Companion Website to hear the correct pronunciation of these terms.

Term

_f_ 1. **cardiologist**

_____ 2. lymphoma

_____ 3. pneumonia

_____ 4. fracture

_____ 5. meningitis

_____ 6. meningocele

_____ 7. epicardium

_____ 8. nephrolithiasis

_____ 9. psychologist

_____ 10. hepatomegaly

_____ 11. pediatrician

_____ 12. bacteriuria

Pronunciation

a. pee dee ah TRI shun

b. men IN goh seel

c. limm FOH mah

d. ep ih KAR dee um

e. FRAK sher

f. **kar dee ALL oh jist**

g. NEFF roh lith EYE ah siss

h. HEPP ah toh MEG ah lee

i. bak ter ee YOO ree ah

j. noo MOH nee ah

k. sigh KALL oh jist

l. MEN in JYE tis

Constructed and Nonconstructed Terms ▶▶▶▶▶

language

1.7 Medical terminology is a functional language. This
_____ has rules of grammar, spelling, and pronunciation, just like any other language. Because medical terminology is the universal language of medicine, its terms must be understood by speakers of many languages in many parts of the world, especially in our age of globalization. For the purpose of learning the language of medical terminology, terms in this specialized language can be separated into two main categories: constructed terms and nonconstructed terms.

constructed terms

word

1.8 Many medical terms are **constructed terms**, which are made up of multiple word parts that are combined to form a new word. In most cases, the word parts are derived from Latin and Greek. The key to learning _____ _____ is to first learn the meaning of the various word parts. It may be helpful to think of constructed terms as if they were written in code. Once you have the key to a code, it becomes a fairly simple process to decode the messages or to use the code to form messages yourself. Similarly, once you learn the meanings of the individual _____ parts, you have the key to the medical terminology code. See Figure 1.1 ■.

Figure 1.1 ■
Medical terms are either constructed words, which are composed of more than one word part, or words you must memorize, which include terms that are a single Latin or Greek word part, eponyms, acronyms, abbreviations, and so on.

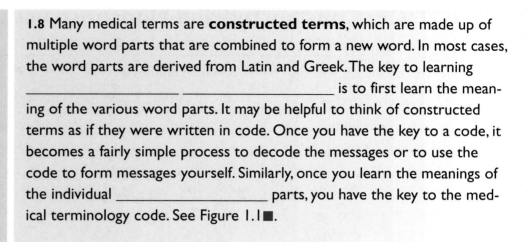

Constructed term

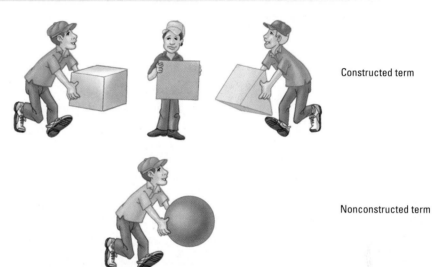

Nonconstructed term

nonconstructed terms

1.9 The second group of medical terms is **nonconstructed terms**, terms that are not formed from individual word parts. Nonconstructed terms include eponyms, which are terms derived from the names of people, for example, *eustachian tube* is derived from the name of Bartolommeo Eustachio; terms derived from other languages, such as the word *plate*, which is derived from the Old French word for a flat object, *plat*; acronyms, which are derived from the initial letters of words in a compound term, for example *LASIK* for *laser-assisted in situ keratomileusis*; and abbreviations, such as *Ab* for *antibody*. To learn _____ _____, you must commit them to memory.

PRACTICE: Constructed and Nonconstructed Terms

The Right Match

Match the term on the left with the correct definition on the right.

_____ 1. nonconstructed terms

_____ 2. constructed terms

_____ 3. medical terminology

_____ 4. eponym

a. term derived from a person's name

b. must be committed to memory

c. made up of word parts

d. the universal language of medicine

The Word Parts ▶▶▶▶

word parts	1.10 When a constructed term is formed, individual _____ _____ are assembled to create a term with a new meaning. This is very useful in medicine, because new discoveries are made frequently, and the need to provide them with relevant names is important. The three primary types of word parts are prefixes, word roots, and suffixes.
prefix	1.11 A **prefix** is a word part that is affixed to the beginning of a word. Its purpose is to expand or enhance the meaning of the word. Let's look at an example of a prefix in action, using the word *construction*. In our sample word, *con-* is the prefix. It means "with, together, jointly." Notice the hyphen following the prefix. You will know that a word part is a _____ by the hyphen that immediately follows it (for example, *con-*).
word root	1.12 A **word root** is a word part that provides the primary meaning of the term. The _____ _____ provides the basis for the term, and is the part to which other word parts are attached. Nearly all terms have a word root, and some have more than one. In our sample word *construction*, *struct* is the word root. It means "make, build."
suffix	1.13 A **suffix** is a word part that is affixed to the end of a word. The _____ often indicates the word's part of speech (noun, verb, adjective, adverb, etc.) or modifies the word's meaning. In our sample word *construction*, the suffix is *-ion*. It indicates that the word is a noun and it means "process." You will know that a word part is a suffix by the hyphen that immediately precedes it (for example, *-ion*).

three

1.14 To summarize using our example, the word *construction* is composed of _____ word parts (Figure 1.2■):

con- + struct + -ion
(prefix + word root + suffix)

We decipher the meaning of medical words by defining each of the word parts. First, we look at the meaning of the suffix, then we look at the meaning of the prefix. Finally, we define the word root. Then we combine the meanings of all the word parts in the way that makes the most sense. Thus, con- + struct + -ion means "process of building together."

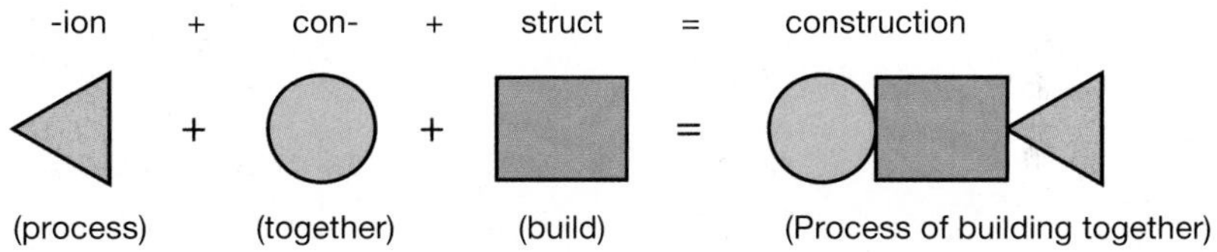

Figure 1.2 ■
Most medical terms are formed by assembling word parts.

-ion	+	con-	+	struct	=	construction
(process)		(together)		(build)		(Process of building together)

word parts

1.15 The word *construction*, then, as we use it in medical terminology, refers to *building words out of word parts*. This is what we do every time we write and speak. This is also what we do when we use medical terminology by speaking and writing medical terms. Understanding how to build words out of _____ _____ is essential to understanding the meaning of medical terms. Equally important is understanding how to deconstruct or break down a medical term into its component word parts. That is exactly what we did when we deciphered the meaning of our sample word *construction*. We broke the word down into its prefix, word root, and suffix parts and then combined the definitions of the word parts to derive the meaning of the term.

word root

1.16 Not every medical term has all three word parts. Many medical terms have more than one word root, such as *gastroenteritis* (GAS troh en ter EYE tis). It breaks down like so:

gastroenteritis
gastr + enter + itis
(word root + word root + suffix)

gastr is a word root that means "stomach"
enter is a _____ _____ that means "small intestine"
-itis is a suffix that means "inflammation"

Thus, the term *gastroenteritis* means "inflammation of the stomach and small intestine." Notice the letter *o* between the two word roots. You will learn about the importance of its use very soon (Frame 1.18).

suffix

1.17 Some medical terms are made simply of a prefix and a suffix. The term *aphasia* is an example.

aphasia
a- + -phasia
(prefix + suffix)

a- is a prefix that means "without or absence of"
-phasia is a _____ that means "speaking"

Thus, the term *aphasia* means "absence of speaking."

combining vowel

1.18 A fourth word part is the **combining vowel**. It is used when a word root requires a connecting vowel to add a suffix that begins with a consonant or another word root when forming a term. The _____ _____ does not add to or alter the meaning of the word root; it simply assists us in pronouncing a term. In most cases, the combining vowel is the letter *o*, and in some cases it is the letter *i* or *e*.

combining form

1.19 Generally, it is best to learn a word root with its combining vowel. This word root plus combining vowel form is called a **combining form**. Whenever possible, the combining forms are presented in this text to ease your building and deconstructing of medical terms, some of which are shown in Figure 1.3■. The method for writing a _____ _____ involves the use of a slash between the word root and the combining vowel, such as

cardi/o
(word root/combining vowel)

The combining vowel in *cardi/o* is *o*.

Figure 1.3 ■
The human body, with many of the common combining forms.

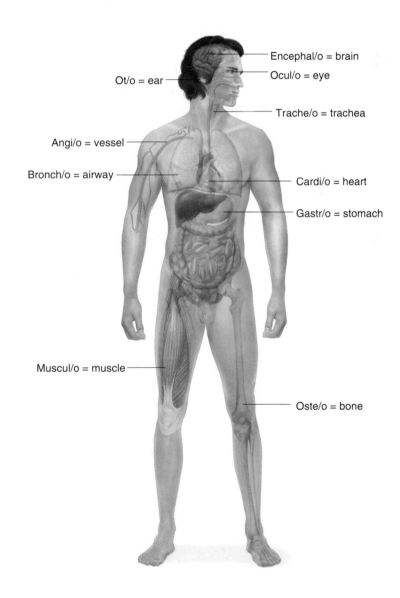

Encephal/o = brain
Ocul/o = eye
Ot/o = ear
Trache/o = trachea
Angi/o = vessel
Bronch/o = airway
Cardi/o = heart
Gastr/o = stomach
Muscul/o = muscle
Oste/o = bone

o

1.20 You learned from Frame 1.18 that the most common combining vowel is the letter _____. As practice, let's take a look at a medical term with which you may already be familiar:

cardiology

This term is made up of three word parts: a word root, a combining vowel, and a suffix. The combining form is *cardi/o* and the suffix is *-logy*. *Cardi/o* means "heart" and *-logy* means "study or science of." Thus, when we define the word parts of the term *cardiology* and then combine their definitions in a logical way, we know it means "the study or science of the heart." It may help to write the constructed form of the term, which is written with slashes separating each word part:

cardi/o/logy

1.21 Let's practice deconstructing medical terms and using word parts to decipher their meaning. Here are some more medical terms that you may already know.

dermatologist
dermat/o + logist
(combining form + suffix)

combining form

Dermat/o is a _____ _____ that means "skin"
-logist is a suffix that means "one who studies"

Thus, the term *dermatologist* means "one who studies the skin." The constructed form is written dermat/o/logist.

1.22 Another example is:

tonsillectomy
tonsill + -ectomy
(word root + suffix)

tonsill is a word root that means "almond or tonsil"
-ectomy is a _____ that means "surgical removal"

suffix

Thus, the term *tonsillectomy* means "surgical removal of tonsil (shaped like an almond)." The constructed form is written tonsill/ectomy.

micro/scop/ic

1.23 Another example is:

microscopic
micro- + scop + -ic
(prefix + word root + suffix)

micro- is a prefix that means "small"
scop is a word root that means "viewing instrument"
-ic is a suffix that means "pertaining to"

Thus, the term *microscopic* means "pertaining to the viewing instrument for investigating small things," or "visible only by means of a microscope." The constructed form is written _____/_____/_____.

PRACTICE: The Word Parts

The Right Match

Match the term on the left with the correct definition on the right.

_____ 1. prefix

_____ 2. word root

_____ 3. *-ectomy*

_____ 4. *o*

_____ 5. *cardi/o*

_____ 6. constructed term

a. the most common combining vowel

b. is a combining form

c. a word part that is affixed to the beginning of a word

d. a term built from word parts

e. a word part that provides the primary meaning of the term

f. is a suffix

Forming Words from Word Parts ▶▶▶▶▶

word parts

1.24 You have learned that constructed medical terms are created from building blocks called word parts, and include word roots, prefixes, suffixes, and combining forms. You will now learn how to form medical terms by using these _____ _____.

combining vowel

1.25 One rule to remember when forming words from word parts is the proper use of the combining vowel. The combining vowel is not always used at the end of a word root to create a combining form. As a general rule, the _____ _____ is used to connect a word root with a suffix that begins with a consonant.

cardi/o/logy

cardioplasty

1.26 For example, let's use the word root for "heart," *cardi*. As you know, cardiology means "study of the heart." The constructed form of this term is written _____/_____/_____. Notice that it contains the combining vowel *o* and the suffix begins with a consonant (*l*). Another term with the word root for "heart" is *carditis*, which means "inflammation of the heart." The constructed form of this term is written card/itis. Notice that the suffix begins with a vowel (*i*), and there is no combining vowel. If you wanted to change the suffix to -*plasty*, which means "surgical repair," to form the term that means "surgical repair of the heart," how would you write the new term? Because the suffix -*plasty* begins with a consonant (*p*), you would include the combining vowel (*o*) to form a new term, which is _____. The constructed form of this term is written cardi/o/plasty.

combining vowel
consonant

1.27 There are exceptions to this rule, so it is not absolute. You will learn these exceptions as you learn the material in this book. For now, just keep in mind that you need to include the _____ _____ when the suffix begins with a _____.

word roots

muscul/o/skelet/al

1.28 A second rule to remember when forming new constructed terms involves combining two word roots. Constructed medical terms use combining vowels to unite two _____ _____.
For example, when describing an injury that involves both the muscular and skeletal systems, the two word roots (*muscul* and *skelet*) are united by placing the combining vowel between them. To make the term complete, the suffix -*al* is added to form the term *musculoskeletal*. Literally, the term means "pertaining to muscles and the skeleton," and its constructed form is written _____/_____/_____/_____.

cardiopulmonary

1.29 Another example of this use of combining vowels occurs when forming the term describing a condition of the heart and lungs. As you know, the word root for heart is *cardi*. The word root for lung is *pulmon*. The suffix -*ary* ("pertaining to") is added to form the term *pulmonary*. A combining vowel is added to unite the two word roots, creating the new term _____, which can be written as cardi/o/pulmon/ary.

epi/derm/is

1.30 A third rule to remember when forming constructed words from word parts occurs when prefixes are added to other word parts. Generally, a prefix requires no change when another word part unites with it to form a new term. For example, *epi-* is a prefix that means "upon, over, above, or on top." When it is combined with the word *dermis,* which means "skin," it forms the new term *epidermis* that means "on top of the skin." The constructed form of this new term is written _____/_____/_____. Notice that the prefix *epi-* did not change.

vertebrae

diagnoses

myocardia

1.31 Finally, because most medical terms are composed of Latin or Greek word parts, changing a singular medical term into a plural form is handled differently than in most English-language words where an *s* is simply added to the end. Here are some helpful points:

- If the term ends in *a,* the plural is usually formed by adding an *e.* For example, the plural form of the term vertebra is _____.
- If the term ends in *is,* the plural form is usually formed by changing the *is* to *es.* For example, the plural form of diagnosis is _____.
- If the term ends in *itis,* the plural form is *itides.* For example, the plural form of gastritis is gastritides.
- If the term ends in *on* or *um,* the plural form drops the *on* or *um* and adds *a.* For example, the plural form of ganglion is ganglia and myocardium is _____.

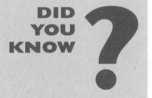

DID YOU KNOW ?

Rules to Remember
- A prefix comes before the word root or combining form.
- A suffix is a word ending and comes after the word root(s) or combining form(s).
- The word root or combining form provides the primary meaning of the term.
- The combining vowel for most word roots is *o.* The vowels *i* and *e* are also used as combining vowels for some word roots. If the combining form is to be joined with another word root or combining form that begins with a consonant, retain the combining vowel. When adding a suffix starting with a vowel to a combining form, drop the combining vowel.
- Prefixes do not require combining vowels to join with other word parts. Rarely, a prefix will drop its ending vowel to combine with another word part.
- Medical terms are deciphered by breaking them into word parts, then defining first the suffix, then the prefix, then the word root(s) or combining forms.

The following list of word parts includes prefixes, word roots/combining forms, and suffixes. These are provided for you to practice constructing and deconstructing medical terms in the exercises that follow. You will be asked to learn these terms and their definitions later in this text. For now, concentrate on practicing the principles of constructed medical terms that you learned in the previous frames.

Prefix	Definition
anti-	against, opposite of
brady-	slow
endo-	within
epi-	upon, over, above, on top
neo-	new
pre-	before

Word Root/ Combining Vowel	Definition
append/o, appendic/o	appendix
bi/o	life
cardi/o	heart
cerebr/o	cerebrum (the largest portion of the brain)
dermat/o	skin
electr/o	electricity
encephal/o	brain
gastr/o	stomach
hem/o	blood
hepat/o	liver
hyster/o	uterus
laryng/o	larynx, voice box
leuk/o	white
mamm/o	breast
mast/o	breast
ment/o	mind
nat/o	birth
neur/o	nerve
path/o	disease
proct/o	rectum or anus
psych/o	mind
rhin/o	nose
tonsill/o	almond, tonsil
vas/o	vessel

Suffix	Definition
-al	pertaining to
-ectomy	surgical excision, removal
-emia	condition of blood
-gram	a record or image
-iatry	treatment, specialty
-ia	condition of
-ic	pertaining to
-itis	inflammation
-logist	one who studies
-logy	study or science of
-pathy	disease
-philia	loving, affinity for
-plasty	surgical repair
-scope	instrument, used for viewing

PRACTICE: Forming Words from Word Parts

The Right Match

Match the term on the left with the correct definition on the right.

_____ 1. combining vowel

_____ 2. -al

_____ 3. prefix

_____ 4. consonant

a. adding this word part to a word root requires no combining vowel

b. a suffix

c. if a suffix begins with this type of letter, use a combining vowel

d. used to connect a word root with another word root or a suffix

Break the Chain

Analyze these medical terms:

a)   Separate each term into its word parts and label each word part using **p** = prefix, **r** = root, **cv** = combining vowel, and **s** = suffix.

b)   For the Bonus Question, write the requested word part or definition in the blank that follows.

The first set has been completed for you as an example.

1.   a)   cardiology

   cardi / o / logy
       r   cv   s

   b)   *Bonus Question:* What is the definition of the suffix? *study or science of*

2.   a)   appendicitis

   _____ / _____
          /

   b)   *Bonus Question:* What is the definition of the suffix? _____

3.   a)   hepatitis

   _____ / _____
        /

   b)   *Bonus Question:* What is the definition of the word root? _____

4.   a)   neonatology

   _____ / _____ / ___ / _____
        /   /   /

   b)   *Bonus Question:* Does this term contain a word root? _____

5.   a)   mammoplasty

   _____ / ___ / _____
         /   /

   b)   *Bonus Question:* What is the definition of the suffix? _____

6.   a)   electrocardiogram

   _____ / ___ / _____ / ___ / _____
         / /   / /

   b)   *Bonus Question:* How many word roots/combining forms does this term have? _____

7.   a)   prenatal

   _____ / _____ / _____
        /   /

   b)   *Bonus Question:* What is the definition of the prefix? _____

Linkup

Link the word parts in the list to create the terms that match the definitions. You may use word parts more than once. Remember to add combining vowels when needed—and that some terms do not use any combining vowel. The first one is completed for you as an example.

Prefixes	Word Roots/ Combining Vowel	Suffixes
endo-	encephal/o	-ectomy
neo-	hyster/o	-gram
	mamm/o	-itis
	mast/o	-logist
	nat/o	-logy
	neur/o	-pathy
	path/o	-plasty
	rhin/o	-scope

	Definition	Term
1.	inflammation of the brain	*encephalitis*
2.	study of newborns	
3.	disease of the nerves	
4.	surgical removal of a breast	
5.	surgical repair of the nose	
6.	instrument for viewing within	
7.	X-ray image of a breast	
8.	one who studies disease	
9.	surgical removal of the uterus	

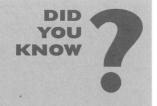

DID YOU KNOW

The Origins of Medical Terms

Just as Greek and Latin have played a critical role in the formation and meaning of words in many languages such as English, French, Italian, Spanish, Portuguese, and others, these two ancient languages have contributed to the development of the language of medicine and many related disciplines. The ancient Greeks are considered the fathers of modern medicine (Figure 1.4■). These early scholars explored and observed the human body and its functions, and they wrote about their discoveries using everyday words from their native language. The Romans advanced medicine with their own experiments and observations. They added Latin terms to the growing body of medical language.

For example, the fallopian tube that connects the ovary with the uterus is known as a *salpinx* (plural, *salpinges*). This is an ancient Greek word meaning "trumpet." The organ in the female body was named for its trumpet-like shape. From this descriptive Greek word, we can build many medical terms such as *salpingitis* ("inflammation of the uterine tube"), *salpingoplasty* ("surgical repair of the uterine tube"), *salpingo-oophorectomy* ("surgical removal of the ovary and uterine tube"), and many others. See Table 1.1 ■ for examples of combining forms that are from Greek and Latin.

Sometimes the origins of medical terms relate to history, poetry, mythology, geography, physical objects, and ideas. For example, the medical term *psychology* has its origins in the meaning of the Greek word *psyche* ("mind, soul"). Further investigation leads to the Greek myth of a princess named Psyche who falls in love with the god of love, Eros. Knowing the myth of Psyche and Eros may help some students remember the meaning of the term *psyche* when they encounter it.

We will briefly explore the origins of medical terms in other "Did You Know?" features throughout the text. Look for these boxes to expand your understanding of medical terminology and provide a useful way to remember meanings.

Figure 1.4 ■
The Greek father of medicine, Hippocrates, who originated many medical terms.
Courtesy of the National Library of Medicine.

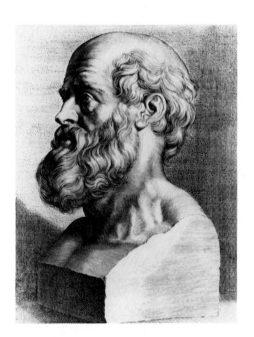

Table 1.1 ■ Word Roots from Greek and Latin

Root	Origin	Definition	Medical Term Example
lith	*lithos*, Greek	stone	*cholelithiasis* condition of having gallstones
maxim	*maximus*, Latin	biggest, highest	*gluteus maximus* the biggest (outermost) gluteus muscle in the buttocks
derm	*derma*, Greek	skin	*dermatitis* inflammation of the skin
path	*pathos*, Greek	disease	*pathogen* disease-causing agent

▶▶▶▶▶ Chapter Review

Word Building

Construct medical terms from the following meanings. (All are built from word parts. Refer to the word parts table on page 14 for word part meanings). The first question has been completed for you as an example.

1. disease within the nose   endorhino*pathy*_____

2. surgical removal of the tonsils   tonsill_____

3. surgical repair of the fallopian tube   salpingo_____

4. inflammation of the skin   _____itis

5. study of the nose   _____logy

6. pertaining to the mind   _____al

7. disease of the nerves   _____pathy

8. inherited defect in blood coagulation   _____philia

9. inflammation of the larynx   laryng_____

10. study of the skin   dermato_____

11. instrument used for viewing the larynx   _____scope

12. study (or science) of life   _____logy

13. inflammation of within the heart   endo_____itis

14. condition of slow heart (beat)   _____cardia

15. pertaining to against life   anti_____

16. surgical repair of the skin   _____plasty

17. study of nerves   neuro_____

18. pertaining to the cerebrum   cerebr_____

19. surgical removal of the stomach   _____ectomy

20. inflammation of the brain   encephal_____

21. instrument used for viewing the uterus   hystero_____

22. surgical repair of the breast   mammo_____

23. surgical removal of the appendix   append_____

24. pertaining to the liver   _____ic

Multimedia Preview ▶▶▶▶▶

Additional interactive resources and activities for this chapter can be found on the Companion Website. For videos, audio glossary, and review, access the accompanying DVD-ROM in this book.

DVD-ROM Highlights

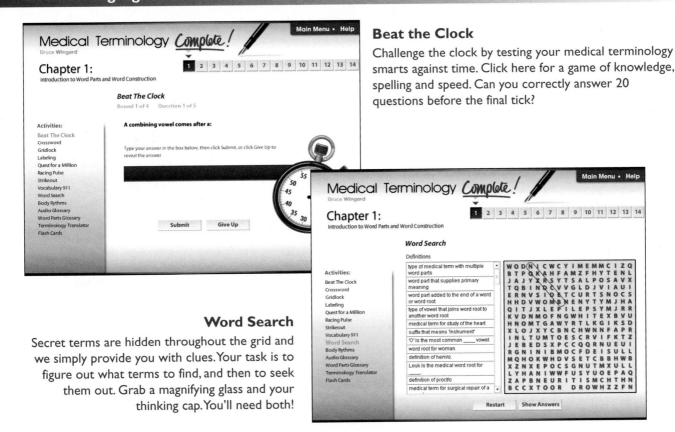

Beat the Clock

Challenge the clock by testing your medical terminology smarts against time. Click here for a game of knowledge, spelling and speed. Can you correctly answer 20 questions before the final tick?

Word Search

Secret terms are hidden throughout the grid and we simply provide you with clues. Your task is to figure out what terms to find, and then to seek them out. Grab a magnifying glass and your thinking cap. You'll need both!

Website Highlights—www.prenhall.com/wingerd

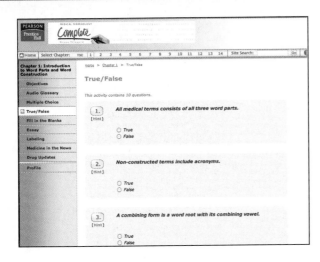

True/False Quiz

Click here to take advantage of the free-access online study guide that accompanies your textbook. You'll find a true/false quiz that provides instant feedback, allowing you to check your score and see what you got right or wrong. By clicking on this URL you'll also access links to download mp3 audio reviews, current news articles, and an audio glossary.

Understanding Suffixes ▶▶▶▶▶

Learning Objectives

After completing this chapter, you will be able to:

- Define and spell the suffixes significant in medical terminology.

- Identify suffixes in medical terms.

- Use suffixes to build medical terms that pertain to medical specialties, conditions, and diseases.

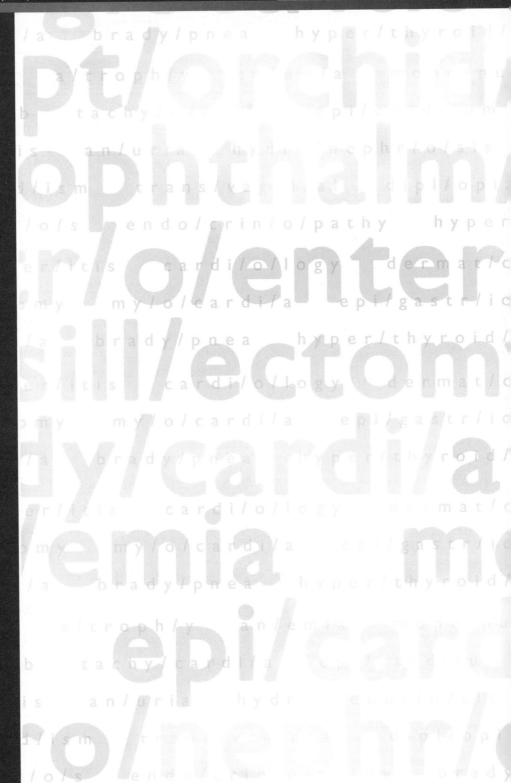

Getting Started with Suffixes ▶▶▶▶▶

Review the following list of common suffixes and their definitions. This will help you to recognize suffixes and their meanings.

Suffixes	Definition
-al	pertaining to
-ic	pertaining to
-ous	pertaining to
-itis	inflammation
-logy	study or science of
-meter	measure, measuring instrument
-pathy	disease
-scope	an instrument used for viewing
-scopy	process of viewing

	2.1 A **suffix** is the word part that is attached to the end of the word root. Like the prefix, the suffix modifies the meaning of a term. The following frames contain examples of suffixes.
-al	**2.2** In the familiar word *abnormal*, which can be shown as: *ab/norm/al* the suffix is _____, which means "pertaining to." It is the suffix because it is placed at the end of the root and it modifies the word meaning.
-itis	**2.3** The medical term *endocarditis* can be shown as *endo/card/itis* It means "inflammation within the heart." The suffix is _____, which means "inflammation." It is a suffix because it is placed at the end of the root and it modifies the word meaning.
-pathy	**2.4** The medical term *arthropathy* can be shown as: *arthr/o/pathy* It means "disease of the joint." The suffix is _____, which means "disease."

-itis	**2.5** The medical term *gastritis* can be shown as: *gastr/itis* It means "inflammation of the stomach." The suffix is _____, and the word root *gastr* means "stomach."

Suffix Introduction

Complete the following frames to expand the suffixes you know.

pertaining to **pertaining to** **pertaining to**	**2.6** The suffixes *-ic, -ous,* and *-al* all share the same meaning, which is "pertaining to." This can be seen in the terms: *hypodermic,* which means _____ _____ below the skin; *fibrous,* which means _____ _____ fiber; and *intradermal,* which means _____ _____ within the skin.
inflammation	**2.7** Because the suffix *-itis* means "inflammation," the term *esophagitis* means _____ of the esophagus.
study of	**2.8** Because the suffix *-logy* means the "study of," the term *cardiology* means the _____ _____ the heart.
measures	**2.9** Because the suffix *-meter* means "measure," a thermometer is an instrument that _____ temperature.
disease	**2.10** Because the suffix *-pathy* means "disease," the term *cardiopathy* means any _____ of the heart.
viewing	**2.11** The suffix *-scope* indicates the instrument that is used for viewing. A laparoscope is an instrument used for _____ the abdomen.

process

2.12 Because the suffix *-scopy* means "process of viewing," the term *laparoscopy* indicates a _____ in which an instrument (in this case, a laparoscope) is used to view the abdomen. (See Figure 2.1 ■.)

Figure 2.1 ■
(a) A lighted endoscope specialized for insertion into the abdomen, called a laparoscope, is used to view reproductive organs. The laparoscope may also be outfitted with surgical devices for excision of structures.
(b) Laparoscopic surgery, as seen from the monitor attached to the laparoscope.
Source: Southern Illinois University/Photo Researchers, Inc.

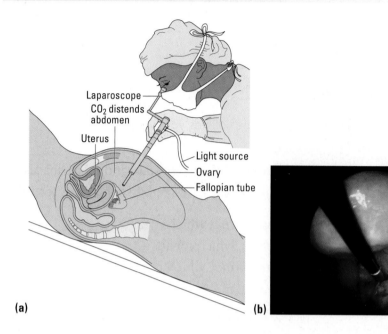

Laparoscope
CO_2 distends abdomen
Uterus
Light source
Ovary
Fallopian tube

(a)　　　(b)

PRACTICE: Suffix Introduction

The Right Match

Match the suffix on the left with the correct definition on the right.

_____ 1. -meter
_____ 2. -al
_____ 3. -scopy
_____ 4. -itis
_____ 5. -logy
_____ 6. -ous
_____ 7. -pathy
_____ 8. -scope
_____ 9. -ic

a. disease
b. pertaining to
c. inflammation
d. pertaining to
e. process of viewing
f. study or science of
g. measure
h. pertaining to
i. an instrument used for viewing

Suffix Linkup

Link the suffixes in the list to create the terms that match the definitions.

Suffix	Definition
-scopy	process of viewing
-meter	measure, measuring instrument

Suffix	Definition
-logy	study or science of
-itis	inflammation

Definition

1. study or science of the heart

2. an instrument that measures temperature

3. a procedure in which an instrument (in this case, a laparoscope) is used to view the abdomen

4. inflammation of the stomach

Term

cardio_____

thermo_____

laparo_____

gastr_____

Suffixes that Indicate an Action or State

Complete the following frames to learn about suffixes that indicate an action or state.

running	**2.13** In the term *syndrome*, the suffix *-drome*, which means "run or running," and the prefix *syn-*, which means "together," combine to literally mean "_____ together." The medical term is formally defined as a group of symptoms that together are characteristic or indicative of a specific disorder, condition, or disease.
-emesis	**2.14** In the term *hematemesis*, the word root *hemat*, which means "blood," is modified by the suffix _____, which means "vomiting." The term *hematemesis* means "vomiting of blood."
softening	**2.15** The suffix *-malacia* means "softening" as in the term *cardiomalacia*, which is the _____ or degeneration of heart tissue, usually from insufficient blood supply or tissue degeneration.
view	**2.16** In the term *biopsy*, the suffix *-opsy* means "view of"; the term is defined as the removal and examination (or _____) of tissue.
oxygen	**2.17** In the term *hypoxia*, the suffix *-oxia* means "oxygen"; the term indicates that the level of _____ in the blood is below normal.
affinity for	**2.18** The suffixes *-phil* and *-philia* mean "loving or affinity for," as in the term *hemophilia*, which literally means "_____ _____ blood" and is a condition of uncontrolled blood loss.

swallowing	**2.19** The suffix -*phagia* means "eating or swallowing." In the term *dysphagia*, the prefix adds to the meaning of the term; together these word parts combine literally to mean "painful or difficult eating or swallowing." The term is defined as a difficulty in _____.
speaking	**2.20** The suffix -*phasia* means "speaking." In the term *aphasia*, the prefix *a-*, which means "without or absence of," adds to the meaning of the term; together these word parts combine to literally mean "without or absence of _____." The term is defined as an absence or impairment of speech.
WORDS TO WATCH OUT FOR !	***-phagia* or *-phasia*?** Don't confuse the suffix -*phagia* with the suffix -*phasia*. Their meanings are very different: -*phagia* means "eating or swallowing"; -*phasia* means "speaking."
growth	**2.21** The suffix -*physis* means "growth." In the term *hypophysis*, it combines with the prefix *hypo-*, which means "below," to literally mean "_____ below." The hypophysis is the pituitary gland, which is located at the base of the brain.
paralysis	**2.22** In the term *quadriplegia*, the suffix -*plegia* means "paralysis." When it is combined with the prefix *quadri-*, the whole term means "_____ of four limbs."
tumor	**2.23** In the term *osteoma*, the suffix -*oma* means "tumor"; when combined with the word root *oste*, the combined word parts mean "_____ of bone."
still	**2.24** The suffix -*stasis* means "standing still." In the term *homeostasis*, the description, standing _____, gives an idea of continual balance; the term is defined as the tendency of an organism or system to maintain internal stability.

PRACTICE: Suffixes that Indicate an Action or State

The Right Match

Match the term on the left with the correct definition on the right.

_____ 1. -plegia
_____ 2. -oma
_____ 3. -emesis
_____ 4. -phasia
_____ 5. -oxia
_____ 6. -physis
_____ 7. -malacia
_____ 8. -philia

a. tumor
b. speaking
c. growth
d. oxygen
e. paralysis
f. softening
g. loving, affinity for
h. vomiting

Suffix Linkup

Link the suffixes in the list to create the terms that match the definitions.

Suffix	Definition
-drome	run, running
-opsy	view of
-phagia	eating or swallowing

Suffix	Definition
-philia	loving, affinity for
-stasis	standing still

Definition

1. a group of symptoms that together are characteristic or indicative of a specific disorder, condition, or disease

2. the removal and examination (or view) of tissue

3. a condition of uncontrolled blood loss

4. a difficulty in swallowing

5. the tendency of an organism or system to maintain internal stability

Term

syn_____

bi_____

hemo_____

dys_____

homeo_____

Suffixes that Indicate a Condition or Disease

Complete the following frames to learn about suffixes that indicate a condition or disease.

pain	**2.25** In the term *arthralgia*, the suffix *-algia*, which means "pain," combines with the root *arthr* to mean "_____ in a joint."
weakness	**2.26** The suffix *-asthenia*, which means "weakness," makes the term *myasthenia* mean the "_____ of muscle."

absence	**2.27** The suffix -*atresia* means "a closure or the absence of a normal body opening," so the term hysteratresia is the _____ of the uterine cavity.
hernia	**2.28** Because the suffix -*cele* means "hernia, swelling, or protrusion," a meningocele is a _____ of the meninges of the brain or spinal column that protrudes through an abnormal opening in the skull or spinal column. (See Figure 2.2■.)

Figure 2.2 ■
Photograph of a child born with spina bifida, with a large meningocele.

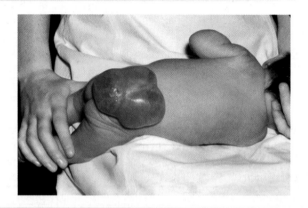

pain	**2.29** Because the suffix -*dynia* means "pain," the term *tenodynia* means "_____ in a tendon."
condition	**2.30** The suffix -*ia* means "condition," so the term *toxemia* means "a _____ in which toxins are found in the blood."
condition	**2.31** The suffix -*osis* also means "condition." In the term *adenosis*, the word root for gland is included to form the meaning "_____ of a gland."
condition	**2.32** Another suffix with the meaning "condition" is -*ism*. Thus, the term *embolism* means "a _____ in which a blood vessel is blocked by an embolus, or clot."
inflammation	**2.33** The suffix -*itis* means "inflammation." Adding this ending to the word root that means "stomach" forms the term *gastritis*, which means "_____ of the stomach."

tumor	**2.34** The suffix -*oma* means "tumor." Adding this suffix to the word root for fat, *lip*, forms the term *lipoma*, which means "_____ of fat tissue."
disease	**2.35** The suffix -*pathy* is very common and means "disease," as in the terms *neuropathy*, *gastropathy*, and *adenopathy*. In the latter, it makes the term mean "_____ of a gland."
abnormal reduction	**2.36** Because -*penia* means "deficiency or abnormal reduction in number," the term *calcipenia* means "an _____ _____ of calcium" in the tissues and fluids of the body.
fear	**2.37** The suffix -*phobia* is well known and means "fear"; hence, hydrophobia means "_____ of water."
growth	**2.38** Because -*plasia* means "formation or growth," *neoplasia* means "new formation or _____," usually referring to a tumor.
bleed	**2.39** Because -*rrhagia* means "condition of profuse bleeding or hemorrhage," the term *rhinorrhagia* means "nose_____."
discharge	**2.40** The suffix -*rrhea* means "excessive discharge," so the term *seborrhea* is an excessive _____ from the sebaceous glands.
rupture	**2.41** Because -*rrhexis* means "rupture," an amniorrhexis is a _____ of the membrane enclosing a fetus known as the amnion.
hardening	**2.42** The suffix -*sclerosis* means "condition of hardening." In the term *arteriosclerosis*, the artery walls are thickening and _____.
sudden involuntary	**2.43** The word *spasm* and the suffix -*spasm* both indicate a sudden, involuntary muscle contraction. Thus, the term *bronchospasm* indicates a _____, _____ contraction of the muscular lining of the bronchi.

PRACTICE: Suffixes that Indicate a Condition or Disease

The Right Match

Match the term on the left with the correct definition on the right.

_____ 1. -spasm
_____ 2. -algia
_____ 3. -rrhexis
_____ 4. -ism
_____ 5. -oma
_____ 6. -sclerosis
_____ 7. -pathy
_____ 8. -dynia
_____ 9. -plasia
_____ 10. -rrhagia
_____ 11. -phobia

a. rupture
b. disease
c. sudden, involuntary muscle contraction
d. formation or growth
e. pain
f. fear
g. condition of hardening
h. condition or disease
i. condition of profuse bleeding, hemorrhage
j. tumor
k. pain

Suffix Linkup

Link the suffixes in the list to create the terms that match the definitions.

Suffix	Definition
-asthenia	weakness
-cele	hernia, swelling, protrusion
-dynia	pain
-ia	condition of
-itis	inflammation
-oma	tumor

Suffix	Definition
-penia	abnormal reduction in number, deficiency
-plasia	shape, formation
-rrhagia	condition of profuse bleeding, hemorrhage
-rrhea	excessive discharge
-rrhexis	rupture

Definition		Term
1.	a nosebleed	rhino_____
2.	pain in a tendon	teno_____
3.	rupture of the amnion	amnio_____
4.	a tumor of fat tissue	lip_____
5.	an abnormal reduction of calcium in the tissues and fluids of the body	calci_____
6.	a condition in which toxins are found in the blood	toxem_____
7.	growth or formation of a tumor	neo_____
8.	debility and weakness of muscle	my_____
9.	an abnormal discharge from the sebaceous glands	sebo_____
10.	hernia or swelling of the meninges of the brain or spinal column that protrudes through a hole in the skull or spinal column	meningo_____
11.	inflammation of the stomach	gastr_____

Suffixes that Indicate Location, Number, or a Quality

Complete the following frames to learn about suffixes that indicate location, number, or a quality.

toward	**2.44** Because the suffix -*ad* means "toward," the term *cephalad* means "_____ the head."
blood	**2.45** The suffixes -*emia* and -*hemia* mean "blood or condition of blood." The prefix *poly*- means "excessive, over, or many" and the root *cyt* means "cell." These word parts combine in the term *polycythemia*, which is a condition in which there is an overproduction of red _____ cells.
fistulae	**2.46** The suffix -*a* indicates that the term is singular; the suffix -*ae* indicates the plural form, as in the singular form *fistula* versus its plural form _____.
pertaining to	**2.47** There are numerous suffixes that mean "pertaining to." They are: • -*ac* • -*al* • -*ar* • -*ary* • -*ic* • -*ous* Here are some examples of terms using these suffixes: • *cardiac*, which means "pertaining to the heart" • *cervical*, which means "pertaining to the cervix" • *ocular*, which means "pertaining to the eyes" • *pulmonary*, which means "_____ _____ the lungs" • *cephalic*, which means "pertaining to the head" • *nervous*, which means "pertaining to the nerves"

PRACTICE: Suffixes that Indicate Location, Number, or a Quality

The Right Match

Match the term on the left with the correct definition on the right.

_____ 1. -ad   a. singular

_____ 2. -emia   b. plural

_____ 3. -a   c. pertaining to

_____ 4. -ac   d. toward

_____ 5. -ae   e. condition of blood

Suffix Linkup

Link the suffixes in the list to create the terms that match the definitions. You may use them more than once.

Suffix	Definition
-a	singular
-ac	pertaining to
-ad	toward
-al	pertaining to
-ar	pertaining to
-ary	pertaining to
-hemia	blood (condition of)
-ic	pertaining to
-ous	pertaining to

Definition	Term
1. pertaining to the heart	cardi_____
2. pertaining to the cervix	cervic_____
3. pertaining to the eyes	ocul_____
4. pertaining to the lungs	pulmon_____
5. pertaining to bacteria	bacteri_____
6. pertaining to the head	cephal_____
7. pertaining to the nerves	nerv_____
8. toward the head	cephal_____
9. a condition in which there is an overproduction of red blood cells	polycyt_____

Suffixes that Indicate a Medical Specialty

Complete the following frames to learn about suffixes that indicate a medical specialty.

treatment	**2.48** Because the suffix *-iatry* means "treatment or specialty," the term *podiatry* refers to the field of health care involving the diagnosis and _____ of disorders, injuries, and diseases of the feet.
studies	**2.49** The suffix *-logist* means "one who studies," so the term *audiologist* describes a specialist who _____ about and practices in evaluating and rehabilitating communication disorders that are caused in part or wholly by hearing disorders.
study	**2.50** Similarly, the suffix *-logy* means "the study of"; hence the term *pathology* is the _____ of diseases and the structural and functional changes they cause.
practice	**2.51** The suffix *-practic* comes from the Greek word *praktikos*, which means "a practice." The suffix means "practice"; hence the term *chiropractic* is the health care _____ involving the diagnosis and treatment of musculoskeletal and nervous system disorders by manipulation of the spinal column and other body structures.

PRACTICE: Suffixes that Indicate a Medical Specialty

The Right Match

Match the term on the left with the correct definition on the right.

_____ 1. -iatry

_____ 2. -logist

_____ 3. -logy

_____ 4. -practic

a. practice

b. the study of

c. treatment, specialty

d. one who studies

Suffix Linkup

Link the suffixes in the list to create the terms that match the definitions.

Suffix	Definition
-iatry	treatment, specialty
-logist	one who studies
-logy	the study of
-practic	practice

Definition

Term

1. a specialist who studies and practices evaluating and rehabilitating communication disorders that are caused in part or wholly by hearing disorders

audio_____

2. the study of diseases and the structural and functional changes caused by them

patho_____

3. the healthcare profession involving the practice (diagnosis and treatment) of musculoskeletal and nervous system disorders by manipulation of the spinal column and other body structures

chiro_____

4. the healthcare field involving the diagnosis and treatment of disorders, injuries, and diseases of the feet

pod_____

Suffixes that Indicate a Procedure or Treatment

Complete the following frames to learn about suffixes that indicate a procedure or treatment.

puncture	**2.52** The suffix -centesis means "surgical puncture"; so the term thoracocentesis describes a medical procedure in which a surgical _____ is made into the chest cavity to remove fluid.
broken apart	**2.53** The suffixes -clasia, -clasis, and -clast all mean to "break apart." So the term osteoclasis describes a surgical procedure in which a bone is artificially fractured (or _____ _____) to correct deformity.
fusion	**2.54** An arthrodesis is a procedure that involves the surgical fixation or fusion of two or more joints using either bone grafts or metal rods. The suffix -desis means "surgical fixation or _____."
excision	**2.55** The suffix -ectomy means "_____," or "surgical removal." For example, a chondrectomy is the excision of cartilage, and a gastrectomy is the excision of the stomach. (See Figure 2.3■.)

Figure 2.3 ■
Gastrectomy. A removal of part of the stomach, called a partial gastrectomy. Surgical repair follows, which is called gastroplasty (Frame 2.62).

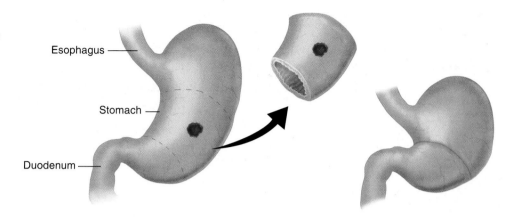

Esophagus

Stomach

Duodenum

recording	**2.56** The suffixes *-gram*, *-graph*, and *-graphy* are closely related: *-gram* means "a record or image," *-graph* means "an instrument for recording," and *-graphy* is a "recording process." When the combining form *angi/o* is added to these suffixes, the resulting terms are: • *angiogram*, a record or X-ray image of arteries • *angiograph*, which is an instrument for _____ arteries using radioactive dye injected into the artery • *angiography*, which is the process of recording an angiogram
measuring	**2.57** Because the suffix *-meter* means "measure or measuring instrument," a thermometer is an instrument used for _____ temperature.
measurement	**2.58** Similarly, the suffix *-metry* means "measurement or process of measuring." Hence, urinometry is the _____ or process of measuring the specific gravity of urine.
fixation	**2.59** The suffix *-pexy* means "surgical fixation or suspension." The term *mastopexy* means "a surgical _____ or lifting of the breasts."
protective	**2.60** The suffix *-phylaxis* means "protection" as in the term *prophylaxis*, which means "_____ treatment to prevent disease."
surgical repair	**2.61** The suffix *-plasty* means "surgical repair," so the term *gastroplasty* means "a _____ _____ of the stomach."
suturing	**2.62** Because *-rrhaphy* means "suturing," the term *angiorrhaphy* means "the _____ of a blood vessel."

instrument **viewing**	**2.63** The suffixes -*scope* and -*scopy* are very similar: -*scope* means "a viewing instrument," and -*scopy* means "the process of viewing." So the term *gastroscope* means "an _____ for examining and treating the stomach," whereas a gastroscopy indicates the _____, or examination, process itself.
surgical	**2.64** The suffix -*stomy* means "surgical creation of an opening," so the term *gastrostomy* means "the _____ creation of an opening into the stomach."
cutting instrument	**2.65** The suffixes -*tome* and -*tomy* are closely related. The suffix -*tome* is a cutting instrument, and -*tomy* is an incision. So the craniotome is the _____ _____ used during a craniotomy.
crush	**2.66** The suffix -*tripsy* means "surgical crushing," as in the term *lithotripsy*, which means "to _____ unwanted stones" that may form in the kidneys or gallbladder.
process	**2.67** The suffix -*ion* means "process," as in the term *ovulation*, which is the _____ of ovulating.

PRACTICE: Suffixes that Indicate a Procedure or Treatment

The Right Match _____

Match the term on the left with the correct definition on the right.

_____ 1. -centesis		a.	measurement or process of measuring
_____ 2. -graphy		b.	surgical creation of an opening
_____ 3. -clast		c.	immobilization
_____ 4. -tomy		d.	process of viewing
_____ 5. -metry		e.	suturing
_____ 6. -desis		f.	recording process
_____ 7. -stomy		g.	break apart
_____ 8. -scopy		h.	incision
_____ 9. -pexy		i.	surgical puncture
_____ 10. -rrhaphy		j.	excision or surgical removal
_____ 11. -ectomy		k.	surgical repair
_____ 12. -plasty		l.	surgical fixation

Suffix Linkup

Link the suffixes in the list to create the terms that match the definitions. You may use them more than once.

Suffix	Definition
-centesis	surgical puncture
-clasis	break apart
-desis	surgical fixation, fusion
-gram	a record or image
-graphy	recording process
-ion	process
-meter	measure, measuring instrument
-pexy	surgical fixation, suspension
-phylaxis	protection
-plasty	surgical repair
-scope	viewing instrument
-tome	cutting instrument
-tripsy	surgical crushing

Definition		Term
1.	a medical procedure in which a surgical puncture is made into the chest cavity to remove fluid	thoraco_____
2.	a surgical procedure in which a joint is artificially fractured (or broken apart) to correct deformity	osteo_____
3.	to surgically crush or pulverize kidney stones or gallstones	litho_____
4.	the cutting instrument used during a craniotomy	cranio_____
5.	a procedure that involves the surgical fixation or fusion of two or more joints using either bone grafts or metal rods	arthro_____
6.	the image or recording or X-ray of arteries	angio_____
7.	the process of recording an angiogram	angio_____
8.	an instrument used for measuring temperature	thermo_____
9.	the process of ovulating	ovulat_____
10.	a surgical fixation or lifting of the breasts	masto_____
11.	protective treatment against disease	pro_____
12.	surgical repair of the stomach	gastro_____
13.	an instrument for examining and treating the stomach	gastro_____

▶▶▶▶▶ Chapter Review

Word Building _____

Construct medical terms from the following meanings. The first question has been completed for you as an example.

1. disease of the joint .... arthro*pathy*_____
2. pertaining to the nerves .... nerv_____
3. group of symptoms that together are characteristic or indicative of
    a specific disorder, condition, or disease .... syn_____
4. surgical procedure in which a bone is artificially fractured (or broken
    apart) to correct deformity .... osteo_____
5. benign tumor made of fat tissue .... lip_____
6. condition of uncontrolled blood loss .... hemo_____
7. specialist who studies about and practices in evaluating and rehabilitating
    communication disorders that are caused in part or wholly by hearing disorders ... audio_____
8. study of diseases and the structural and functional changes they cause ... patho_____
9. vomiting of blood .... hemat_____
10. painful or difficult eating or swallowing .... dys_____
11. protective treatment against disease .... pro_____
12. surgical puncture into the chest cavity to remove fluid .... thoraco_____
13. health care field involving the diagnosis and treatment of disorders,
    injuries, and diseases of the feet .... pod_____
14. softening or degeneration of heart tissue .... cardio_____
15. to surgically crush unwanted stones that may form in the kidneys or
    gallbladder .... litho_____
16. pain in a tendon .... teno_____
17. surgical repair of the stomach .... gastro_____
18. condition in which toxins are found in the blood .... toxem_____
19. hernia of the meninges of the brain or spinal column that protrudes
    through a hole in the skull or spinal column .... meningo_____
20. level of oxygen in the blood is below normal .... hyp_____
21. instrument for examining and treating the stomach .... gastro_____
22. pertaining to the cervix .... cervic_____
23. health care practice (diagnosis and treatment) of musculoskeletal and nervous
    system disorders by manipulation of the spinal column and other body structures ... chiro_____
24. procedure that involves the surgical fixation or fusion of two or more joints
    using either bone grafts or metal rods .... arthro_____
25. removal and examination (or view) of tissue .... bi_____

26. debility and weakness of muscle   my_____

27. instrument that measures temperature   thermo_____

28. inflammation of the esophagus   esophag_____

29. process of using an instrument to view the abdomen   laparo_____

30. without or absence of speaking   a_____

31. literally, "growth below"   hypo_____

32. paralysis of four limbs   quadri_____

33. pain in a joint   arthr_____

34. abnormal reduction of calcium   calci_____

35. new formation or growth   neo_____

36. condition of profuse bleeding of the nose (nosebleed)   rhino_____

37. record or X-ray image of arteries   angio_____

38. process of recording an angiogram   angio_____

39. pertaining to below the skin   hypoderm_____

40. tendency of an organism or system to maintain internal stability   homeo_____

41. absence of the uterine cavity   hyster_____

42. condition of a gland   aden_____

43. condition in which a blood vessel is blocked by a clot   embol_____

44. excessive discharge from the sebaceous glands   sebo_____

45. condition of hardening of the artery walls   arterio_____

46. sudden, involuntary contraction of the bronchi   broncho_____

47. toward the head   cephal_____

48. plural form of *fistula*   fistul_____

49. pertaining to the heart   cardi_____

50. pertaining to the eyes   ocul_____

51. excision of the stomach   gastr_____

52. surgical fixation of the breasts   masto_____

53. suturing of a blood vessel   angio_____

54. surgical creation of an opening into the stomach   gastro_____

55. process of ovulating   ovulat_____

56. fear of wate   hydro_____

Multimedia Preview ▶▶▶▶▶

Additional interactive resources and activities for this chapter can be found on the Companion Website. For videos, audio glossary, and review, access the accompanying DVD-ROM in this book.

DVD-ROM Highlights

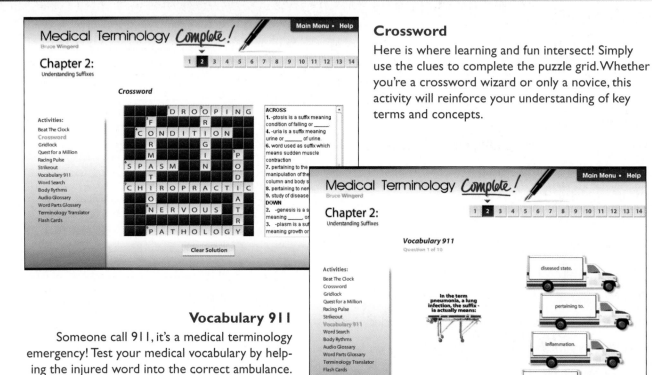

Crossword

Here is where learning and fun intersect! Simply use the clues to complete the puzzle grid. Whether you're a crossword wizard or only a novice, this activity will reinforce your understanding of key terms and concepts.

Vocabulary 911

Someone call 911, it's a medical terminology emergency! Test your medical vocabulary by helping the injured word into the correct ambulance.

Website Highlights—www.prenhall.com/wingerd

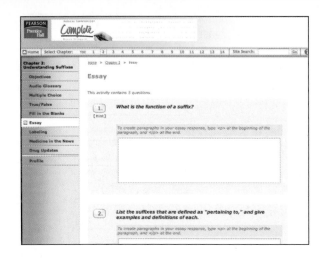

Essay Questions

Click here to take advantage of the free-access online study guide that accompanies your textbook. You'll find a series of short answer essay questions that correspond to the concepts in this chapter. By clicking on this URL you'll also access links to download mp3 audio reviews, current news articles, and an audio glossary.

Understanding Prefixes ▶▶▶▶▶

Learning Objectives

After completing this chapter, you will be able to:

- Define and spell the prefixes commonly used in medical terminology.

- Identify prefixes in medical terms.

- Use prefixes to build medical terms.

Getting Started with Prefixes ▶▶▶▶▶

Review the following list of some prefixes and their definitions. This will help you become more familiar with prefixes.

Prefixes	Definition
a-	without or absence of
ab-	away from
bi-	two
endo-	within
hyper-	excessive, abnormally high, above
hypo-	deficient, abnormally low, below
intra-	within
post-	to follow after
pre-	to come before
sub-	under, beneath, below

fix	**3.1** A **prefix** is the word part that is placed before the root to modify its meaning. The word *prefix* literally means "to _____ at the beginning of a word." The following frames contain some examples of prefixes.
prefix	**3.2** The familiar word *abnormal*, which can be shown as: *ab/norm/al* includes the prefix *ab-*, which means "away from." It is the _____ because it is placed before the root to modify the word's meaning.
intra-	**3.3** The medical term *intravenous*, which can be shown as: *intra/ven/ous* means "pertaining to within a vein." The prefix is _____, which means "within." It is the prefix because it is placed before the root to modify the word's meaning.
hyper-	**3.4** The word *hypertension* can be shown as: *hyper/tens/ion* The prefix is _____, which means "excessive, abnormally high, or above."

Prefix Introduction

Complete the following frames to expand the prefixes you know.

convulsions	**3.5** The prefix *anti-* means "against or opposite of" as in the term *anti-convulsive*, which is a type of drug used to stop _____.
a-	**3.6** The one-letter prefix that means "without or absence of" is _____. An example of its use is found in the term *aphasia*, which means "absence of speech."
together	**3.7** The prefix *con-* means "with, together, or jointly." For example, when twins are conjoined the *con-* prefix indicates that the twins are joined _____.
conception	**3.8** *Contra-* means "counter or against" as in the term *contraception*, which literally means "against _____."
WORDS TO WATCH OUT FOR !	**contra- or con-?** Don't confuse the prefix *contra-* with the prefix *con-*. Their meanings are very different. *Contra-* means "counter or against"; the prefix *con-* means "with, together, or jointly."
changed	**3.9** *Meta-* means "after or change" as in the term *metabolism*, which is the process by which foods are _____ into elements the body can use.

PRACTICE: Prefix Introduction

The Right Match _____

Match the term on the left with the correct definition on the right.

_____ 1. meta-

_____ 2. a-

_____ 3. contra-

_____ 4. con-

_____ 5. anti-

a. against or opposite

b. after or change

c. without or absence of

d. counter or against

e. with, together, or jointly

Prefix Linkup

Link the prefixes in the list to create the terms that match the definitions.

Prefix	Definition
a-	*without or absence of*
con-	*with or together*
contra-	*counter or against*
meta-	*after or change*

Definition

1. prevention of conception

2. the process by which foods are changed into elements the body can use

3. when twins are joined together

4. the absence of speech

Term

_____ception

_____bolism

_____joined

_____phasia

Prefixes that Indicate Number or Quantity

Complete the frames below to learn about prefixes that indicate number or quantity.

both	3.10 The prefix *ambi-* means "both"; the term *ambidextrous* is the ability to use _____ hands equally.
bifocal	3.11 The prefix *bi-* means "two." For example, _____ means "pertaining to two focal points," as in eyeglasses that correct for both near vision and far vision.
two	3.12 The term *bicuspid* means "having _____ points."
second	3.13 Another way to say "two" is "second." Therefore, a woman who has given birth for the _____ time is bipara.
double	3.14 The prefix *di-* means "double." Therefore, diplegia is _____ plegia, or paralysis of two limbs.
double	3.15 The prefix *dipl-* also means "double." In the term *diplopia,* the prefix *dipl-* indicates that a person with the condition perceives a single object as two images; it is also called _____ vision.
one	3.16 Because the prefix *hemi-* means "half," hemiplegia is a paralysis of half the body; in other words, on _____ side of the body.

one	**3.17** The prefix *mono-* means "one." Monoplegia means "paralysis of _____ limb or muscle/muscle group."
numerous	**3.18** The prefix *multi-* means "many, more than once, or numerous." Multiple myeloma is a disease of the bone marrow in which _____ myelomas, which are small tumors, are found in the bone marrow of different bones.
once	**3.19** When a woman's chart indicates *multipara*, it means that she has given birth multiple times, or more than _____.
never	**3.20** The terms *nullipara* and *nulligravida* share the prefix *nulli-*, which means "none." Nullipara means "the condition of never having given birth or no births"; nulligravida means "_____ having been pregnant or no pregnancies."
little	**3.21** The prefixes *oli-* and *oligo-* mean "little." The secretion of less than 400 mL of urine in a 24-hour period is called *oliguria*; it is also commonly described as "scanty" urine output. Similarly, oligospermia is a condition in which the body produces _____, or an insufficient amount of, sperm.
all	**3.22** Because the prefix *pan-* means "all," the term *pandemic* refers to a disease that is prevalent universally in an area. Also, pansinusitis is inflammation of _____ paranasal sinuses on one or both sides of the nose.
poly-	**3.23** The term *polyphagia* includes the prefix _____. The prefix means "excessive, over, or many." The term means "excessive eating."
excessive	**3.24** Polydipsia is _____ thirst.
excessive	**3.25** Polyuria is the _____ excretion of urine.
many	**3.26** Polyarteritis is the inflammation of _____ medium and small arteries where they branch.
first	**3.27** The prefix *primi-* means "first." A woman who has given birth for the _____ time is a primipara.

primi-	**3.28** A woman who is pregnant for the first time is a _____ gravida.
four	**3.29** Quadriplegia and tetraplegia both mean "paralysis of four limbs." Therefore, *quadri-* and *tetra-* are both prefixes that mean _____.
partially	**3.30** The prefix *semi-* means "half or partial." The term *semiconscious* means "_____ conscious."
three	**3.31** The prefix *tri-* means "three," as in *tricycle*. The term *tripara* means "a woman who has given birth _____ times."
three	**3.32** The tricuspid valve consists of _____ cusps, which are membranous flaps that control blood flow between the right atrium and the right ventricle of the heart.
one	**3.33** The prefix *uni-* means "one," similar to *mono-*. Therefore, a unipara woman has given birth to _____ child.

PRACTICE: Prefixes that Indicate Number or Quantity

The Right Match

Match the term on the left with the correct definition on the right.

_____ 1. di-		a.	excessive, over, or many
_____ 2. ambi-		b.	half
_____ 3. quad-		c.	first
_____ 4. hemi-		d.	half or partial
_____ 5. bi-		e.	two
_____ 6. primi-		f.	double
_____ 7. tri-		g.	both
_____ 8. pan-		h.	little or insufficient
_____ 9. semi-		i.	four
_____ 10. uni-		j.	one
_____ 11. multi-		k.	one
_____ 12. poly-		l.	null or none
_____ 13. mono-		m.	all
_____ 14. nulli-		n.	many, more than once, or numerous
_____ 15. oligo-		o.	three

Prefix Linkup

Link the prefixes in the list to create the terms that match the definitions. You may use them more than once.

Prefix	Definition
ambi-	both
mono-	one
nulli-	none
oligo-	little
poly-	excessive, over, or many
tri-	three

Definition   Term

1. paralysis of one limb or muscle/muscle group   _____plegia

2. never having been pregnant or no pregnancies   _____gravida

3. the ability to use both hands equally   _____dextrous

4. excessive eating   _____phagia

5. the valve that consists of three cusps that control blood flow between   _____cuspid
   the right atrium and the right ventricle

6. a condition where the body produces an insufficient amount of sperm   _____spermia

Prefixes that Indicate Location or Timing

Complete the following frames to learn about prefixes that indicate location or timing.

away	**3.34** The prefix *ab-* means "away from," so the term *abduction* means "_____ from the midline of the body."
toward	**3.35** The prefix *ad-* means "toward," so the term *adduction* means "_____ the midline of the body."
anatomy	**3.36** The prefix *ana-* means "up, toward"; the word root *tom* means "to cut"; and the suffix *-y* means "process of." So the term _____ means "process of cutting up."
before	**3.37** Prenatal and antenatal share the root *nat*, which means "birth." Both terms mean "before birth," so both prefixes, *pre-* and *ante-*, have the same meaning, which is "_____" or "to come before."
through	**3.38** The term *dialysis* literally means "to loosen through" because the prefix *dia-* means "_____" and the suffix *-lysis* means "to loosen." The term *dialysis* refers to the procedure that removes uric acid and urea from circulating blood.

apart **away**	**3.39** The prefix *dis-* means "apart or away." In the term *dislocation*, the prefix indicates that the dislocated part is _____ or _____ from its normal position in the body.
outside	**3.40** *Ec-* and *ecto-* mean "outside or out." An ectopic pregnancy is one in which the fertilized egg implants somewhere _____ the uterus.
within	**3.41** The prefix *endo-* means "within." Thus, the term *endogastric* means "_____ the stomach." (See Figure 3.1■.)

Figure 3.1 ■
(a) Endogastric procedure using an endoscope to observe the internal stomach lining.
(b) Image of a peptic ulcer on the stomach lining.

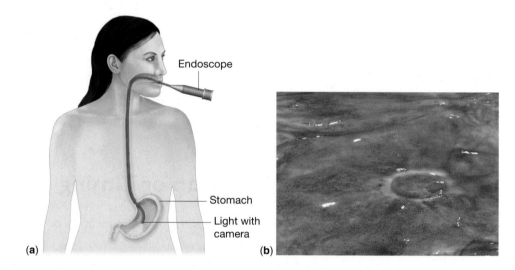

Endoscope

Stomach

Light with camera

(a)   (b)

over	**3.42** The prefixes *ep-* and *epi-* mean "upon, over, above, or on top." The epidermis is the outermost layer of skin because it is _____ the dermis layer.
inward	**3.43** Esotropia is a condition where the eye deviates _____ because the prefix *eso-* means "inward."
away from	**3.44** The prefixes *ex-* and *exo-* mean "outside or away from," so in the condition *exotropia,* the eye deviates _____ _____ its normal position.
extra-	**3.45** The common prefix shared by *extracellular*, *extracorporeal*, and *extrauterine* is _____, which means "outside."
below	**3.46** *Infer-* has the meaning "below," as in the term *inferior.* The term *inferior* indicates a position _____ another point of reference.

between	**3.47** Because the prefix *inter-* means "between," the term *intervertebral* indicates a position _____ the vertebrae.
intra-	**3.48** Intracellular and intrauterine share the prefix _____, which also means "within."
within	**3.49** Because *intra-* means "within," the term *intradermal* means "_____ the layers of the skin."
abnormal	**3.50** The prefix *para-* means "alongside or abnormal." In the term *paracusis*, it indicates _____ hearing or a disorder in hearing.
around	**3.51** The prefix *peri-* means "around." In the term *pericardium*, this prefix indicates that the membrane called the pericardium covers the area _____ the heart.
after	**3.52** The prefix *post-* means "to follow after," thus the term *postpartum* means "to follow _____ birth."
after	**3.53** Postnatal and postpartum share the prefix *post-*, which means "to follow after." Both terms mean "to follow _____ birth."
hypo- **subcutaneous**	**3.54** The prefixes *sub-* and *hypo-* both mean "beneath, below." To build a term that means "beneath the skin," add the prefix _____ to the word root for skin, *dermis*. The resulting term is *hypodermis*. An alternate term for the area beneath the skin attaches *sub-* to another word for skin, *cutaneous*. The resulting term is _____. (See Figure 3.2■.)

Figure 3.2 ■
Skin layers. The epidermis is on top of the dermis, and the hypodermis (or subcutaneous layer) is below the dermis.

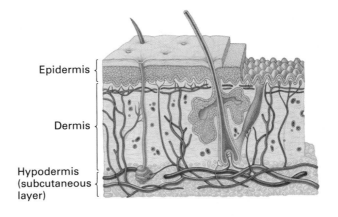

Epidermis

Dermis

Hypodermis
(subcutaneous
layer)

above	**3.55** The prefixes *super-* and *supra-* share the meaning "above"; in the term *superior* it indicates a position _____ another point of reference.
together	**3.56** The prefixes *sym-* and *syn-* also share a meaning. In this case they mean "together or joined." For example, a syndrome is a group of symptoms or signs that occur _____ .

PRACTICE: Prefixes that Indicate Location or Timing

The Right Match _____

Match the term on the left with the correct definition on the right.

_____ 1. ab-	a.	before
_____ 2. dia-	b.	up
_____ 3. ad-	c.	apart or away
_____ 4. endo-	d.	outside
_____ 5. ante-	e.	away, away from
_____ 6. extra-	f.	outside or away from
_____ 7. ep-, epi-	g.	toward
_____ 8. ana-	h.	within
_____ 9. infer-	i.	inward
_____ 10. ec-, ecto-	j.	through
_____ 11. para-	k.	upon, over, above, or on top
_____ 12. dis-	l.	to follow after
_____ 13. peri-	m.	between
_____ 14. ex-, exo-	n.	alongside, abnormal
_____ 15. intra-	o.	below
_____ 16. eso-	p.	around
_____ 17. sub-	q.	outside or out
_____ 18. post-	r.	before
_____ 19. pre-	s.	together or joined
_____ 20. super-, supra-	t.	beneath, below
_____ 21. sym-, syn-	u.	above

Prefix Linkup

Link the prefixes in the list to create the terms that match the definitions. You may use them more than once.

Prefix	Definition
ab-	away from
ana-	up, toward
ante-	before
dia-	through
ecto-	outside, out
exo-	outside, away from
infer-	below
para-	alongside, abnormal
pre-	to come before
sub-	under, beneath, below
syn-	together, joined

Definition

1. to cut up
2. away from the midline of the body
3. a pregnancy in which the fertilized egg implants somewhere outside the uterus
4. a procedure that removes uric acid and urea from circulating blood
5. a condition in which the eye deviates away from its normal position
6. a position below another point of reference
7. a disorder in hearing
8. beneath the skin
9. a group of symptoms or signs that occur together
10. before birth

Term

_____tomy

_____duction

_____pic

_____lysis

_____tropia

_____ior

_____cusis

_____cutaneous

_____drome

_____natal

Prefixes that Indicate a Specific Quality about a Term

Complete the following frames to learn about prefixes that indicate a specific quality about a term.

without	**3.57** Because the prefix *a-* means "without or absence of," the term *aseptic* means "sterile," or "pertaining to _____ living pathogenic organisms."
a-	**3.58** Similarly, *asymptomatic* means "pertaining to not having symptoms," because the prefix _____ means "without."
without	**3.59** The prefix *an-* also means "without or absence of." Thus, the term *anoxia* means "_____ oxygen."

slow	**3.60** Because *brady-* means "slow," the term *bradycardia* means "condition of _____ heart."
slowing	**3.61** The term *bradykinesia* combines *brady-* with the root *kines* to mean "condition of _____ or decreasing movement."
around	**3.62** The term *circumference* contains the prefix *circum-*, which means "around." The term *circumcision* literally translates as a "cut _____." Circumcision is a surgery to remove the foreskin around the penis.
dys-	**3.63** The term *dyslexia* has the prefix _____ which means "bad, abnormal, painful, or difficult." It is a learning disability involving impaired reading, spelling, and writing ability.
good	**3.64** The prefix *eu-* means "normal or good." It is a prefix in the terms *euthanasia*, and *eupepsia*, where it alters the meaning of the root to include the meaning of "normal or _____."
different	**3.65** *Heter-* and *hetero-* both mean "different." In medicine, tropia is an abnormal deviation of the eye. Adding the prefix *hetero-* adds to the meaning of the term to indicate the eyes are oriented in _____ directions.
hyper-	**3.66** The terms *hyperacidity, hyperemesis, hyperkinesia,* and *hyperthermia* share the common prefix _____, which means "excessive, abnormally high, or above."
excessive	**3.67** Hyperthyroidism is a condition of _____ levels of thyroid hormones in the body.
low	**3.68** The prefix *hypo-* means "deficient, abnormally low, or below." Hypothyroidism is a condition of abnormally _____ levels of thyroid hormones in the body, causing high blood calcium, reduced energy, and weight gain.
hyper-	**3.69** The prefix *hypo-* has a meaning that is the opposite of the prefix _____.

abnormally	**3.70** In the term *hypocalcemia*, *hypo-* indicates that the levels of calcium in the blood are _____ low.
low	**3.71** The term *hypothermia* means a "state of abnormally _____ body temperature."
large	**3.72** The prefix *macro-* means "large." The word root *cephal* means "head" and the suffix *-y* means "process of," so the term *macrocephaly* means "process of _____ head."
bad	**3.73** The prefix *mal-* means "bad," so *malabsorption* literally means "_____ absorption."
large	**3.74** The prefix *mega-* is familiar to many people and is in common use today. It shares the meaning "large or great" with the prefix *megalo-*. So the term *megalocyte* literally means "_____ cell."
small	**3.75** The prefix *micro-* means "small." Microcephaly means "process of _____ head."
neo-	**3.76** The term *neonate* refers to a newborn, specifically a baby within the first 28 days of life. The prefix _____ means "new," and the root *nat* means "birth."
false	**3.77** The prefix *pseudo-* means "false," as in the term *pseudocyesis*, which means "_____ pregnancy."
rapid	**3.78** The prefix *tachy-* means "rapid, fast." Tachycardia is an abnormally _____ heart rate that is usually defined as more than 100 beats per minute in adults.
through **across** **cross** **across**	**3.79** The prefix *trans-* means "through, cross/across, or beyond," as in *transvaginal*, which means "_____ or _____ the vagina," *transexual*, which means to "_____ over to another gender," and *transverse*, which means to "lie _____ or in a crosswise direction."

PRACTICE: Prefixes that Indicate a Specific Quality about a Term

The Right Match _____

Match the term on the left with the correct definition on the right.

_____	1. a-, an-	a.	bad
_____	2. hypo-	b.	slow
_____	3. neo-	c.	small
_____	4. tachy-	d.	false
_____	5. trans-	e.	around
_____	6. dys-	f.	normal or good
_____	7. macro-	g.	deficient, abnormally low, below
_____	8. hyper-	h.	without or absence of
_____	9. circum-	i.	different
_____	10. brady-	j.	rapid, fast
_____	11. micro-	k.	bad, abnormal, painful, or difficult
_____	12. eu-	l.	large or great
_____	13. mal-	m.	large
_____	14. pseudo-	n.	through, cross/across, or beyond
_____	15. heter-, hetero-	o.	new
_____	16. mega-, megalo-	p.	excessive, abnormally high, above

Prefix Linkup

Link the prefixes in the list to create the terms that match the definitions. You may use them more than once.

Prefix	Definition
a-	without or absence of
brady-	slow
circum-	around
dys-	bad, abnormal, painful, or difficult
hyper-	above, excessive, abnormally high
mal-	bad
megalo-	large, great
neo-	new
pseudo-	false
trans-	through, cross/across, or beyond

Definition

1. false pregnancy

2. sterile, having no living pathogenic organisms

3. a newborn; specifically, a baby within the first 28 days of life

4. abnormally slow heart rate

5. a surgery to remove the foreskin around the penis

6. cross over to another gender

7. a learning disability involving impaired reading, spelling, and writing ability

8. a condition of excess levels of thyroid hormones in the body

9. bad absorption

10. large cell

Term

_____cyesis

_____septic

_____nate

_____cardia

_____cision

_____sexual

_____lexia

_____thyroidism

_____absorption

_____cyte

▶▶▶▶ Chapter Review

Word Building

Construct medical terms from the following meanings. The first question has been completed for you as an example.

1. excessive or abnormally high sensitivity to painful stimuli   _____*hyper*_algesia

2. a substance that stops convulsions   _____convulsive

3. process by which foods are changed into useful elements   _____bolism

4. condition of seeing a single object as two images   _____opia

5. paralysis of half the body   _____plegia

6. has given birth more than once   _____para

7. has never given birth   _____para

8. universally prevalent   _____demic

9. paralysis of corresponding parts on both sides of the body   _____plegia

10. inflammation of many medium and small arteries   _____arteritis

11. having given birth for the first time   _____para

12. toward the midline of the body   _____duction

13. procedure that removes uric acid and urea from blood   _____lysis

14. body part that is apart or away from its normal position   _____located

15. pregnancy in which the fertilized egg implants somewhere outside the uterus   _____pic

16. within the layers of the skin   _____dermal

17. membrane that covers around the heart   _____cardium

18. a group of symptoms or signs occurring together   _____drome

19. pertaining to not having symptoms   _____symptomatic

20. a state of sterility, having no living pathogens   _____sepsis

21. slowing or decreasing movement   _____kinesia

22. removal of the foreskin around the penis   _____cision

23. "normal" or "good" death   _____thanasia

24. abnormally low levels of calcium in the blood   _____calcemia

25. false pregnancy   _____cyesis

26. rapid heart rate greater than 100 beats per minute   _____cardia

27. twins that are joined together   _____joined

28. literally, "against conception"   _____ception

29. ability to use both hands equally   _____dextrous

30. pertaining to two focal points   _____focal

31. paralysis of one limb or muscle/muscle group   _____plegia

32. insufficient (or "little") amount of sperm   _____spermia

33. paralysis of four limbs   _____plegia

34. partially conscious   _____conscious

35. a woman who has given birth three times   _____para

36. a woman who has given birth to one child   _____para

37. away from the midline of the body   _____duction

38. process of cutting up   _____tomy

39. before birth   _____natal

40. within the stomach   _____gastric

41. layer of skin that is over the dermis layer   _____dermis

42. condition in which the eye deviates inward   _____tropia

43. condition in which the eye deviates away from its normal position   _____tropia

44. outside the cellular area   _____cellular

45. position below another point of reference   _____ferior

46. position between the vertebrae   _____vertebral

47. abnormal hearing or a disorder in hearing   _____cusis

48. to follow after birth   _____partum

49. area beneath the skin   _____cutaneous

50. position above another point of reference   _____ior

51. without, or absence of, oxygen   _____oxia

52. learning disability that involves impaired reading, spelling, and writing ability   _____lexia

53. eyes oriented in different directions   _____tropia

54. literally, "process of large head"   _____cephaly

55. literally, "bad absorption"   _____absorption

56. literally, "large cell"   _____cyte

57. literally, "process of small head"   _____cephaly

58. baby within the first 28 days of life (newborn)   _____nate

59. through the vagina   _____vaginal

Multimedia Preview ▶▶▶▶▶

Additional interactive resources and activities for this chapter can be found on the Companion Website. For videos, audio glossary, and review, access the accompanying DVD-ROM in this book.

DVD-ROM Highlights

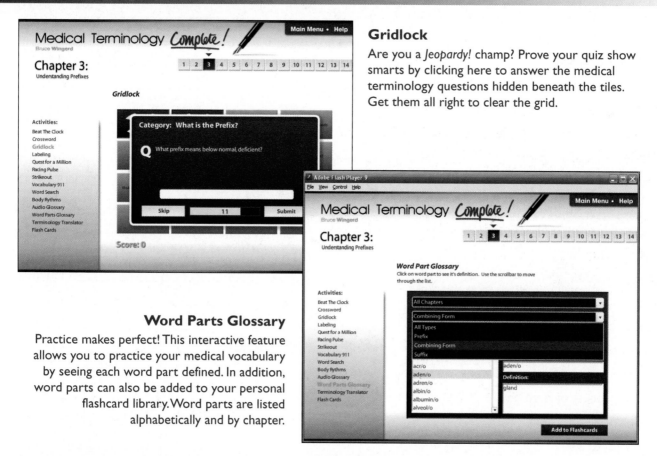

Gridlock

Are you a *Jeopardy!* champ? Prove your quiz show smarts by clicking here to answer the medical terminology questions hidden beneath the tiles. Get them all right to clear the grid.

Word Parts Glossary

Practice makes perfect! This interactive feature allows you to practice your medical vocabulary by seeing each word part defined. In addition, word parts can also be added to your personal flashcard library. Word parts are listed alphabetically and by chapter.

Website Highlights—www.prenhall.com/wingerd

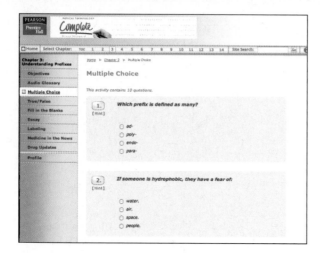

Multiple-Choice Quiz

Take advantage of the free-access online study guide that accompanies your textbook. You'll find a multiple-choice quiz that provides instant feedback, allowing you to check your score and see what you got right or wrong. By clicking on this URL you'll also access links to download mp3 audio reviews, current news articles, and an audio glossary.

The Human Body in Health and Disease ▶▶▶▶

Learning Objectives

After completing this chapter, you will be able to:

- Define and spell the word parts used to create terms for the human body.

- Identify the building blocks, organ systems, and cavities of the body.

- Identify the anatomical planes, regions, and directional terms used to describe areas of the body.

- Break down and define the important terms associated with the anatomy and physiology of the human body.

- Define the introductory terms associated with medical terminology.

- Identify the five major diagnostic imaging procedures.

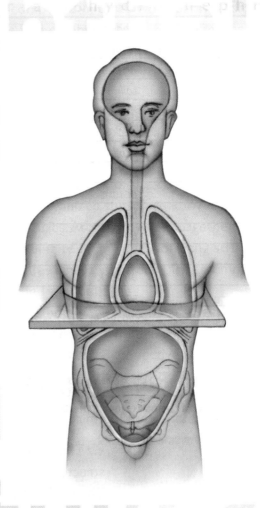

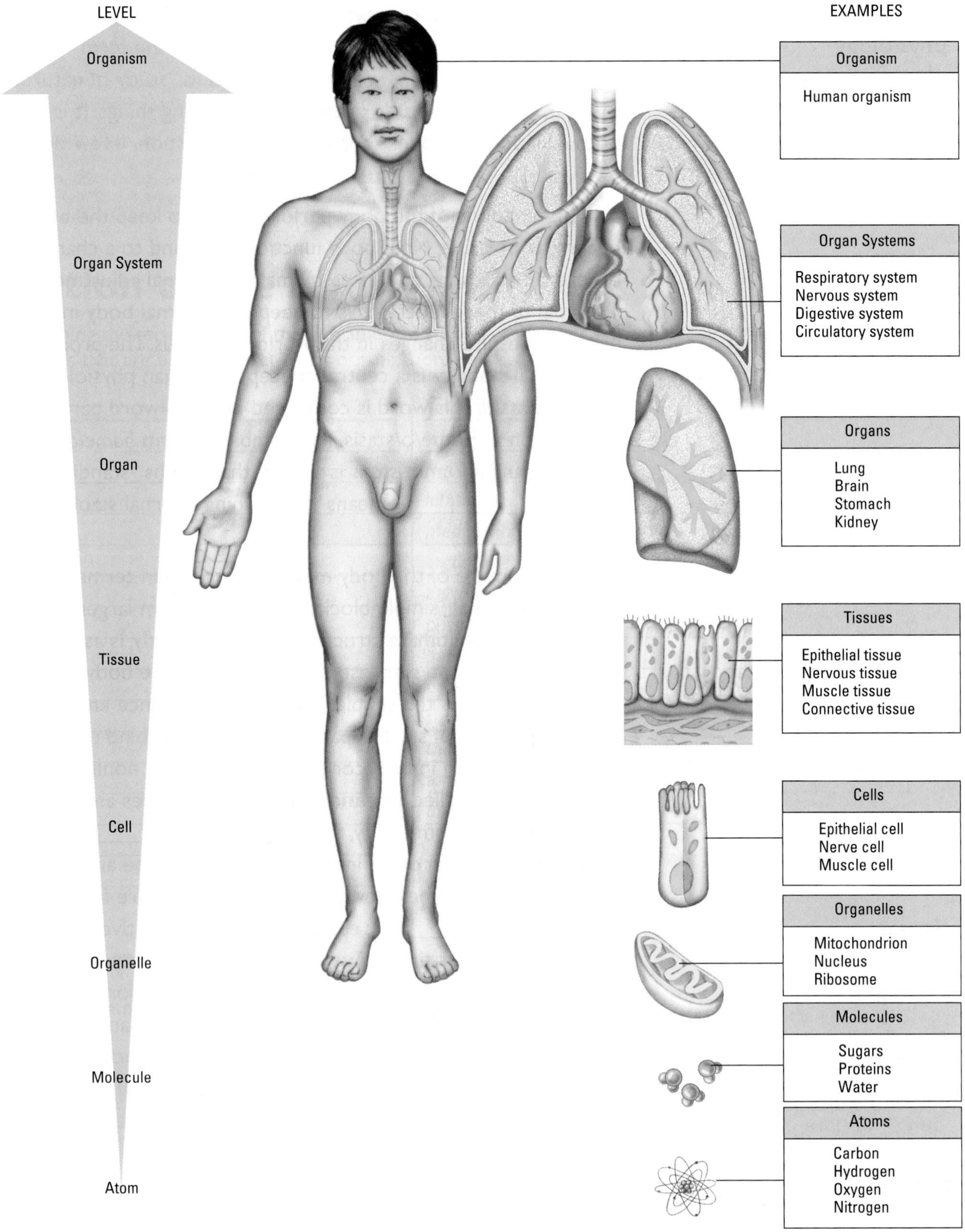

LEVEL

Organism

Organ System

Organ

Tissue

Cell

Organelle

Molecule

Atom

EXAMPLES

Organism
Human organism

Organ Systems
Respiratory system
Nervous system
Digestive system
Circulatory system

Organs
Lung
Brain
Stomach
Kidney

Tissues
Epithelial tissue
Nervous tissue
Muscle tissue
Connective tissue

Cells
Epithelial cell
Nerve cell
Muscle cell

Organelles
Mitochondrion
Nucleus
Ribosome

Molecules
Sugars
Proteins
Water

Atoms
Carbon
Hydrogen
Oxygen
Nitrogen

Figure 4.1 ■
Building blocks of the body. Complexity increases in the direction of the arrow.

Table 4.1 ■ Systems of the Body

System	Major Organs	General Function
Cardiovascular	Major arteries (in red) — Heart — Major veins (in blue)	Transport substances to and from body cells
Lymphatic	Tonsils — Thymus — Lymphatic vessels — Spleen — Lymph nodes	Remove unwanted substances and recycle fluid to the blood
Respiratory	Pharynx — Nose — Larynx — Trachea — Bronchial — Right lung — Left lung	Exchange gases between the external environment and blood

(continued)

Figure 4.4 ■
Body cavities. (a) Lateral view of a sagittal section through the body. (b) Anterior view of a frontal section through the body.

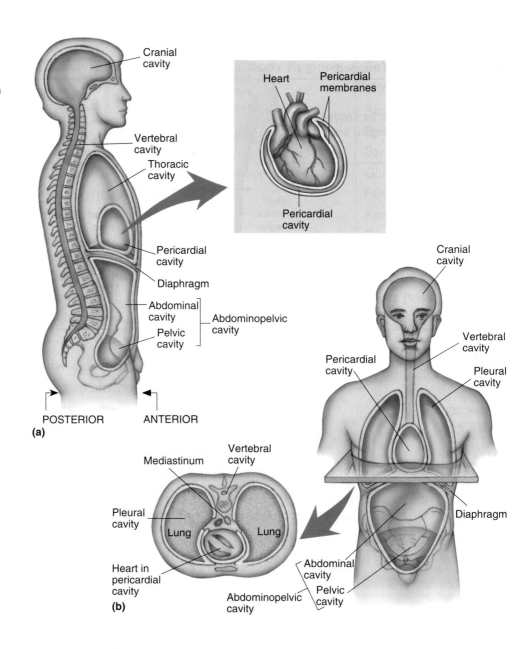

ventral cavity	4.13 The _____ _____ in the anterior part of the body is much larger than the dorsal cavity. A muscular partition called the **diaphragm** (DYE ah fram) divides the ventral cavity into an upper and lower cavity. The cavity that is superior to the diaphragm is the
inferior	**thoracic cavity**, and the cavity _____ to the diaphragm is the **abdominopelvic cavity**. You learned in Frame 4.9 that the term *thoracic* is composed of two word parts and is written thorac/ic. The term *abdominopelvic* contains four word parts and is written abdomin/o/pelv/ic. As the names suggest, the thoracic cavity lies within the chest, and the
abdominopelvic cavity	_____ _____ lies within the abdominal and pelvic areas.

pericardial cavity

pleural cavity

4.14 The thoracic cavity contains several smaller cavities. The **pericardial cavity** lies along the midline of the thoracic cavity. The term *pericardial* consists of three word parts, peri/cardi/al, and literally means "pertaining to around the heart." Thus, the _____ _____ contains the heart. The other cavities within the thoracic cavity are the two **pleural cavities**. The term *pleural* is written pleur/al and contains two word parts, *pleur*, which means "lung," and -*al*, which means "pertaining to." Thus, each _____ _____ contains one lung.

mediastinum

mee dee ah STY num

4.15 In addition to the pericardial cavity and the two pleural cavities, the thoracic cavity includes a potential space in the area including the heart and the space above, or superior to, the heart. Because it lies along the midline and is deep to the breastbone or sternum, it is called the **mediastinum**. The three word parts forming this term can be shown as media/stin/um, which literally means "pertaining to middle of sternum." The _____ contains the large blood vessels located above the heart and a gland called the thymus gland.

abdominal

pelvic

4.16 As you have learned, the abdominopelvic cavity is the large cavity of the abdominal and pelvic regions. It contains an upper and lower area, which are not divided by a partition. The upper area is the **abdominal cavity**, which contains the liver, stomach, pancreas, spleen, and most of the small and large intestines. Recall that _____ literally means "pertaining to the abdomen." At the level of the iliac crest (the tips of the hip bones), the **pelvic cavity** begins and continues to the base of the abdominopelvic cavity. The pelvic cavity contains the urinary bladder, internal reproductive organs, and parts of the small and large intestines. The word _____ may be separated into its two word parts, pelv/ic, and literally means "pertaining to a bowl," describing this bowl-shaped cavity very accurately.

PRACTICE: Anatomy and Physiology Introduction

The Right Match

Match the combining form on the left with the correct definition on the right.

_____	1. abdomin/o		a.	skull
_____	2. anter/o		b.	neck
_____	3. brachi/o		c.	tail
_____	4. caud/o		d.	back
_____	5. cephal/o		e.	distant
_____	6. cervic/o		f.	front
_____	7. cran/o, crani/o		g.	abdomen
_____	8. cyt/o		h.	arm
_____	9. dist/o		i.	cell
_____	10. dors/o		j.	head
_____	11. femor/o		k.	below
_____	12. gastr/o		l.	groin
_____	13. glute/o		m.	loin or lower back
_____	14. hom/o, home/o		n.	tool
_____	15. ili/o		o.	stomach
_____	16. infer/o		p.	middle
_____	17. inguin/o		q.	hip, groin
_____	18. lumb/o		r.	buttock
_____	19. medi/o		s.	thigh
_____	20. organ/o		t.	same
_____	21. pelv/o		u.	to cut
_____	22. physi/o		v.	chest, thorax
_____	23. poster/o		w.	navel
_____	24. proxim/o		x.	nature
_____	25. super/o		y.	belly
_____	26. thorac/o		z.	back
_____	27. tom/o		aa.	bowl
_____	28. ventr/o		ab.	above
_____	29. umbilic/o		ac.	near

Word Root Linkup _____

Link the word roots in the list to create the terms that match the definitions. You may use them more than once.

Word Root	Definition
abdomin	abdomen
cardi	heart
chondri	cartilage

Word Root	Definition
pelv	bowl
physi	nature

Definition

Term

1. refers to the study of the nature of living things

    _____/o/logy

2. the area of the abdomen

    _____/al

3. below the cartilage

    hypo/_____/ac

4. pertaining to around the heart

    peri/_____/al

5. literally means "pertaining to a bowl," describing this bowl-shaped cavity very accurately

    _____/ic

Medical Terms Introduction

As a second step in learning the terminology of the human body, in this section you will explore introductory medical terms and diagnostic procedures. Following are two combining forms that you will see in this section.

Combining Form	Definition
chron/o	time
path/o	disease

Complete the following frames to learn the basic medical terms and diagnostic procedures.

disease
dih ZEEZ

4.17 The body's goal is to keep itself alive and healthy. Each system performs functions that endeavor to keep the body in a constant, stable state by adjusting to changes. As you learned in Frame 4.4, this is the process of maintaining homeostasis. When body functions fail to maintain homeostasis, a condition of instability results that is called **disease**. In general, the term _____ refers to a state of the body in which homeostasis has faltered due to any cause.

pathology
path AHL oh jee

4.18 The study of disease is a field of medicine called **pathology**. This term is derived from the Greek word for suffering or disease, *pathos*, creating the combining form *path/o*. The term is completed by adding the suffix *-logy*, which means "study of." A **pathologist** is a physician who specializes in _____, or the study of disease.

diagnosis
DYE ag NO sis

4.19 When examining a patient who is complaining of an illness, the health-care professional must first identify the illness before it can be treated. Identification of the illness is called a **diagnosis**. This is a constructed word containing the word parts *dia-*, which means "through," and *-gnosis*, which means "knowledge." The _____ must be established before a treatment program can be made.

symptoms
SIMP tumz

4.20 To make a diagnosis, a healthcare professional listens to the patient to learn about clues that might suggest the nature of the illness. Experiences of the patient resulting from a disease are called **symptoms**. They are usually sensations—such as pain, heat, cold, or pressure—but can also be the loss of sensations, such as numbness or loss of appetite. Other _____ include dizziness, loss of balance, and mental confusion.

sign

4.21 Before a diagnosis can be made, a healthcare professional often examines the patient for physical signs of disease. A **sign** is a finding that can be discovered by an objective examination. For example, a thermometer inserted into the mouth or ear canal will indicate the presence of an elevated body temperature, or **fever**, which is a common _____ of an infectious disease.

acute
ah KYOOT

4.22 As part of a diagnosis, a disease is commonly classified as having either an expected brief duration or a long duration. The term **acute** describes a disease of short duration, often with a sharp or severe effect. For example, a head cold is usually an _____ disease because of its short duration. The medical term for a head cold is acute **coryza** (kor EYE zah). Some acute diseases can be life threatening, so keep in mind that the term does not imply a mild disease.

DID YOU KNOW ?

Acute

The term **acute** is derived from the Latin word *acutus*, which means "sharp." It describes how a symptom or sign that is of short duration strikes quickly, such as would result from a stinging stab from a sharp instrument.

chronic
KRON ik

4.23 A term frequently used to describe diseases that are of long duration is **chronic**. Derived from the Greek word for time, *kronos*, _____ diseases usually develop slowly and last for many years. An example of a chronic disease is the skin condition **psoriasis** (soh RYE ah siss), which lasts a lifetime.

infection
in FEKK shun

4.24 Diseases may also be classified on the basis of their cause or origin. One of the most common forms of disease is **infection**, in which parasitic organisms such as bacteria, viruses, and fungi attack body cells. The presence of _____ results in the development of **infectious disease**.

trauma
TRAW mah

4.25 Disease may also be caused by physical injury or **trauma**. For example, a fractured bone is a common _____ arising from an automobile collision. It is a disease because it upsets homeostasis of the affected bone. Disease resulting from trauma is called **traumatic disease**.

prognosis
prog NOH sis

4.26 Once a reliable diagnosis is made, the healthcare professional may predict the probable course of the disease and its probable outcome. This prediction is called a **prognosis**. Similar to the term _diagnosis_, _____ is a constructed word containing the word parts _pro-_, which means "before," and _-gnosis_, which means "knowledge."

diagnostic imaging

4.27 As you may suspect, making an accurate diagnosis is an essential part of medicine. As a result of improving technologies, making a diagnosis has become efficient and reliable. The most important improvements have been in the way instruments are able to observe the internal structure and functions of the body without the need for open surgical procedures. These noninvasive procedures are called **diagnostic imaging**. The five major types of _____ _____ are endoscopy, CAT scan, PET scan, MRI, and ultrasound.

endoscopy
end AH skoh pee

4.28 The use of a long, flexible tube that can be inserted into a patient is called **endoscopy**. This constructed term includes two word parts: _endo-_, which means "within," and _-scopy_, which means "process of viewing." During the _____, a healthcare professional may observe the internal cavities and organs of the patient with the attachment of a camera at the far end of the tube (Figure 4.5■). The tube may also contain surgical attachments, enabling a surgeon to manipulate internal body parts while viewing a monitor.

Figure 4.5 ■
Endoscopy. A surgical procedure using
an endoscope to view and remove an
internal mass is in progress.
Source: Getty Images—Stone Allstock.

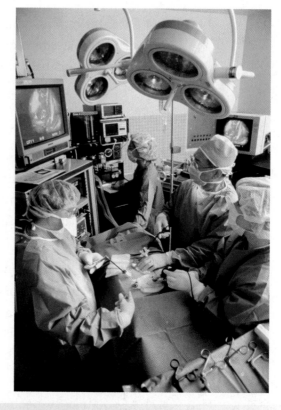

CAT scan

4.29 A **CAT scan** is a diagnostic procedure that combines multiple X-rays
and computer enhancement to produce three-dimensional images of internal body structures (Figure 4.6■). The term _____ _____ is
an acronym for **computed axial tomography scanning**. As a result of
the computer enhancement, cross-sectional images or "slices" of body regions are produced. CAT scans are useful when cross-sectional images of
organs in the chest or abdomen, muscles, and joints are needed. Speed and
relatively low cost make CAT scans the standard for evaluation of trauma
to most areas of the body.

Figure 4.6 ■
CAT scan. The CAT scan image is
visible on the monitor.
Source: Getty Images, Inc.—Taxi.

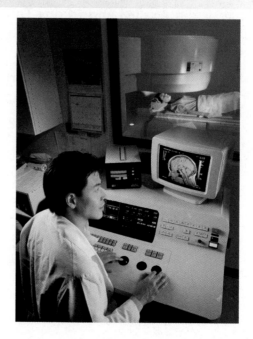

PET scan

4.30 A **PET scan** is a procedure that detects the journey of a radioactive-labeled substance, such as glucose (sugar), through the body. The PET scan instrument contains scanners that respond to the labeled glucose, and computers that create an image to track the pathway of the glucose as it is metabolized by body cells. As a result, the _____ _____ reveals areas of the body that have an unusually high metabolic rate, such as tumors (Figure 4.7■). The term *PET* is an acronym for **positron emission tomography**.

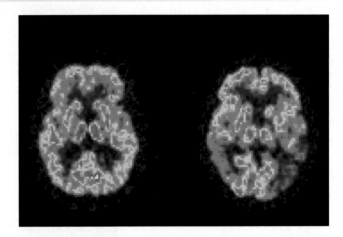

Figure 4.7 ■
PET scan. Two images of the brain, showing increased metabolic activity of cells in orange.
Source: Getty Images, Inc.—Photodisc.

MRI

4.31 Among all of the diagnostic imaging techniques available, the **MRI** has generated the most excitement in the medical community because it offers the clearest, most complete images of internal anatomy. The term *MRI* is an acronym for **magnetic resonance imaging**. The instrument includes magnets that respond to hydrogen atoms in the body by sending signals to a computer, which analyzes the information to produce three-dimensional images (Figure 4.8■). The _____ can be used to diagnose many forms of cancer, joint disease, and trauma.

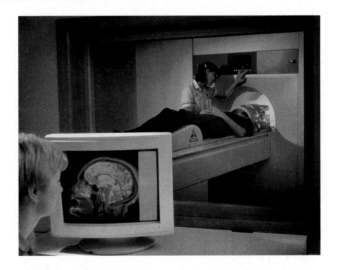

Figure 4.8 ■
MRI. The patient is exiting the MRI instrument from the adjacent computer room with an MRI of the head visible on the monitor.
Source: Geoff Tompkinson/Photo Researchers, Inc.

ultrasound imaging

4.32 Ultrasound imaging, or **sonography**, involves the pulsation of harmless sound waves through a body region. As the waves travel through tissues of varying density, they produce echoes that can be detected by a probe and interpreted by a computer (Figure 4.9■). Because of its harmless nature, _____ _____ has proven useful in prenatal care by providing an early glimpse of the developing fetus (a child before birth) in the uterus.

Figure 4.9 ■
Ultrasound imaging. The use of sound waves produces a computer-enhanced image of this couple's child on the monitor, giving the parents an exciting early view of their child and health-care professionals a valuable tool for mapping the progress of the child. *Source: Photo Researchers, Inc.*

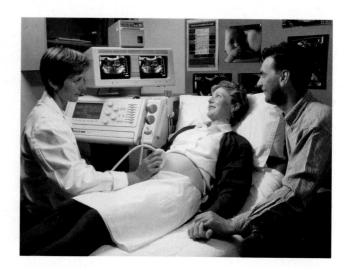

▶▶▶▶▶ Chapter Review

Word Building _____

Construct medical terms from the following meanings. (Some are built from word parts, some are not.) The first question has been completed for you as an example.

1. identification of an illness   dia/*gnosis*_____
2. maintaining internal stability   home/o/_____
3. middle of the sternum   _____/stin/um
4. of long duration   _____/ic
5. the study of disease   _____/o/logy
6. a disease of short duration   _____ (do this one on your own!)
7. divides the body into superior and inferior portions   _____ plane
8. body cavity inferior to the diaphragm   _____/_____/_____ic cavity
9. procedure using a long flexible tube   _____/scopy
10. term for a finding following an objective examination   _____
11. formed from similarly grouped cells   _____
12. area of the chest   _____ region
13. MRI   magnetic _____ imaging
14. on top of the stomach   _____/_____/ic
15. pertaining to the lung   _____/al
16. divides the body vertically into right and left portions   _____ plane
17. pertaining to the navel   _____/al
18. a common cause of disease   _____
19. study of body structure   _____/tom/y
20. study of nature   _____o/logy
21. pertaining to the back   _____/al
22. pertaining to the belly   _____/al
23. pertaining to above   _____/ior
24. pertaining to the front   _____/ior
25. pertaining to the middle   medi/_____
26. pertaining to below   infer/_____
27. region of below the stomach   _____/gastr/ic
28. region of the loin   lumb/_____
29. cavity that contains the heart   _____/cardi/al
30. cavity that contains the urinary bladder, internal repro-   _____/ic
    ductive organs, and parts of the small and large intestines
31. a state of the body in which homeostasis has faltered   _____
32. physical injury that may cause disease   _____

Multimedia Preview ▶▶▶▶▶

Additional interactive resources and activities for this chapter can be found on the Companion Website. For videos, audio glossary, and review, access the accompanying DVD-ROM in this book.

DVD-ROM Highlights

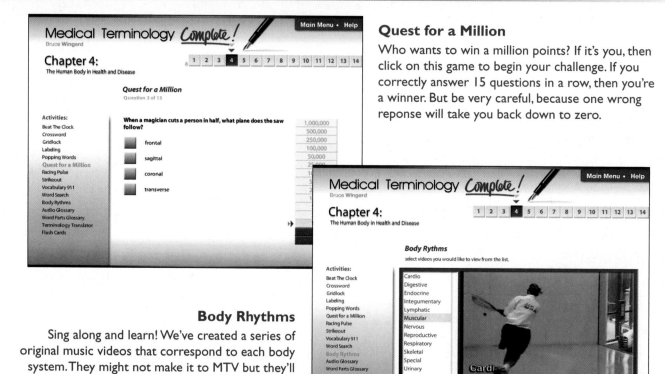

Quest for a Million

Who wants to win a million points? If it's you, then click on this game to begin your challenge. If you correctly answer 15 questions in a row, then you're a winner. But be very careful, because one wrong reponse will take you back down to zero.

Body Rhythms

Sing along and learn! We've created a series of original music videos that correspond to each body system. They might not make it to MTV but they'll help you remember basic anatomy and give you a fun study break at the same time.

Website Highlights—www.prenhall.com/wingerd

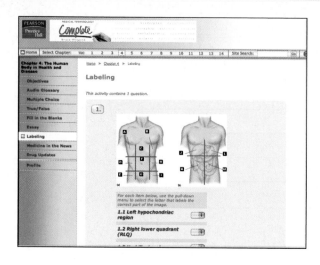

Labeling Exercise

Click here to take advantage of the free-access online study guide that accompanies your textbook. You'll find a figure labeling quiz that corresponds to this chapter. By clicking on this URL you'll also access links to download mp3 audio reviews, current news articles, and an audio glossary.

The Integumentary System ▶▶▶▶▶

Learning Objectives

After completing this chapter, you will be able to:

- Define the word parts used to create medical terms of the integumentary system.

- Break down and define common medical terms used for symptoms, diseases, disorders, procedures, treatments, and devices associated with the integumentary system.

- Build medical terms from the word parts associated with the integumentary system.

- Pronounce and spell common medical terms associated with the integumentary system.

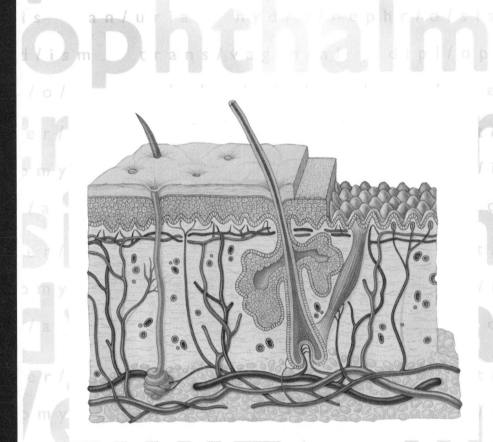

Anatomy and Physiology Terms ▶▶▶▶▶

Review the combining forms that specifically apply to the anatomy and physiology of the integumentary system. Note that the combining forms are colored red to help you identify them when you see them again later in the chapter.

Combining Form	Definition	Combining Form	Definition
aden/o	gland	follicul/o	follicle
aut/o	self	kerat/o	horny tissue
cutane/o	skin	onych/o	nail
cyan/o	blue	seb/o	sebum, oil
derm/o, dermat/o	skin		

integumentary

IN teg yoo MEN tar ee

epidermis

5.1 The _____ system forms the entire surface area of the body. It is dominated by the largest organ of the body, the **skin**. The skin is composed of two distinct layers: an inner, deep layer composed of connective tissue known as the **dermis**, and an outer layer of epithelium called the **epidermis**. The term *dermis* means "skin," and the term _____ means "on top of skin." The integumentary system also includes smaller accessory organs embedded within the skin, such as **hair follicles**, **nails**, **sebaceous glands**, **sweat glands**, and **sensory receptors**.

FUNCTION ▶▶▶

protection

5.2 The primary function of the integumentary system is protection. _____ is provided against outside temperature changes, dehydration, and infectious microorganisms that may cause disease. In addition, the sweat glands, blood vessels, and a layer of fat help the skin to regulate internal body temperature, while receptors in your skin provide the ability to detect changes in the environment, giving the skin the added function of sensation.

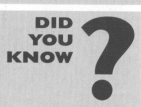

DID YOU KNOW ?

This text has a special color-coding system to help you recognize the individual word parts. Each time a word part is presented, it appears in a specific color:
- Prefixes are **blue**
- Word roots and combining forms are **red**
- Suffixes are **purple**

It's a rainbow of colors to delight your eyes and stimulate your brain. Follow the rainbow to success in medical terminology!

5.3 In the next section, you will review anatomy terms by completing the illustration labels. Use the anatomy terms that appear in the left column to fill in the corresponding blanks in Figures 5.1■ and 5.2■.

1. **epidermis**
2. **sebaceous**
3. **hair**
4. **follicle**

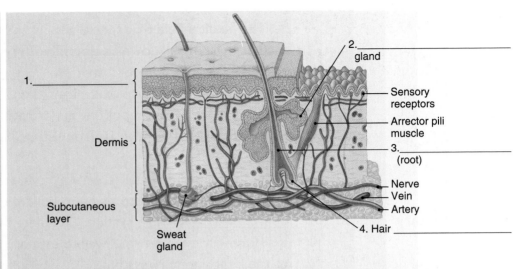

1. _____

2. _____ gland

Sensory receptors

Arrector pili muscle

3. _____ (root)

Nerve
Vein
Artery

4. Hair _____

Dermis

Subcutaneous layer

Sweat gland

Figure 5.1 ■
Anatomy of the skin. Illustration of a section of skin showing key structures.

5. **cuticle**
6. **nail**
7. **body**
8. **root**

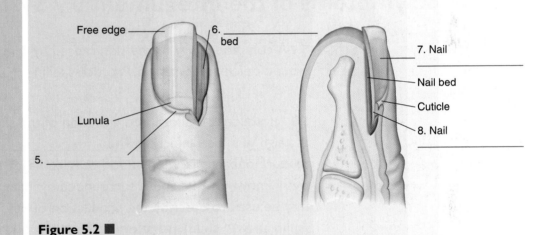

Free edge

6. _____ bed

7. Nail _____

Nail bed

Cuticle

8. Nail _____

Lunula

5. _____

Figure 5.2 ■
Nail structure, side view and cross-sectional view.

Medical Terms of the Integumentary System ▶▶▶▶▶

organ

skin

protection

5.4 The integumentary system can experience many types of challenges to its homeostasis. As the outermost organ of the body, the skin is more exposed to the extremes of the external environment than any other _____, subjecting it to temperature fluctuations, physical injury, and invasion by unwanted microorganisms. Many types of inherited and acquired diseases may also afflict the _____. In many cases, it is the first part of the body to display signs and symptoms of an internal disorder because it is the body part with which we are most familiar—we often see, feel, and touch our skin throughout the day. The _____ that it provides to your overall health is significant: A loss of skin can lead to severe consequences due to dehydration and infection, even death.

dermat/o/logy	**5.5** The medical field that specializes in the health and disease of the integumentary system is known as **dermatology** (derm ah TOL oh jee). This term is a constructed word, written _____/_____/_____, using the combining form that means "skin," *dermat/o*, to carry the primary meaning. A physician specializing in dermatology is commonly known as a **dermatologist** (derm ah TOL oh jist).
integumentary	**5.6** In the following sections, we will review the prefixes, combining forms, and suffixes that combine to build the medical terms of the _____ system. Complete the frames and review exercises that follow. You are on your way to mastery of the medical terms related to the integumentary system!

Signs and Symptoms of the Integumentary System

KEY TERMS A-Z

abrasion ah BRAY zhun	**5.7** A common injury to the skin caused by scraping produces a superficial wound called an **abrasion**. Practice spelling this term: _____.
abscess AB sess	**5.8** An **abscess** is a localized elevation of the skin containing a cavity, which is a sign of a local infection. The _____ cavity contains a mixture of bacteria, white blood cells, damaged tissue, and fluids collectively known as **pus** and is surrounded by inflamed tissue. Several words may be used to describe the production of pus. They are **suppuration** (suhp ah RAY shun), **purulence** (PEWR yoo lens), and **pyogenesis** (PIE oh JENN eh SISS).
cellulite SELL yoo light	**5.9 Cellulite** is a local uneven surface of the skin and is a sign of subcutaneous fat deposition. _____ is relatively common in women on the thighs and buttocks.
cicatrix SIK ah trix	**5.10** An injury to the skin resulting in a break through the epidermis and into the dermis or deeper layers of skin requires the process of healing. During this process, epidermal cells migrate to the wound and produce new cells while cells within the dermis produce additional protein fibers. If the wound is too large for the epidermal cells to close the breakage, additional protein fibers (collagen) will be produced to seal the wound. In this case, the wound becomes closed by the formation of **scar tissue**. A clinical term for "scar" is **cicatrix**. _____ is a Latin word that means "scar." The plural form is **cicatrices** (sik ah TRYE sees).

comedo KOM ee doh	**5.11** The clinical term for "pimple" is **comedo**. It is a local elevation of the skin arising from the buildup of oil from sebaceous (oil) glands. Bacteria feed on the oil, attracting the movement of white blood cells and their products and resulting in the localized inflammation. In Latin, the word _____ means "glutton," referring to the fact that the lesion is caused by the action of "gluttonous" bacteria. The plural form is **comedones** (KOM ee DOH neez).
contusion kon TOO zhun	**5.12** Commonly known as a bruise, a **contusion** (kon TOO zhun) is a discoloration and swelling of the skin that is symptomatic of an injury, such as a blow to the body. A _____ is a common symptom following a physical trauma, such as an automobile accident.
cyanosis sigh ah NO siss	**5.13** The combining form for the color blue is *cyan/o*. Adding the ending *-osis*, which means "condition of," produces the term _____. It is a blue tinge of color to an area of the skin and is a sign of a cardiovascular disturbance. Cyanosis is usually apparent most clearly in the lips and fingertips.
cyst sist	**5.14** Derived from the Greek word *kystis* that means "bladder," a **cyst** is a closed sac or pouch on the surface of the skin that is filled with liquid or semisolid material. Notice that the *c* in the term _____ sounds like an *s*.
edema eh DEE mah	**5.15** An injury often leads to inflammation, which includes swelling. Swelling occurs when fluid accumulates in a confined space, such as beneath the skin. The clinical term for fluid accumulation is **edema**. Caused by the leakage of fluid across capillary walls, _____ is a common sign of injury and infection.
erythema air ih THEE mah	**5.16** The Greek word for "blush" is *erythema*. We use the same word for any redness of the skin. It is a common sign of injury or infection. The correct spelling is the same as the original Greek word; it is spelled _____.

fissure
FISH er

5.17 The clinical term for a narrow break or slit in the skin is **fissure**. It is derived from the Latin word for a split or crack, *fissura*, and is illustrated in Figure 5.3■ with other signs of skin disease. Write the correct spelling of this term: _____.

Figure 5.3 ■
Common skin signs. Each of the illustrations depicts a section through skin.

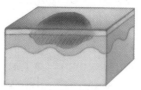
A macule is a discolored spot on the skin; freckle

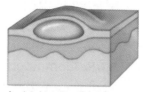
A wheal is a localized, evanescent elevation of the skin that is often accompanied by itching; urticaria

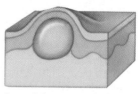
A papule is a solid, circumscribed, elevated area on the skin; pimple

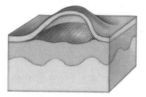
A vesicle is a small fluid filled sac; blister. A bulla is a large vesicle.

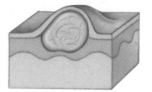
A pustule is a small, elevated, circumscribed lesion of the skin that is filled with pus; varicella (chickenpox)

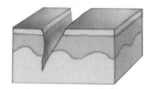
A fissure is a crack-like sore or slit that extends through the epidermis into the dermis; athlete's foot

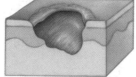
An erosion or ulcer is an eating or gnawing away of tissue; decubitus ulcer

furuncle
FOO rung kl

5.18 If an abscess is associated with a hair follicle, the local swelling on the skin is called a **furuncle**. A photograph of a _____ is provided in Figure 5.4■.

Figure 5.4 ■
Furuncle.
Courtesy of Jason L. Smith, MD.

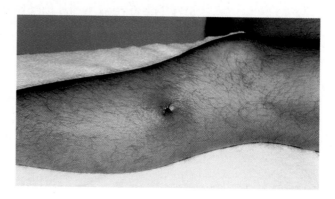

induration in doo RAY shun	**5.19** A local hard area on the skin, or perhaps elsewhere in the body, is known as **induration**. This word is derived from the Latin word *induratio*, which means "the process of becoming firm or hard." An _____ is usually a sign of an excessive deposit of collagen or calcium.
jaundice JAWN diss	**5.20** The French word for "yellow" is *jaune*. It is the origin of the clinical term for an abnormal yellow coloration of the skin and eyes, **jaundice**. In most cases, _____ is a sign of liver or gallbladder disease. The yellowing results from an abnormal release of bile pigments by the liver.
keloid KEE loyd	**5.21** You have learned that a cicatrix may be formed when skin is torn (see Frame 5.10). An overgrowth of scar tissue that forms an elevated lesion on the skin is known as a **keloid**. This large scar, or _____, is often discolored, which sets it apart from adjacent, normal skin (Figure 5.5■).

Figure 5.5 ■
Keloid.
Courtesy of Jason L. Smith, MD.

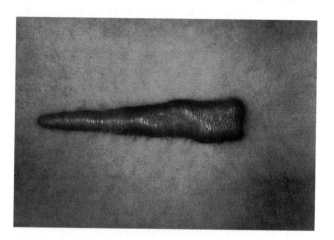

laceration LASS err AY shun	**5.22** A **laceration** is the common result of an injury caused by a tear or perhaps a cut by a sharp object with an irregular surface. A _____ penetrating the dermis and extending for more than one inch often requires stitching to close the wound.
macule MAK yool	**5.23** A discolored flat spot on the skin surface, such as a freckle, is clinically called a **macule**. A _____ is a sign of sun damage to the skin, and the tendency to develop them is genetically determined. A macule is illustrated in Figure 5.3.

nevus
NEE vus

5.24 Similar to a macule but darker in color, a **nevus** is a pigmented spot that is commonly called a mole (Figure 5.6■). It is actually a sign of a benign tumor, and if its edges become irregular or the color changes, the _____ should be examined as a suspect malignancy known as a **melanoma** (see Frame 5.51).

Figure 5.6 ■
Nevus.
Courtesy of Jason L. Smith, MD.

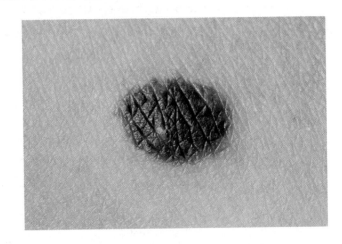

pallor
PAL or

5.25 Pallor is an abnormally pale color of the skin. Derived from the Latin word *pallor* that means "paleness," _____ is a sign of an internal condition causing a decreased flow of blood to the skin.

Papule
PAP yool

5.26 A **papule** is a general term describing any small, solid elevation on the skin (see Figure 5.3). An example of a _____ is a comedo, or pimple.

petechia
peh TEE kee ah

5.27 A **petechia** is a sign of a circulatory disorder. It occurs when a small blood vessel supplying the dermis of the skin ruptures. In people with light skin color, a _____ is observable as a small red dot on the skin.

pruritus
proo RYE tuss

5.28 The symptom of itchy skin is known as **pruritus**. As you might suspect, _____ means "an itching" in Latin.

WORDS TO WATCH OUT FOR !

Pruritus

You might think at first glance that *pruritus* ("an itching") is a constructed term that uses the suffix *-itis*, meaning "inflammation." This isn't the case, however. Make a note of the spelling of this nonconstructed Latin term. The correct spelling of pruritus has a *u* near the end.

purpura
PER pew rah

5.29 The Greeks used the word *porphyra* to name a shellfish that releases a purple dye. In time, it was changed to name the color purple. Dermatologists use a form of the word, **purpura**, for a symptom of purple-red skin discoloration. _____ is usually the result of a hemorrhage (broken blood vessel) that spreads blood through the skin.

pustule
PUS tyool

5.30 You learned from Frame 5.8 that pus is a fluid containing bacteria, white blood cells, and their products. A general term for an elevated area of the skin filled with pus is **pustule**. An example of a _____ is a blackhead, a comedo (pimple) with pus. A pustule is illustrated in Figure 5.3.

ulcer
ULL ser

5.31 An **ulcer** is an erosion through the skin or mucous membrane (see Figure 5.3). The term is derived from the Latin word for "a sore," *ulcus*. A common form of ulcer arises from lack of movement when lying supine for an extended period of time. It is called a **decubitus** (dee KYOO bih tus) _____.

urticaria
er tih KARE ree ah

5.32 A common allergic skin reaction to medications, foods, infection, or injury produces small fluid-filled skin elevations, known as **urticaria**. Also known as hives, _____ may be accompanied by pruritus.

verruca
ver ROO kah

5.33 A wart is a sign of infection by a papilloma virus. The wart, or **verruca**, is an effort by the skin to rid itself of the virus and is observed as a skin elevation with a thickened epidermis. A _____ can be treated with antiviral medication.

vesicle
VESS ih kl

5.34 A **vesicle** is a small elevation of the epidermis that is filled with fluid (see Figure 5.3). A blister is an example of a _____ that results from injury to the skin.

wheal
WEEL

5.35 A temporary, itchy elevation of the skin, often with a white center and red perimeter, is called a **wheal**. A _____ is a symptom of an allergic reaction of the skin and is illustrated in Figure 5.3.

PRACTICE: Signs and Symptoms of the Integumentary System

The Right Match

Match the term on the left with the correct definition on the right.

_____	1. cellulite	a.	localized skin swelling that is a sign of inflammation
_____	2. abscess	b.	abnormal yellow coloration of the skin
_____	3. cicatrix	c.	a local uneven surface of the skin caused by fat deposition
_____	4. abrasion	d.	an erosion through the skin or mucous membrane
_____	5. jaundice	e.	itchy skin
_____	6. nevus	f.	clinical term for scar
_____	7. pruritus	g.	a pigmented spot on the skin; a mole
_____	8. ulcer	h.	scraping injury to the skin
_____	9. cyst	i.	a wart
_____	10. erythema	j.	elevated area of the skin filled with pus
_____	11. furuncle	k.	temporary, itchy elevation of the skin
_____	12. pustule	l.	redness of the skin
_____	13. verruca	m.	abscess associated with a hair follicle
_____	14. wheal	n.	a closed sac or pouch filled with liquid or semisolid material
_____	15. comedo	o.	any small, solid elevation on the skin
_____	16. vesicle	p.	a discolored flat spot on the skin, such as a freckle
_____	17. urticaria	q.	an overgrowth of scar tissue
_____	18. pallor	r.	small fluid-filled skin elevations caused by an allergic reaction
_____	19. papule	s.	abnormally pale skin color
_____	20. keloid	t.	a small elevation of the epidermis that is filled with fluid
_____	21. macule	u.	pimple

Diseases and Disorders of the Integumentary System

Review some of the word parts that specifically apply to the diseases and disorders of the integumentary system that are covered in the following section. Note that the word parts are color coded to help you identify them: prefixes are blue, combining forms are red, and suffixes are purple.

Prefix	Definition
ec-	outside, out
par-	alongside, abnormal

Combining Form	Definition
actin/o	radiation
aden/o	gland
albin/o	white
carcin/o	cancer
cellul/o	small cell
chym/o	juice
crypt/o	hidden
derm/o, dermat/o	skin
follicul/o	small follicle
hidr/o	sweat
kerat/o	horny tissue
leuk/o	white
melan/o	black
myc/o	fungus
onych/o	nail
pedicul/o	body louse
scler/o	thick, hard
trich/o	hair
xer/o	dry

Suffix	Definition
-a	singular
-ia	condition of
-ic	pertaining to
-ism	condition
-itis	inflammation
-malacia	softening
-oma	tumor
-osis	condition of
-pathy	disease
-rrhea	excessive discharge

KEY TERMS A-Z

acne
AK nee

5.36 Acne is an uncomfortable condition of the skin resulting from bacterial infection of sebaceous glands and ducts (Figure 5.7■). The skin disease known as _____ is characterized by the presence of numerous open comedones (blackheads) and closed comedones (whiteheads) in affected parts of the face, and also often involves the neck, back, and chest. Acne is the most common skin disease of adolescence, due to the rapid growth of sebaceous glands during this period of life.

Figure 5.7 ■
Acne.
Courtesy of Jason L. Smith, MD.

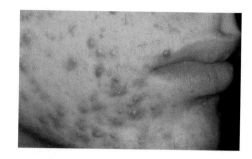

actinic keratosis ak TIN ik * kair ah TOH siss	**5.37 Actinic keratosis** is a precancerous condition of the skin caused by exposure to sunlight. It forms skin lesions resulting from overgrowths of the epidermis, usually with scaly surfaces. The term _____ is a constructed word, actin/ic kerat/osis, in which *actinic* is Greek for "pertaining to light rays" and *keratosis* means "a condition of keratin." In general, any form of keratosis produces a sign of scaly skin.
albinism AL bin izm	**5.38** A genetic condition characterized by the reduction of the pigment melanin in the skin is known as **albinism**. The term _____ uses the combining form *albin/o*, which is derived from the Latin word for "white," *albus*. It is a constructed word, albin/ism, which means "a condition or disease of white." The term **albino** refers to the person affected with albinism.
alopecia al oh PEE she ah	**5.39** A loss or lack of scalp hair is a clinical sign known as baldness, or **alopecia**. Alopecia may be a sign of an infection of the scalp, high fevers, drug reactions, or emotional stress. The common appearance of _____ in men, often called **male-pattern baldness**, is the result of a genetically controlled factor that prevents the development of hair follicles in certain areas of the scalp.
burn	**5.40** A **burn** is an injury to the skin caused by excessive exposure to fire, electricity, chemicals, or sunlight. The level of injury caused by the _____ is determined by the amount of surface area damaged, called **total body surface area** (TBSA), and the **depth** of the damage. A burn becomes life threatening when a large TBSA has become damaged, exposing the body to infection and exposure. In the past, burn depth classified burns into first degree, second degree, third degree, and fourth degree categories. More recently, burn depth is recorded as **partial thickness, full thickness**, and **deep**. These classifications are illustrated in Figure 5.8■.

Figure 5.8 ■
Classification of burn injury by depth in skin.

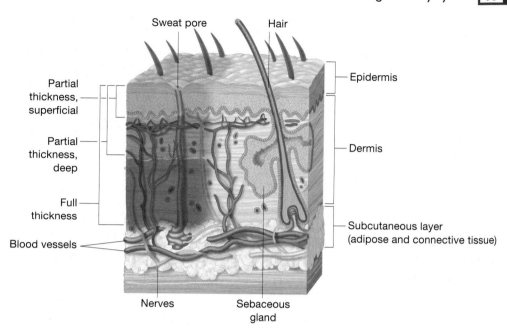

5.41 A **carbuncle** is a skin infection composed of a cluster of boils (Figure 5.9■). The most common source of infection is staphylococci bacteria, or "staph." The term _____ is derived from the Latin word *carbo*, which means "live coal" and refers to the hot pain associated with this disease.

carbuncle
KAR bung kl

Figure 5.9 ■
Carbuncle.
Courtesy of Jason L. Smith, MD.

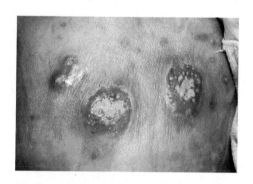

5.42 Remember that the combining form *carcin/o* means "cancer." When you add the suffix that means "tumor," it forms the word _____. Several forms of cancer, or carcinoma, affect the skin. **Basal cell carcinoma** (Figure 5.10■) and **squamous cell carcinoma** are tumors arising from the epidermis that usually remain localized, although the lesions do spread and can become serious if they are not treated. Squamous cell carcinomas, in particular, can be dangerous. The third major form of skin cancer is **melanoma**, which will be described later in Frame 5.51.

carcinoma
kar sih NOH mah

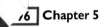

Figure 5.10 ■
Basal cell carcinoma.
Courtesy of Jason L. Smith, MD.

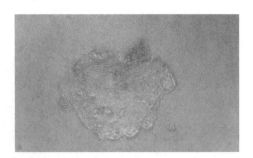

cellulitis

sell you LYE tiss

5.43 Cellulitis is an inflammation of the connective tissue in the dermis (Figure 5.11■). It is caused by an infection that spreads from the skin surface or hair follicles to the dermis and sometimes the subcutaneous tissue. It is usually bacterial in origin. The term _____ is a constructed word, cellul/itis, which literally means "inflammation of small cells." The related term used for follicle infection, **folliculitis** (foh LIK yoo LYE tiss), is also a constructed word. It means "inflammation of little follicles."

Figure 5.11 ■
Cellulitis.
Courtesy of Jason L. Smith, MD.

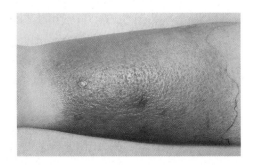

dermatitis

der mah TYE tiss

5.44 Dermatitis is a generalized inflammation of the skin, involving edema (Frame 5.15) of the dermis (Figure 5.12■). In addition to swelling, symptoms may include pruritus (Frame 5.28), urticaria (Frame 5.32), vesicles (Frame 5.34), and wheals (Frame 5.35), or some combination of these. The major types of _____ include **contact dermatitis**, caused by physical contact with a triggering substance such as poison ivy; **seborrheic** (SEB or EE ik) **dermatitis**, which is an inherited form characterized by excessive sebum production; and **actinic dermatitis**, caused by sunlight exposure. **Eczema** (EK zeh mah) is a superficial form of dermatitis, with flakiness of the epidermis as the primary sign. Dermatitis is a constructed word, dermat/itis, which literally means "inflammation of the skin."

Figure 5.12 ■
Dermatitis.
Courtesy of Jason L. Smith, MD.

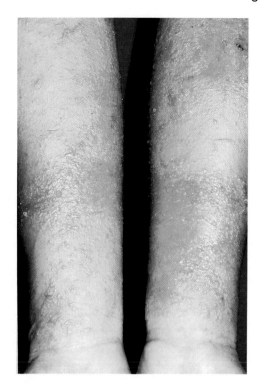

ecchymosis
ek ih MOH siss

5.45 Ecchymosis is a condition of the skin caused by leaking blood vessels in the dermis, producing purplish patches of purpura (Frame 5.29) larger in size than petechiae (Frame 5.27). The term _____ is a constructed word, ec/chym/osis, which literally means "condition of leaking out."

herpes
HER peez

5.46 A skin eruption producing clusters of deep blisters is known as **herpes.** The vesicles (Frame 5.34) appear periodically, affecting the borders between mucous membranes and skin. There are several types of _____, all of which are caused by herpes simplex virus (HSV). The major types are **oral herpes**, caused by herpes virus type 1 (Figure 5.13■), **genital herpes**, caused by herpes virus type 2, and **shingles**, caused by the herpes zoster virus. It is an infectious disease, transferable when the vesicles burst open and physical contact is made between the carrier and another person. In the absence of lesions, it may also be transferable by body fluid contact.

Figure 5.13 ■
Herpes. The blisters often last for several days to one week and form in response to periodic outbreaks of the virus.
Courtesy of Jason L. Smith, MD.

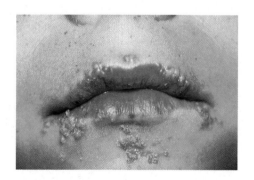

hidradenitis
high drad en EYE tiss

5.47 In the condition **hidradenitis**, the individual suffers from excessive perspiration. It is due to the inflammation of sweat glands, which can become worsened by bacterial infection. The word _____ is a constructed term, hidr/aden/itis, with two word roots: _hidr_, which means "sweat," and _aden_, which means "gland." Thus, the literal meaning of the term is "inflammation of sweat gland."

impetigo
imp eh TYE goh

5.48 Impetigo is a contagious skin infection (Figure 5.14■). Similar to oral herpes due to the development of small vesicles (Frame 5.34) usually forming around the lips, it is often caused by bacteria and is characterized by the presence of golden crusts following the rupture of the vesicles. The term _____ is a Latin word meaning "scabby eruption."

Figure 5.14 ■
Impetigo.
Courtesy of Jason L. Smith, MD.

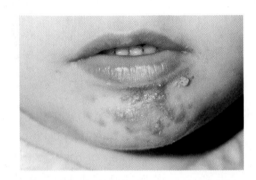

Kaposi's sarcoma
KAP oh seez * sar KOH mah

5.49 Kaposi's sarcoma is a form of skin cancer arising from the connective tissue of the dermis (Figure 5.15■). It is indicated by the presence of brown or purple patches on the skin and appears among some elderly patients. _____ _____ is also a common condition associated with HIV infection and AIDS.

Figure 5.15 ■
Kaposi's sarcoma.
Courtesy of Jason L. Smith, MD.

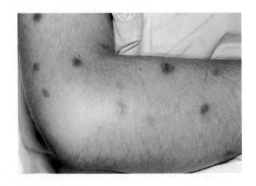

leukoderma
loo koh DER mah

5.50 As some people age, their skin becomes lighter in color due to reduced activity of the pigment-producing cells in the skin, the melanocytes. This condition is called **leukoderma**. The term _____ is a constructed word, leuk/o/derm/a, which literally means "white skin."

melanoma
mell ah NOH mah

5.51 The most life-threatening skin cancer is **malignant melanoma**, which is shown in Figure 5.16■. It arises from the cells normally providing the pigment **melanin** (MELL ah nin) to the skin, called **melanocytes** (mell AN oh sites). _____ is a constructed term, melan/oma, which literally means "black tumor." Once established in the skin, the tumor grows rapidly and metastasizes (goes elsewhere in the body). About one-half of cases arise from nevi (moles).

Figure 5.16 ■
Melanoma.

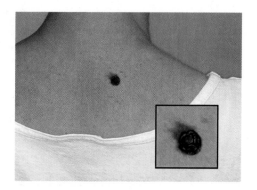

onychocryptosis
ON ih koh krip TOH siss

5.52 The combining form for nail is _onych/o_ and is used in the construction of terms relating to nail diseases. In general, a disease of the nail is an **onychopathy** (ON ih KOHP a thee). In the nail condition called **onychocryptosis**, a nail becomes buried in the skin due to abnormal growth. It is commonly called an "ingrown nail." The term _____ is a constructed word, onych/o/crypt/osis, and means "condition of hidden nail."

onychomalacia
ON ih koh mah LAY she ah

5.53 In the condition **onychomalacia**, a nail is abnormally soft. It is often a sign of calcium or vitamin D deficiency. The term _____ is a constructed word, onych/o/malacia, which means "softening of the nail."

onychomycosis
ON ih koh my KOH siss

5.54 The condition _____ is a fungal infection of one or more nails (Figure 5.17■). Notice that the word root for fungus, _myc_, is included in this constructed term, onych/o/myc/osis, to form its meaning into "condition of fungus of the nail."

Figure 5.17 ■
Onychomycosis.
Courtesy of Jason L. Smith, MD.

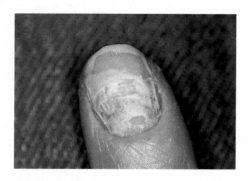

paronychia
pair oh NIK ee ah

5.55 In **paronychia**, the prefix *par-*, which means "alongside," is included to build the term. Thus, the constructed word par/onych/ia means "condition of alongside the nail." As you might guess, _____ is an infection around the nail (Figure 5.18■).

Figure 5.18 ■
Paronychia.
Source: Leonard Morse/Medical Images, Inc.

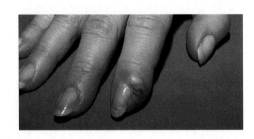

pediculosis
peh dik yoo LOH siss

5.56 The Latin word for a parasitic body louse is *pediculus*, which is the origin of the combining form of *pedicul/o*. When this combining form is combined with the suffix for "condition of," it forms the constructed word _____. Pediculosis occurs mostly on the scalp, where it is called head lice, but it may also be found in the pubic region (called pubic lice) and other parts of the body (called body lice). Pediculosis can be treated effectively with medicated shampoo.

psoriasis
soh RYE ah siss

5.57 Psoriasis is a painful, chronic disease of the skin characterized by the presence of red lesions covered with silvery epidermal scales (Figure 5.19■). Believed to be an inherited inflammatory disease of the skin, _____ is a Greek word meaning "to itch" and is spelled exactly like the clinical term.

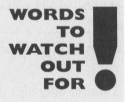

WORDS TO WATCH OUT FOR !

Psoriasis

Psoriasis is a very commonly misspelled term. It is one of the medical terms that is spelled with a silent *p* (terms with the word root *psych* are the others). One way to remember to include the *p* is to think of the **p**atches of red lesions that characterize this condition.

Figure 5.19 ■
Psoriasis.
Courtesy of Jason L. Smith, MD.

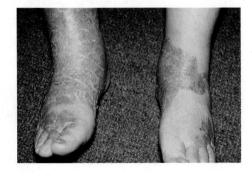

scabies
SKAY bees

5.58 The condition **scabies** is a skin eruption caused by the female itch mite, which burrows into the skin to extract blood. From the Latin word *scabere* that means "scratch," _____ produces the symptoms of dermatitis, such as erythema (Frame 5.16), swelling, and pruritus (Frame 5.28).

scleroderma
sklair oh DER mah

5.59 Scleroderma uses the combining form *scler/o*, which means "hard." It is an abnormal thickening or hardness of the skin, caused by overproduction of collagen in the dermis. The term _____ is a constructed word, scler/o/derm/a, which means "skin hardness."

systemic lupus erythematosus
sis TEM ik * LOO pus *
air ih them ah TOH siss

5.60 Systemic lupus erythematosus, abbreviated **SLE**, is a chronic, progressive disease of connective tissue in many organs including the skin. The early stages of _____ _____ _____, often commonly referred to as just *lupus*, are marked by red patches on the skin of the face and joint pain.

DID YOU KNOW ?

Lupus

The Latin word for *wolf* is *lupus*. The disease *lupus* was named by the appearance of the reddish face rash that reminded early physicians of a wolf.

tinea
TIN ee ah

5.61 Tinea is a fungal infection of the skin. It is often called "ringworm" due to the ring-shaped pattern on the skin that forms in response to the fungi (Figure 5.20■). In fact, the term _____ is the Latin word for "worm" or "larval moth." The three major forms of tinea are **tinea capitis**, which forms on the scalp and can lead to alopecia (Frame 5.39); **tinea pedis**, which forms on the feet and is also known as athlete's foot; and **tinea corporis**, which may occur elsewhere on the body.

Figure 5.20 ■
Tinea. Although it is a fungal infection, tinea is often called ringworm.
Courtesy of Jason L. Smith, MD.

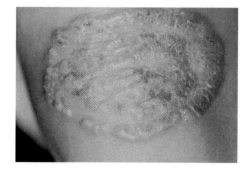

trichomycosis
TRIK oh my KOH siss

5.62 A general term for a disease affecting the hair is **trichopathy** (trye KOH path ee), which combines the word root for hair (*trich*) and the suffix for disease (*-pathy*). The condition **trichomycosis** is a fungal infection of hair. In this constructed term, trich/o/myc/osis, the word roots for *hair* and *fungus* are combined to form the term _____.

xeroderma
zee roh DER mah

5.63 The combining form *xer/o* means "dry"; when this is combined with the combining form that means "skin," it forms the word _____. Therefore, the disease **xeroderma** is characterized by abnormally dry skin. It is caused by hyposecretion (abnormally low secretion) of the oil glands and is an inherited condition. It is a constructed term, xer/o/derm/a, which literally means "dry skin."

PRACTICE: Diseases and Disorders of the Integumentary System

The Right Match

Match the term on the left with the correct definition on the right.

_____ 1. tinea
_____ 2. acne
_____ 3. burn
_____ 4. herpes
_____ 5. alopecia
_____ 6. impetigo
_____ 7. scabies
_____ 8. psoriasis

a. results from bacterial infection of sebaceous glands and ducts
b. characterized by red lesions covered with silvery epidermal scales
c. baldness
d. contagious bacterial skin infection with a yellowish crust
e. caused by excessive exposure to fire, chemicals, or sunlight
f. skin eruption caused by the female itch mite
g. viral skin eruption that produces clusters of deep blisters
h. fungal infection of the skin

Break the Chain _____

Analyze these medical terms:

- a) Separate each term into its word parts; each word part is labeled for you (**p** = prefix, **r** = root, **cf** = combining form, and **s** = suffix).

- b) For the Bonus Question, write the requested word part or definition in the blank that follows.

The first set has been completed for you as an example.

1. a) dermatitis

     dermat / itis
        r   s

   b) *Bonus Question:* What is the definition of the suffix? *inflammation* _____

2. a) melanoma

     _____ / _____
        r   s

   b) *Bonus Question:* What is the definition of the suffix? _____

3. a) onychomycosis

     _____ / ___ / ___ / _____
         cf   r   s

   b) *Bonus Question:* What is the definition of the *second* word root? _____

4. a) pediculosis

     _____ / _____
        r   s

   b) *Bonus Question:* What is the definition of the suffix? _____

5. a) scleroderma

     _____ / ___ / _____ / _____
         cf   r   s

   b) *Bonus Question:* What is the definition of the combining form? _____

6. a) trichomycosis

     _____ / ___ / _____ / _____
         cf   r   s

   b) *Bonus Question:* What is the definition of the combining form? _____

7. a) cellulitis

     _____ / _____
        r   s

   b) *Bonus Question:* What is the definition of the suffix? _____

8. a) leukoderma

     _____ / ___ / _____ / ___
         cf   r   s

   b) *Bonus Question:* What is the definition of the *second* word root? _____

Treatments, Procedures, and Devices of the Integumentary System

Review some of the word parts that specifically apply to the treatments, procedures, and devices of the integumentary system that are covered in the following section. Note that the word parts are color coded to help you identify them: prefixes are blue, combining forms are red, and suffixes are purple.

Prefix	Combining Form	Definition	Suffix	Definition
(none)	abras/o	to rub away	-ectomy	surgical removal
	aut/o	self	-ion	process
	derm/o, dermat/o	skin	-plasty	surgical repair
	rhytid/o	wrinkle	-tome	a cutting instrument

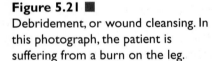

KEY TERMS A-Z

biopsy
BYE op see

5.64 A **biopsy** is a minor surgery involving the removal of tissue for evaluation. Abbreviated **bx**, a _____ is usually a necessary step toward making a diagnosis of a suspected tumor of the skin.

debridement
day breed MON

5.65 Wounds are often complicated by physical contact with a dirty object, including the ground. To clean the wound, a procedure called **debridement** is often used (Figure 5.21■). A French word meaning "unbridled," _____ involves excision of foreign matter and unwanted tissue.

Figure 5.21 ■
Debridement, or wound cleansing. In this photograph, the patient is suffering from a burn on the leg.

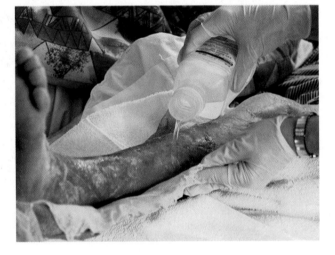

dermabrasion
DERM ah BRAY zhun

5.66 Remember that the combining form *derm/o* means skin. When combined with the suffix that means "process" and the combining form that means "to rub away," *abras/o*, it forms the word _____.
Dermabrasion is a form of **cosmetic surgery**, in which the skin is surgically changed to improve appearance. During dermabrasion, abrasives similar to sandpaper are used to remove unwanted scars and other elevations, and may also be used to remove tattoos. Alternatives to dermabrasion include **chemical peels**, in which a chemical agent is used to remove the outer epidermal layers to treat acne, wrinkles, and sun-damaged skin.

dermatoautoplasty
DER mah toh AW toh PLASS tee

dermatome
DER mah tohm

5.67 Some burns and similar injuries cause extensive damage to a large area of skin, challenging the normal healing process. In these cases, the surgical procedure of **dermatoautoplasty** may be used to improve healing. This is a constructed term that can be written as dermat/o/aut/o/plasty. In this term, note the combining form that means "self," *aut/o*. This is because the surgery involves using the patient's own skin as a graft, usually after it has grown in a media solution. _____ is also called an **autograft**. Alternatively, a skin graft from another person may be used. This procedure is called **dermatoheteroplasty** (DER mah toh HETT er oh PLASS tee), or **allograft**. During both procedures, an instrument called a **dermatome** (DER mah tohm) is used to cut thin slices of skin for grafting. A _____ may also be used to excise (surgically remove) small skin lesions. Recall that the suffix -*tome* means "a cutting instrument."

dermatoplasty
DER mah toh plass tee

5.68 The general term for a surgical procedure of the skin is **dermatoplasty**. This term uses the combining form that means "skin" with the suffix, -*plasty*, which means "surgical repair." In _____, skin tissue is transplanted to the body surface.

emollient
ee MALL ee ant

5.69 An _____ is a chemical agent that softens or smooths the skin. Topical and oral **antibiotics** (ahn tye bye OT iks) are used to manage infections, such as acne and carbuncles. **Retinoids** (RET ih noydz) may also be used to manage certain forms of acne because they cause the upper layers of the epidermis to slough away. Acne and related disorders may also be treated by **ultraviolet light therapy**, which causes a similar effect on the epidermis.

rhytidectomy
rit ih DEK toh mee

5.70 Plastic surgery is a popular form of skin treatment, which is used for skin repair following a major injury, correction of a congenital defect, or cosmetic improvement. Several of the terms related to plastic surgery use the combining form *rhytid/o*, which means "wrinkle." Plastic surgeries that are primarily cosmetic include **rhytidoplasty** (RIT ih doh PLASS tee), which is the surgical repair of skin wrinkles (Figure 5.22■); _____, during which wrinkles are surgically removed; and **liposuction** (LIE poh suk shun), which is the removal of subcutaneous fat (fat immediately deep to the skin) by insertion of a device that applies a vacuum to pull the fat tissue out of the body.

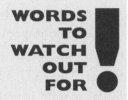
WORDS TO WATCH OUT FOR !

The "Y" in Rhytid

It may be tempting to spell the term *rhytidectomy* with an *i* instead of a *y*. One way to remember to use a *y* is to think of the word *elderly*. As you've learned, the word root *rhytid* means *wrinkle*. Elderly people commonly have wrinkles, and the word *elderly* ends with a *y*.

Figure 5.22 ■
Rhytidoplasty. This is a common form of plastic surgery in which the skin is pulled and sutured to decrease skin wrinkles.
Source: Kim Steele/Getty Images, Inc—PhotoDisc.

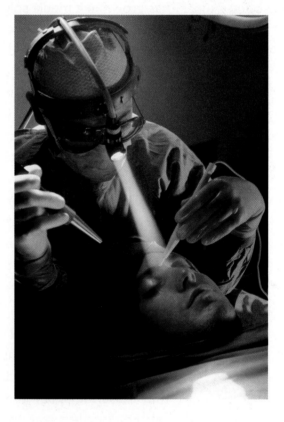

PRACTICE: Treatments, Procedures, and Devices of the Integumentary System

The Right Match

Match the term on the left with the correct definition on the right.

_____ 1. biopsy

_____ 2. emollient

_____ 3. debridement

_____ 4. cosmetic surgery

_____ 5. autograft

a. chemical agent that softens or smooths the skin

b. wound-cleaning procedure

c. surgically changing the skin to improve appearance

d. surgery that uses a patient's own skin as a graft

e. the removal of tissue for evaluation

Linkup

Link the word parts in the list to create the terms that match the definitions. You may use word parts more than once. Remember to add in combining vowels when needed—and that some terms do not use any combining vowel. The first one is completed for you as an example.

Combining Form	Suffix
abras/o	-ectomy
aut/o	-ion
derm/o, dermat/o	-plasty
rhytid/o	-tome

Definition

1. use of abrasives to remove unwanted scars and tattoos

2. the surgical repair of skin wrinkles

3. surgical repair of the skin

4. surgery that involves the use of the patient's own skin to improve healing

5. an instrument that is used to cut thin slices of skin for grafting

Term

dermabrasion

_____

_____

_____

_____

Abbreviations of the Integumentary System

The abbreviations that are associated with the integumentary system are summarized here. Study these abbreviations, and review them in the exercise that follows.

Abbreviation	Definition	Abbreviation	Definition
BCC	basal cell carcinoma	SqCCa	squamous cell carcinoma
bx	biopsy	TBSA	total body surface area
SLE	systemic lupus erythematosus		

PRACTICE: Abbreviations

Fill in the blanks with the abbreviation or the complete medical term.

Abbreviation

1. _____

2. BCC

3. _____

4. SqCCa

5. _____

Medical Term

biopsy

_____

systemic lupus erythematosus

_____

total body surface area

▶▶▶▶ Chapter Review

Word Building

Construct medical terms from the following meanings. The first question has been completed for you as an example.

1. literally means "black tumor"   melan_oma_____

2. inflammation of connective tissue   _____itis

3. disease of the nail   _____pathy

4. fungal infection of a nail   onycho_____

5. abnormally dry skin   _____derma

6. a skin wound caused by scraping   abras_____

7. an infection arising from a follicle   _____cle

8. disease that affects the hair   tricho_____

9. blisters that later form a yellowish crust   _____igo

10. a small, solid circumscribed skin elevation   nev_____

11. a discolored flat spot   _____ule

12. derived from the Latin word "to soften"   emoll_____

13. one who specializes in skin ailments   _____logist

14. overgrowth of scar tissue   kel_____

15. an ingrown nail   _____kryptosis

16. a precancerous condition caused by sunlight   actinic kerat_____

17. abnormally light skin   _____derma

Clinical Application Exercises

Medical Report

Read the following medical report, then answer the questions that follow.

Metropolis County Hospital

5500 University Avenue
Metropolis, TX

Phone: (211) 594-4000
Fax: (211) 594-4001

Medical Consultation: Dermatology

Date: 7/07/2007

Patient: Sally Garcia

Patient Complaint: Redness, swelling, pruritus, and pain reported on the skin of the right upper arm, with skin elevations that open with scratching that is producing scars

History: 22-year-old Hispanic female has complained of occasional skin elevations that cause discomfort from pruritus. No treatments have been provided previously. Patient reports that she works in an environment that is unusually humid and dusty.

Family History: Father, age 72, with melanoma; older brother with seborrheic dermatitis spreading to the scalp to contribute to alopecia.

Allergies: None

Evidences: Generalized inflammation of right upper arm spreading to shoulder and thorax with vesicle formation. Open vesicles are forming cicatrices and keloids.

Treatment: Debridement of damaged tissue and administration of oral antibiotic therapy. Future surgery with autograft may be advised for keloid removal.

Jane K. Hernandez, M.D.

---

1. What is the actual cause of the cicatrices on the skin? _____

   _____

2. If the symptom of pruritus returns after the initial treatment, how might the formation of new scar tissue be

   prevented? _____

   _____

3. Why do you think antibiotic therapy is included in the treatment? _____

   _____

Medical Report Case Study

The following case study provides further discussion regarding the patient in the medical report. Fill in the blanks with the correct terms. Choose your answers from the following list of terms. (Note that some terms may be used more than once.)

actinic keratosis	dermatitis	keloids
biopsy	dermatoautoplasty	pruritus
cicatrices	dermatology	ulcers
debridement	dermatome	vesicles
dermabrasion	erythroderma	

At the (a) _____ clinic where patients with skin ailments are referred, Sally Garcia, a patient

with an unusual skin condition, was observed. The skin condition included a generalized inflammation, or

(b) _____, which included abnormal redness, swelling, and pain. Skin damage caused by sunlight,

a precancerous condition known as (c) _____, was ruled out as a diagnosis, along with all known

forms of skin cancer. Rather, an infectious agent was the likely cause. After several days of general inflammation, fluid-filled

skin elevations, or (d) _____, appeared. The elevations gave the patient symptoms of itching or

(e) _____. Scratching the elevations produced open sores, or (f) _____, which

upon healing left scars, or (g) _____. In some areas, the scar tissue became overgrown, forming

(h) _____. An evaluation of the scar tissue included surgical removal of the affected skin, or

(i) _____, using a (j) _____. Treatment included the removal of diseased tissue, or

(k) _____, and antibiotic treatments were prescribed. Because some scar tissue affected the face,

abrasives were used during the (l) _____ procedure. However, when this treatment failed, an auto-

graft was applied in the (m) _____ procedure, with improved results.

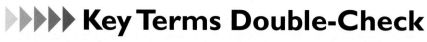

Key Terms Double-Check

Remember that the chapter's key terms appeared alphabetically within each section of this chapter. This exercise helps you to check your knowledge AND review for tests.

    1. First, fill in the missing word in the definitions for the chapter's key terms.

    2. Then, check your answers using Appendix F.

    3. If you got the answer right, put a check mark in the right column.

    4. If your answer was incorrect, go back to the frame number provided and review the content.

Use the checklist to study the terms you don't know until you're confident you know them all.

Key Term	Frame	Definition	Know It?
1. abrasion	5.7	a _____ scraping injury to the skin	☐
2. abscess	5.8	localized skin inflammation that may be accompanied by _____	☐
3. acne	5.36	bacterial infection of sebaceous glands and ducts resulting in numerous _____	☐
4. actinic keratosis	5.37	precancerous condition of the skin caused by exposure to _____	☐
5. albinism	5.38	genetic condition characterized by reduction of the skin pigment _____	☐
6. alopecia	5.39	baldness; may be a sign of an _____ of the scalp, high fevers, or emotional stress	☐
7. biopsy	5.64	minor surgery involving the removal of tissue for evaluation; abbreviated _____	☐
8. burn	5.40	caused by excessive exposure to fire, chemicals, or sunlight, and measured by _____ _____ _____ _____, and depth of the damage	☐
9. carbuncle	5.41	a skin infection composed of a cluster of _____	☐
10. carcinoma	5.42	skin cancer; varieties include _____ cell carcinoma and squamous cell carcinoma	☐
11. cellulite	5.9	a local uneven surface of the skin caused by _____	☐
12. cellulitis	5.43	inflammation of the _____ tissue in the dermis caused by an infection	☐
13. cicatrix	5.10	clinical term for scar _____	☐
14. comedo	5.11	skin blemish that is caused by a buildup of sebaceous oils; _____	☐
15. contusion	5.12	commonly known as a _____	☐
16. cyst	5.14	a closed sac or pouch filled with _____	☐
17. debridement	5.65	excision of _____ matter and unwanted tissue with irrigation	☐

Key Term	Frame	Definition	Know It?
18. dermabrasion	5.66	form of _____ _____ in which the skin is surgically changed to improve appearance	☐
19. dermatitis	5.44	a generalized inflammation of the skin involving _____	☐
20. dermatoautoplasty	5.67	surgery in which the patient's own skin is used as a graft, also called an _____	☐
21. dermatome	5.67	an instrument used to cut thin slices of skin for _____	☐
22. dermatoplasty	5.68	_____ repair of the skin	☐
23. ecchymosis	5.45	condition caused by leaking blood vessels in the dermis, producing purplish patches of _____	☐
24. edema	5.15	condition of fluid accumulating in a _____ _____, such as beneath the skin	☐
25. emollient	5.69	a chemical _____ that softens or smooths the skin	☐
26. erythema	5.16	any _____ of the skin	☐
27. fissure	5.17	the clinical term for a _____ _____ or slit in the skin	☐
28. furuncle	5.18	abscess associated with a hair _____	☐
29. herpes	5.46	viral skin eruption that produces clusters of deep blisters; major types are _____, genital, and shingles	☐
30. hidradenitis	5.47	excessive _____ due to the inflammation of sweat glands	☐
31. impetigo	5.48	contagious bacterial skin infection with a _____ crust	☐
32. induration	5.19	local _____ areas on the skin	☐
33. jaundice	5.20	abnormal _____ coloration of the skin and eyes	☐
34. Kaposi's sarcoma	5.49	a form of skin cancer arising from the connective tissue of the dermis; common among people with _____	☐
35. keloid	5.21	an overgrowth of elevated scar tissue that is often different from adjacent, _____ skin	☐
36. laceration	5.22	result of an injury caused by a _____, or perhaps a cut	☐
37. leukoderma	5.50	condition in which skin becomes lighter in color due to _____ activity of the pigment-producing cells	☐
38. macule	5.23	a discolored flat spot on the skin surface, such as a(n) _____	☐
39. melanoma	5.51	dangerous skin cancer meaning "_____ tumor"	☐
40. nevus	5.24	a pigmented spot on the skin; a(n) _____	☐
41. onychocryptosis	5.52	a nail buried in the skin due to abnormal growth, commonly called _____ nail	☐
42. onychomalacia	5.53	abnormally _____ nails; often a sign of calcium or vitamin D deficiency	☐

Key Term	Frame	Definition	Know It?
43. onychomycosis	5.54	_____ infection of one or more nails	☐
44. pallor	5.25	abnormal _____ color of the skin	☐
45. papule	5.26	any small, solid elevation on the skin, such as a(n) _____	☐
46. paronychia	5.55	an infection alongside the _____	☐
47. pediculosis	5.56	head _____; may also be found in the pubic region and other parts of the body	☐
48. petechia	5.27	rupture of a small blood vessel supplying the _____ of the skin	☐
49. pruritus	5.28	symptom of _____ skin	☐
50. psoriasis	5.57	characterized by red lesions covered with silvery epidermal _____	☐
51. purpura	5.29	symptom of purple-red skin discoloration usually the result of a broken _____ _____	☐
52. pustule	5.30	elevated area of the skin filled with _____	☐
53. rhytidectomy	5.70	_____ _____ in which skin wrinkles are surgically removed	☐
54. scabies	5.58	skin eruption caused by the female itch _____	☐
55. scleroderma	5.59	abnormal _____ or hardness of the skin, caused by inflammation	☐
56. systemic lupus erythematosus	5.60	chronic, progressive disease of connective tissue affecting the skin and many other organs; commonly known as _____	☐
57. tinea	5.61	fungal infection of the skin often called _____	☐
58. trichomycosis	5.62	fungal infection of _____	☐
59. ulcer	5.31	an erosion through the skin or mucous membrane; a bed sore is a(n) _____ ulcer	☐
60. urticaria	5.32	allergic skin reaction to foods, infection, or injury that produces small fluid-filled _____	☐
61. verruca	5.33	a wart that is a sign of infection by a papilloma _____.	☐
62. vesicle	5.34	small skin elevation filled with fluid; a(n) _____	☐
63. wheal	5.35	a temporary, itchy _____ of the skin	☐
64. xeroderma	5.63	characterized by abnormally _____ skin	☐

Multimedia Preview ▶▶▶▶▶

Additional interactive resources and activities for this chapter can be found on the Companion Website. For animations, videos, audio glossary, and review, access the accompanying DVD-ROM in this book.

DVD-ROM Highlights

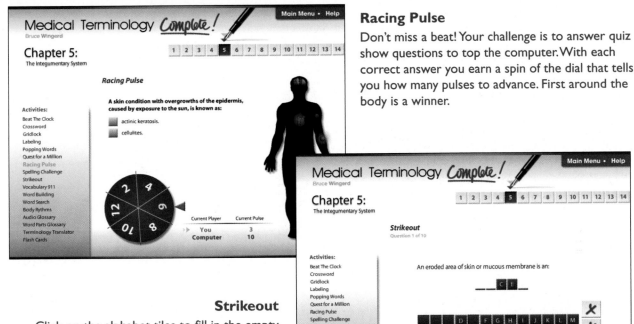

Racing Pulse

Don't miss a beat! Your challenge is to answer quiz show questions to top the computer. With each correct answer you earn a spin of the dial that tells you how many pulses to advance. First around the body is a winner.

Strikeout

Click on the alphabet tiles to fill in the empty squares in the word or phrase to complete the sentence. This game quizzes your vocabulary and spelling. But choose your letters carefully because three strikes and you're out!

Website Highlights—www.prenhall.com/wingerd

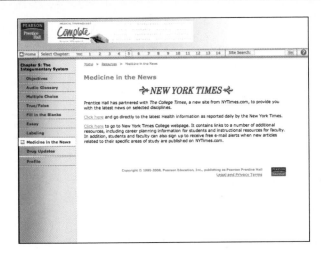

Medicine in the News

Click here to take advantage of the free-access online study guide that accompanies your textbook. You'll be able to stay current with a link to medical news articles updated daily by *The New York Times*. By clicking on this URL you'll also be able to access a variety of quizzes with instant feedback, links to download mp3 audio reviews, and an audio glossary.

The Skeletal and Muscular Systems ▶▶▶▶▶

Learning Objectives

After completing this chapter, you will be able to:

- Define and spell the word parts used to create medical terms for the skeletal and muscular systems.

- Break down and define common medical terms used for symptoms, diseases, disorders, procedures, treatments, and devices associated with the skeletal and muscular systems.

- Build medical terms from word parts associated with the skeletal and muscular systems.

- Pronounce and spell common medical terms associated with the skeletal and muscular systems.

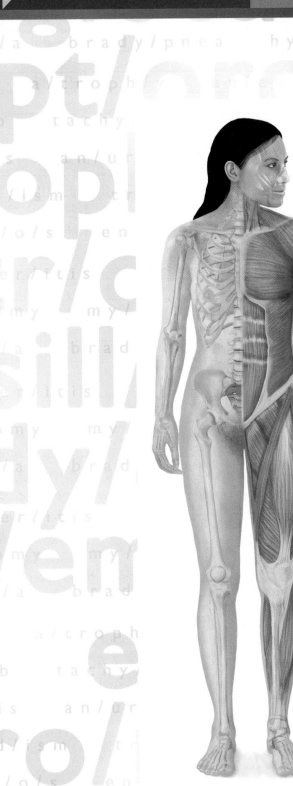

Anatomy and Physiology Terms ▶▶▶▶

The following table provides the combining forms that specifically apply to the anatomy and physiology of the skeletal and muscular systems. Note that the combining forms are colored red to help you identify them when you see them again later in the chapter.

Combining Form	Definition	Combining Form	Definition
arthr/o, articul/o	joint	my/o, myos/o	muscle
burs/o	purse or sac, bursa	oste/o	bone
carp/o	wrist	pariet/o	wall
chondr/o	gristle, cartilage	patell/o	patella
condyl/o	knuckle of a joint	petr/o	stone
cost/o	rib	phalang/o	phalanges
cran/o, crani/o	skull, cranium	phys/o	growth
fasci/o	fascia	pub/o	pubis
femor/o	thigh, femur	radi/o	radius
fibr/o	fiber	sacr/o	sacrum
fibul/o	fibula	skelet/o	skeleton
ili/o	flank, hip, groin, ilium of the pelvis	spondyl/o, vertebr/o	vertebra
ischi/o	haunch, hip joint, ischium	stern/o	chest, sternum
menisci/o	meniscus	synov/o, synovi/o	synovial
muscul/o	muscle	tars/o	tarsal bone
myel/o	bone marrow	ten/o, tendon/o	tendon

musculoskeletal
MUS kyoo loh skehl eh tahl

6.1 The skeletal and muscular systems are combined to form the _____ system. Notice how this constructed term is assembled with four word parts: muscul/o/skelet/al. As you know, the bones and muscles work together to support the body and produce body movement. In fact, nearly every one of the 206 bones in your body receives an attachment to one or more muscles.

FUNCTION ▶▶▶▶

bones

6.2 Each bone is an organ, composed of mainly connective tissue receiving blood vessels, lymphatics, and nerves. Bones function in the support of soft internal organs, the storage of mineral salts including calcium and phosphorus, and the production of blood cells within the red bone marrow, in addition to serving as an attachment site for muscles. Each muscle is an organ also, composed mainly of skeletal muscle tissue and connective tissue. As a muscle shortens in length by contraction, it pulls on the tendons connecting it to _____ to produce body movement. Muscle contraction also produces heat, assisting the body in regulating body temperature.

6.3 Use the anatomy terms that appear in the left column to fill in the corresponding blanks in Figures 6.1■ through 6.3■.

1. **compact bone**
2. **periosteum**
3. **diaphysis**
4. **epiphysis**

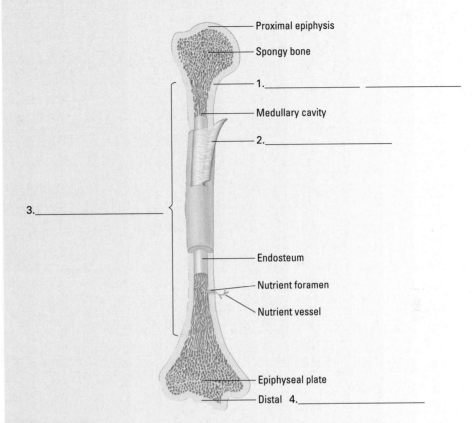

Proximal epiphysis

Spongy bone

1._____ _____

Medullary cavity

2._____

3._____

Endosteum

Nutrient foramen

Nutrient vessel

Epiphyseal plate

Distal 4._____

Figure 6.1 ■
Parts of a bone.

5. cranium
6. clavicle
7. humerus
8. phalanges
9. sacrum
10. femur

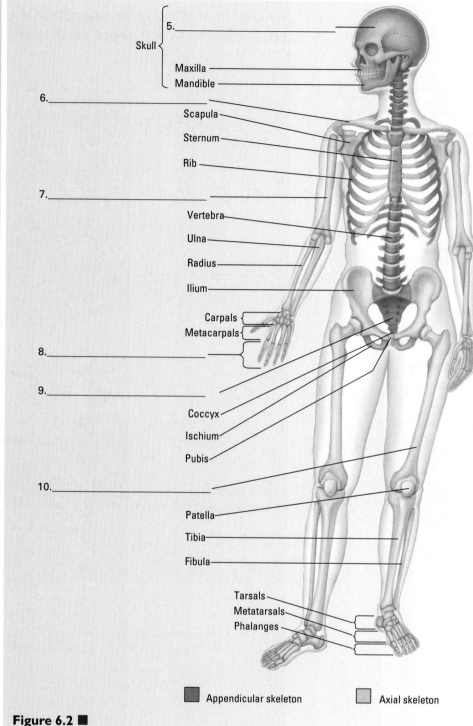

5. _____

Skull {
Maxilla
Mandible

6. _____

Scapula
Sternum

Rib

7. _____

Vertebra
Ulna
Radius
Ilium

Carpals {
Metacarpals {

8. _____

9. _____

Coccyx
Ischium
Pubis

10. _____

Patella
Tibia
Fibula

Tarsals
Metatarsals
Phalanges

Appendicular skeleton   Axial skeleton

Figure 6.2 ■
The bones of the skeleton. The skeleton, anterior view.

11. **biceps**
12. **rectus**
13. **gastrocnemius**
14. **deltoid**
15. **sternocleidomastoid**

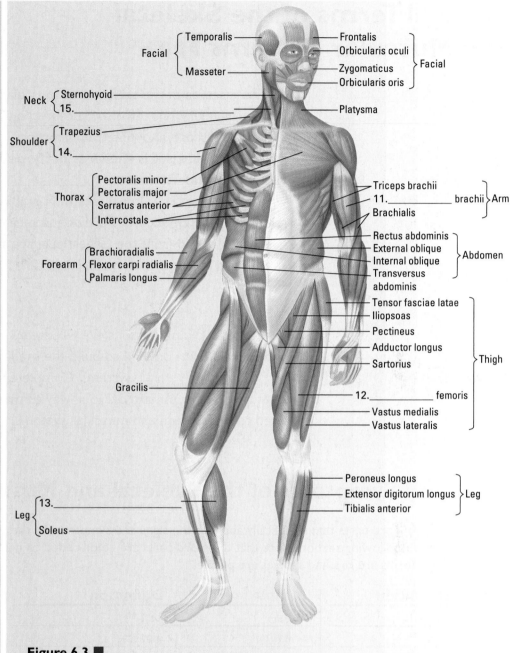

Figure 6.3 ■
The major muscles of the human body, anterior side.

Medical Terms of the Skeletal and Muscular Systems ▶▶▶▶

orthopedic
OR thoh PEE dik

6.4 The diseases of the skeletal and muscular systems are often the result of physical injury, but can also be caused by infections, tumor development, endocrine disease, and inherited disorders. The branch of medicine focusing on these diseases is known as **orthopedics**, which is commonly abbreviated to **ortho**. The term _____ is a constructed word, written orth/o/ped/ic. It includes the combining form *orth/o*, which is derived from the Greek word *orthos* and means "straight," and the word root *ped*, which is also from the Greek language and means "foot." A physician specializing in this field of medicine is called an **orthopedist** (OR thoh PEE dist).

muscular
MUS kyoo lar

6.5 In the following sections, we will review the prefixes, combining forms, and suffixes that combine to build the medical terms of the skeletal and _____ systems. Complete the frames and review exercises that follow. You are on your way to mastery of the medical terms related to the skeletal and muscular systems!

Signs and Symptoms of the Skeletal and Muscular Systems

Following are the word parts that specifically apply to the signs and symptoms of the skeletal and muscular systems that are covered in the following section. Note that the word parts are color-coded to help you identify them: prefixes are blue, combining forms are red, and suffixes are purple.

Prefix	Definition
a-	without
brady-	slow
dys-	bad, abnormal, painful, difficult
hyper-	excessive, abnormally high, above

Combining Form	Definition
arthr/o	joint
kinesi/o	motion
my/o	muscle
tax/o	reaction to a stimulus, movement
ten/o	tendon
troph/o	development

Suffix	Definition
-algia, -dynia	condition of pain
-a	singular
-ia	condition of
-y	process of

KEY TERMS A-Z

arthralgia
ahr THRAL jee ah

6.6 Referring to the preceding word parts table, you'll see that the suffix *-algia* means "condition of pain." Add that to the combining form that means "joint," and it forms the word that means "condition of joint pain," or _____. This is often the first symptom of joint or bone disease. It is also a common complaint following injury to a joint. The constructed form of this word is arthr/algia.

ataxia
ah TAK see ah

6.7 The word root *tax* means "a reaction to a stimulus" or "movement." By adding the prefix *a-* ("without"), the meaning of the term becomes negative. When the suffix *-ia* (condition of) is added, it forms the word _____, which is the inability to coordinate muscles during a voluntary activity. Ataxia is a sign of a nervous system disorder that is often inherited. The constructed form of this word is a/tax/ia.

atrophy
AT roh fee

6.8 Stabilizing a broken limb by casting it in plaster is a common treatment for bone fractures. It prohibits movement of the limb to promote the healing process. Unfortunately, the lack of movement leads to a reduction in muscle strength due to disuse, a sign of reduced muscle size known as **atrophy**. The muscle reduction is reversible when healing is complete and muscle activity is restored. The term _____ also uses the prefix *a-* to make the meaning of the word root negative. The word root *troph* means "development" and *-y* means "process of." The three word parts that form the word can be written as a/troph/y.

bradykinesia
BRAD ee kih NEE see ah

6.9 An abnormally slow movement is a clinical sign of an underlying bone, muscle, or nervous disorder. It is known as _____, which literally means "condition of slow motion." This term is a constructed word that can be written as brady/kines/ia, in which *brady-* means "slow," *kinesi* is the word root for "motion," and the suffix *-ia* means "condition of." (Note that the "i" in the word root is dropped when using a suffix that begins with an "i.")

decalcification
DEE kal sih fih KAY shun

6.10 The abnormal reduction of calcium in bone is a clinical sign known as **decalcification**, which is often caused by a hormonal disorder upsetting the calcium balance between the bloodstream and bone. In many patients, _____ can be treated with a combination of hormonal therapy, a diet rich in calcium and vitamin D, and mild exercise.

dyskinesia
diss kih NEE see ah

6.11 Difficulty in movement is a common sign of a musculoskeletal disorder. Remember from the word *bradykinesia* that the word root *kinesi* means "motion," and the suffix *-ia* means "condition of." When the prefix *dys-* is added, it forms the word _____, which literally means "bad, abnormal, painful, or difficult motion." The constructed form of this term can be written as dys/kines/ia.

dystrophy
DISS troh fee

6.12 A general term to describe a deformity arising during development is _____, which literally means "process of (-y) bad, abnormal, painful, or difficult (dys-) development (troph)." It is a constructed term that can be written as dys/troph/y. It is a sign of a congenital disease that occurs in different forms. For example, there are several types of muscular dystrophies, each of which appears during early childhood to produce musculoskeletal dysfunction.

hypertrophy
high PER troh fee

6.13 The sign of excessive muscle growth or development is known as _____. Although it is an abnormality, it is often induced by exercise enthusiasts by adding tension to weight-training activities. Muscular hypertrophy is produced by the addition of protein to muscle fibers, which is stimulated by strenuous muscle activity. The constructed form of this word is hyper/troph/y, in which hyper- means "excessive," troph means "development," and -y means "process of."

myalgia
my AL jee ah

6.14 During strenuous exercise, muscle cell activity may exceed the capacity of the cell to obtain and use oxygen during metabolism. When this occurs, the "oxygen debt" will cause the cell to metabolize without oxygen (called anaerobic respiration), resulting in the buildup of lactic acid in the muscle tissue. Because lactic acid causes muscle pain, a common symptom of strenuous exercise is _____, which literally means "condition of muscle (my) pain (-algia)." Its constructed form is my/algia. This form of myalgia is temporary, lasting about one day. Chronic forms of myalgia usually suggest an underlying musculoskeletal disease.

tenodynia
TEN oh DINN ee ah

6.15 Tendon pain, or **tenodynia**, is a common symptom of "weekend athletes": people who work inactive jobs during the workweek and become very active on their days off. The symptom of _____ usually indicates minor injury to one or more tendons, often lasting weeks or months. The suffix -dynia means "condition of pain," and ten/o means "tendon." The constructed form of this term is ten/o/dynia. Another suffix with the meaning of "condition of pain" is -algia. If tenodynia is intense, it may indicate tearing of the tendons that requires medical intervention.

PRACTICE: Signs and Symptoms of the Skeletal and Muscular Systems

Break the Chain

Analyze these medical terms:

   a) Separate each term into its word parts; each word part is labeled for you (**p** = prefix, **r** = root, **cf** = combining form, and **s** = suffix).

   b) For the Bonus Question, write the requested definition in the blank that follows.

The first set has been completed for you as an example.

1. a) arthralgia   *arthr / algia*
                              r   s

   b) *Bonus Question:* What is the definition of the suffix? *condition of pain*

2. a) ataxia   ____/_____/___
                         p   r   s

   b) *Bonus Question:* What is the definition of the word root? _____

3. a) atrophy   ____/_____/___
                          p   r   s

   b) *Bonus Question:* What is the definition of the word root? _____

4. a) bradykinesia   _____/_____/_____
                                 p   r   s

   b) *Bonus Question:* What is the definition of the prefix? _____

5. a) dyskinesia   _____/_____/_____
                               p   r   s

   b) *Bonus Question:* What is the definition of the word root? _____

6. a) dystrophy   _____/____/___
                              p   r   s

   b) *Bonus Question:* What is the definition of the suffix? _____

7. a) hypertrophy   _____/____/__
                                p   r   s

   b) *Bonus Question:* What is the definition of the prefix? _____

8. a) myalgia   _____/_____
                            r   s

   b) *Bonus Question:* What is the definition of the word root? _____

9. a) tenodynia   _____/__/_____
                               cf   s

   b) *Bonus Question:* What is the definition of the suffix? _____

Diseases and Disorders of the Skeletal and Muscular Systems

Following are the word parts that specifically apply to the diseases and disorders of the skeletal and muscular systems that are covered in the following section. Note that the word parts are color-coded to help you identify them: prefixes are blue, combining forms are red, and suffixes are purple.

Prefix	Definition
a-	without
epi-	upon, over, above, or on top
para-	alongside or abnormal
poly-	many
quadri-	four

Combining Form	Definition
ankyl/o	crooked
arthr/o	joint
burs/o	purse or sac, bursa
carcin/o	cancer
carp/o	wrist
chondr/o	cartilage
condyl/o	knuckle of a joint
fibr/o	fiber
kyph/o	hump
leuk/o	white
lith/o	stone
lord/o	bent forward
menisc/o, menisci/o	meniscus
myel/o	bone marrow
myos/o	muscle
ost/o, oste/o	bone
por/o	hole
sarc/o	flesh or meat
scoli/o	curved
spondyl/o	vertebra
synov/o, synovi/o	synovial
ten/o, tend/o	tendon

Suffix	Definition
-asthenia	weakness
-cele	hernia, swelling, protrusion
-emia	condition of blood
-genesis	origin, cause
-itis	inflammation
-malacia	softening
-oma	tumor
-osis	condition of
-plasia	formation or growth
-plegia	paralysis
-ptosis	drooping

achondroplasia
ah kon droh PLAY zee ah

6.16 A **dwarf** is an individual with abnormally short limbs and stature. A disease that causes dwarfism is _____, which combines the prefix a- (without), the combining form *chondr/o* (cartilage), and the suffix -plasia (formation) to form the meaning "without cartilage formation." The constructed form of this term is a/chondr/o/plasia. It is genetically determined and involves the abnormal lack of growth of long bones. See Figure 6.4■.

Figure 6.4 ■
Achondroplasia. The three people in
this photograph have achondroplasia,
which is characterized by reduced
height and short limbs.
Source: Photo Researchers, Inc.

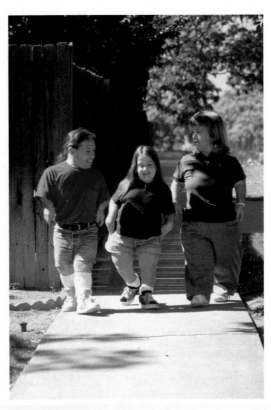

ankylosis
an kill OH siss

6.17 In the disease that literally means "condition of crooked,"
_____, joints are abnormally stiff, and movement is diffi-
cult. Ankylosis is a condition that may follow another disease, such as
arthritis, which may damage the joint structure. The constructed form of
ankylosis is ankyl/osis.

arthritis
ahr THRYE tiss

6.18 The general disorder resulting in inflammation and degeneration of a
joint is known as _____. It literally means "joint inflamma-
tion," which is easy to see in the constructed form of the term, arthr/itis, in
which *arthr* means "joint," and the suffix *-itis* means "inflammation." There
are two major forms of arthritis, each with a different cause.
Osteoarthritis (OA) is a common condition as people age, in which the
joint structures become worn over time and gradually replaced by bone.
See Figure 6.5■. **Rheumatoid arthritis (RA)** is an autoimmune disease
in which joint structures become eroded by the action of the body's own
white blood cells.

Figure 6.5 ■
Arthritis. (a) Photograph of osteoarthritis within the joints of the fingers.
Source: L. Samsuri/Custom Medical Stock Photo.
(b) Progressive changes of rheumatoid arthritis: 1. inflammation of synovial membrane; 2. progressive inflammation and beginning of cartilage destruction; 3. complete loss of synovial membrane; 4. complete joint loss.

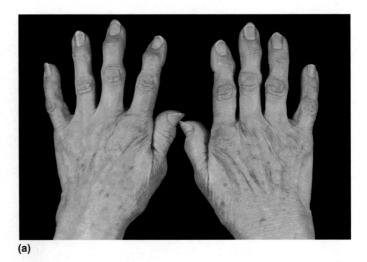

(a)

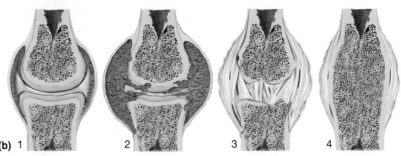

(b) 1   2   3   4

Inflammation

The Latin word *inflammatio* is the origin of this term, which literally means "to ignite or set ablaze." Because the symptoms of inflammation are heat, swelling, redness, and pain, this term is aptly named!

arthrochondritis
AHR throh kon DRY tiss

6.19 In the joint disease **arthrochondritis**, the articular cartilage within synovial joints undergoes inflammation, resulting in joint pain during movements. Unlike arthritis, _____ is usually a temporary condition caused by a localized infection. As a constructed term, it can be written *arthr/o/chondr/itis* by putting together the combining form *arthr/o* (joint) with the word root *chondr* (cartilage) and the suffix *-itis* (inflammation).

bunion
BUN yun

6.20 A **bunion** is an abnormal enlargement of the joint at the base of the big toe. A _____ is caused by an inflammation of a bursa near the big toe.

Bunion

The term *bunion* is derived from the Old French word *buigne,* which means "a swelling caused by a blow to the head." However, the modern meaning is limited to a swelling of the big toe.

bursitis
ber SIGH tiss

6.21 Remember that the suffix *-itis* means "inflammation," and the word root *burs* means "purse or sac," and refers to a saclike bursa that cushions certain joints. So the inflammation of a bursa is known as _____. The constructed form of this term is written as burs/itis.

bursolith
BER soh lith

6.22 A calcium deposit within a bursa of the foot is known as a **bursolith**. The diagnosis of a _____ is confirmed with an X-ray, and is typically surgically removed. The word root *lith* is derived from the Greek *lithos*, which means "a stone." The constructed form of this term is written as burs/o/lith. (Note that no suffix is used in this term.)

carpal tunnel syndrome
KAR pahl * TUN ul * SIN drohm

6.23 People working at computer stations for extended periods of time increase their risk of a repetitive stress injury of the wrist. Commonly known as _____ _____ _____, or **CTS**, it is characterized by inflammation of the wrist (**tenosynovitis**, see Frame 6.57) that causes pressure against the median nerve, resulting in local pain and restricted movement.

carpoptosis
KAR pop TOH siss

6.24 Also known as "wrist drop," the condition **carpoptosis** is a weakness of the wrist resulting in difficulty supporting the hand. _____ is a constructed term, which can be written as carp/o/ptosis. It literally means "drooping of the wrist" (*-ptosis* is the suffix that means "drooping" and the combining form *carp/o* means "wrist").

cramps

6.25 Prolonged, involuntary muscular contractions cause pain wherever they occur, often striking the stomach wall or thigh muscles after strenuous exercise. The painful contractions are called _____.

DJD

6.26 A general term describing a disease of joints in which the cartilage undergoes degeneration is called **degenerative joint disease**, abbreviated _____. This type of disease is progressive, becoming worse in time. During the process of joint degeneration, the articular cartilage degrades and is often replaced with bone. Arthritis (Frame 6.18) is the most common form of DJD.

Duchenne's muscular dystrophy
doo SHENZ * MUS kyoo lar * DIS troh fee

6.27 Children are occasionally born with a disease causing skeletal muscle degeneration, resulting in progressive muscle weakness and deterioration. Abbreviated **DMD**, it is called **Duchenne's muscular dystrophy**. Unfortunately, _____ _____ _____ has no known cure.

epicondylitis
ep ih kon dih LYE tiss

6.28 When the suffix that means "inflammation" is combined with the word root *condyl* ("knuckle of a joint") and the prefix *epi-* ("upon, over, above, or on top"), it forms the term _____. The epicondyles are small bony elevations on the humerus near the elbow joint. In epicondylitis this area of the elbow becomes inflamed, usually due to an injury. The constructed form of this term is written as epi/condyl/itis.

fibromyalgia
FIE broh my AHL jee ah

6.29 A disease of unknown origin that produces widespread pain of musculoskeletal structures of the limbs, face, and trunk is known as **fibromyalgia**. This term is constructed of the combining form *fibr/o*, the word root *my*, and the suffix *-algia*, which together mean "condition of pain of the fibers and muscles." _____ can be written as fibr/o/my/algia. Also known as **fibromyalgia syndrome**, there is some evidence that it may be, at least in part, caused by sleep deprivation.

fracture
FRAK sher

6.30 The clinical term for a break in a bone is _____. There are numerous types of fractures, many of which are described further in Table 6.1 ■ and illustrated in Figure 6.6■.

Table 6.1 ■ Categories of Fractures

Category	Definition
Colles' (KOH leez)	a break in the distal part of the radius
comminuted (KOM ih noo ted)	a break resulting in fragmentation of the bone
compression (kom PREH shun)	a crushed break, often due to weight or pressure applied to a bone during a fall
displaced	a break causing an abnormal alignment of bone pieces
epiphyseal (eh PIFF ih see al)	a break at the location of the growth plate, which can affect growth of the bone
greenstick	a slight break in a bone that appears as a slight fissure in an X-ray
nondisplaced	a break in which the broken bones retain their alignment
Pott's	a break at the ankle that affects both bones of the leg
spiral	a spiral-shaped break often caused by twisting stresses along a long bone

Figure 6.6 ■
Common bone fractures.

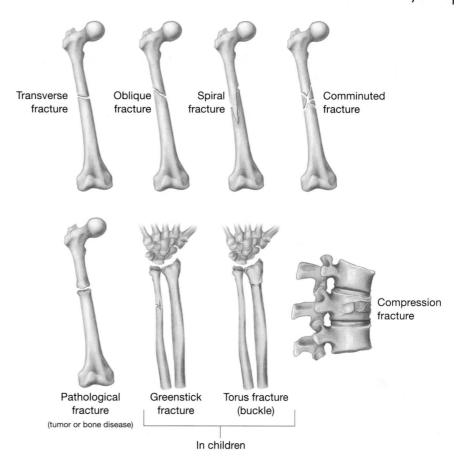

Transverse fracture

Oblique fracture

Spiral fracture

Comminuted fracture

Pathological fracture
(tumor or bone disease)

Greenstick fracture

Torus fracture (buckle)

Compression fracture

In children

gout
GOWT

6.31 In **gout**, a person experiences sharp pain in the joints of the toes, especially the big toe. See Figure 6.7■. The pain of _____ is often exacerbated by a diet high in protein because the disorder is caused by an abnormal accumulation of uric acid crystals in the joints, which are waste products of protein metabolism.

Figure 6.7 ■
Gout. Also known as gouty arthritis, it often strikes the big toe, as seen in this photograph.
Source: Reprinted from the Clinical Slide Collection on the Rheumatic Diseases. © 1991, 1995. Used by permission of the American College of Rheumatology.

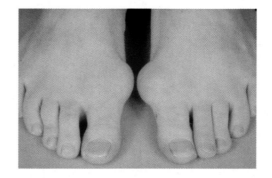

Gout

The term *gout* is derived from the Latin word *gutta*, which means "a drop." The foot pain that characterizes gout was thought to be caused by a body fluid dripping internally onto the joint. It was a malady common to European aristocracy prior to the 20th century, made worse by poor dietary habits that included diets high in protein and low in fresh vegetables and fruits.

herniated disk
    HER nee ay ted * disk

6.32 The rupture of an intervertebral disk is called **herniated disk**. It causes pressure against spinal nerves, which generates back pain. A _____ _____ is a back injury often caused by a sudden movement or an attempt to lift a heavy object. See Figure 6.8■.

Figure 6.8 ■
Herniated disk. A herniated disk is a protrusion of the disk's gelatinous center, called the nucleus pulposus, which often pushes into the spinal cord to cause pain and loss of movement (left illustration). The illustration on the right shows the back surgery necessary to access the injury.

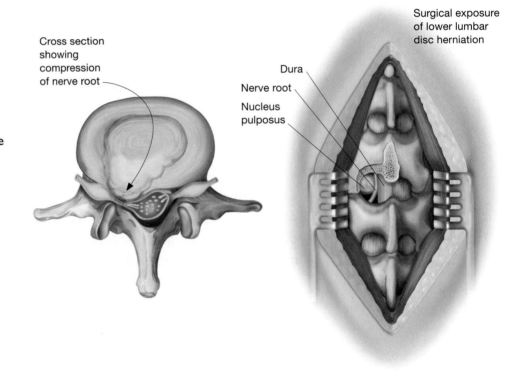

Cross section showing compression of nerve root

Surgical exposure of lower lumbar disc herniation

Dura
Nerve root
Nucleus pulposus

6.33 Spinal curvatures are normal and help us to stand erect. However, some individuals suffer from a deformity of the spine that alters the normal curves. The three primary spinal deformities are **kyphosis**, **lordosis**, and **scoliosis**. A _____ occurs when the upper thoracic curve bends posteriorly, causing an abnormal hump at the upper back (*kyph* means "hump") that often accompanies osteoporosis (see Frame 6.46). A _____ is an exaggerated anterior spinal curve in the lumbar area (*lord* means "bent forward"). A _____ is a lateral curvature of the spine with a congenital origin, usually in the thoracic or lumbar regions (*scoli* means "curved"). See Figure 6.9■. All three terms for abnormal spinal curvatures are constructed terms. For example, scoliosis can be written as scoli/osis.

kyphosis
kih FOH siss

lordosis
lor DOH siss

scoliosis
SKOH lee OH siss

Figure 6.9 ■
Spinal disfigurements. (a) Kyphosis, or humpback, in which the upper thoracic curve bends posteriorly; lordosis, an exaggerated anterior curve in the lumbar region; and scoliosis, a lateral curvature.
(b) Photograph of a woman with kyphosis.
Source: Phototake NYC.
(c) Photograph of a relatively severe scoliosis.
Source: Photo Researchers, Inc.

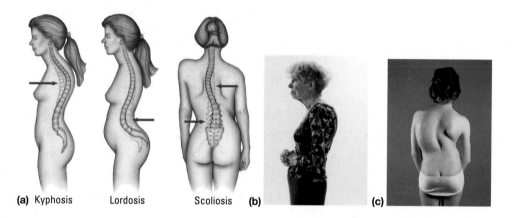

(a) Kyphosis   Lordosis   Scoliosis   (b)   (c)

6.34 The congenital disease called **Marfan's syndrome** results in excessive cartilage formation at the epiphyseal plates (growth plates), forming abnormally long limbs and a tall, thin body form. The heart valves of those suffering from _____ _____ are also deformed, resulting in valvular heart disease. Some forensic scientists have postulated that Abraham Lincoln suffered from this syndrome.

Marfan's syndrome
mahr FAHNZ * SIN drohm

6.35 A meniscus is a crescent-shaped band of cartilage that supports certain joints, such as the knee and shoulder. Inflammation of a meniscus results in joint pain and is called _____. As a constructed term, it is written as menisc/itis.

meniscitis
MEN ih SIGH tiss

6.36 Myasthenia gravis is characterized by a progressive failure of muscles to respond to nerve stimulation. The term _____ _____ means "serious muscle weakness." The word *gravis* means "serious," and you may recognize *myasthenia* as a constructed term that can be written as my/asthenia.

myasthenia gravis
my ass THEE nee ah * GRAHV iss

myeloma my ah LOH mah	**6.37** The red bone marrow is the site of blood cell formation. A malignant tumor arising from this tissue is known as **myeloma**. The term literally means "tumor of red bone marrow," in which *myel* means "bone marrow" and *-oma* means "tumor." The constructed form of _____ is written as myel/oma.
myocele MY oh seel	**6.38** A muscle is surrounded by a layer of tough connective tissue, known as fascia. An injury to a muscle may cause the muscle to tear through the fascia, causing a protrusion. This condition is known as a **myocele**. The constructed form of the term _____ is written as my/o/cele, which is composed of the combining form for muscle, *my/o*, and the suffix *-cele*, which means "protrusion."
myositis my oh SYE tiss	**6.39** A common result of muscle injury is a local inflammation known as **myositis**. Combining *myos* (muscle) and *-itis* (inflammation), the constructed form of _____ is written as myos/itis.
osteitis OSS tee EYE tiss	**6.40** When injured or exposed to infection, bone tissue often responds with inflammation. This condition, which combines the suffix that means "inflammation" and *oste*, the word root meaning "bone," is known as _____, which literally means "inflammation of bone." The constructed form is written as oste/itis.
osteitis deformans OSS tee EYE tiss * day FOR manz	**6.41** Also called **Paget's disease**, **osteitis deformans** results in bone deformities due to the acceleration of bone loss. Common symptoms of _____ _____ include severe bone pain and frequent fractures. Recent evidence suggests this disease is caused by a virus.

6.42 Bone cancer arising from epithelial tissue that has invaded a bone is generally known as **osteocarcinoma**. An **osteosarcoma** is bone cancer arising from connective tissue, usually within the bone itself. Although both forms of neoplasms are life threatening, the osteosarcoma is a more aggressive form of bone cancer. The constructed form of the cancer arising from epithelial tissue, or _____, is oste/o/carcin/oma, and that of bone cancer arising from connective tissue, or _____, is oste/o/sarc/oma. Both terms share the suffix -oma (tumor) and the combining form oste/o (bone). What differentiates them are their word roots, with _carcin_ meaning "cancer" and _sarc_ meaning "flesh or meat." A third form of malignant bone cancer arises from the cells of the red bone marrow and is called **leukemia** (loo KEE mee ah). This term literally means "condition of white blood," named because of the high levels of deformed white blood cells in a blood sample that are a diagnostic of the disease.

osteocarcinoma
OSS tee oh kar sin OH mah

osteosarcoma
OSS tee oh sar KOH mah

6.43 An inherited disease resulting in impaired bone growth and fragile bones is known as **osteogenesis imperfecta**. The term means "imperfect bone development." Tragically, _____ _____ is progressive, leading to severe bone pain, skeletal deformities, and frequent fractures.

osteogenesis imperfecta
OSS tee oh jen eh siss *
im per FEK tah

6.44 The suffix -_malacia_ means "softening," and the combining form oste/o means "bone." A disease resulting in the softening of bones is generally known as _____. It is a constructed term that is written as oste/o/malacia. The cause is usually a hormonal imbalance, resulting in the gradual loss of calcium to bone tissue.

osteomalacia
OSS tee oh mah LAY she ah

6.45 The word root _myel_ means "bone marrow." Inflammation of the red bone marrow is a painful disease known as _____, which literally means "inflammation of red bone marrow and bone." The usual cause is a bacterial infection. Osteomyelitis is a constructed term that can be written as oste/o/myel/itis.

osteomyelitis
OSS tee oh my eh LYE tiss

osteoporosis
OSS tee oh por ROH siss

6.46 The abnormal loss of bone density is a common result of aging, especially among postmenopausal women. The condition is called **osteoporosis** and results in a loss of posture and flexibility. See Figure 6.10■. The term _____ literally means "condition of holes in bone." The constructed term includes four word parts and is written as oste/o/por/osis. (The word root *por* means "hole.")

Figure 6.10 ■
Osteoporosis. (a) A section through normal spongy bone.
(b) A section through a bone with osteoporosis reveals a reduction of bone spicules and additional space.
(c) Spinal curvatures resulting from osteoporosis of the vertebral column with advancing age.

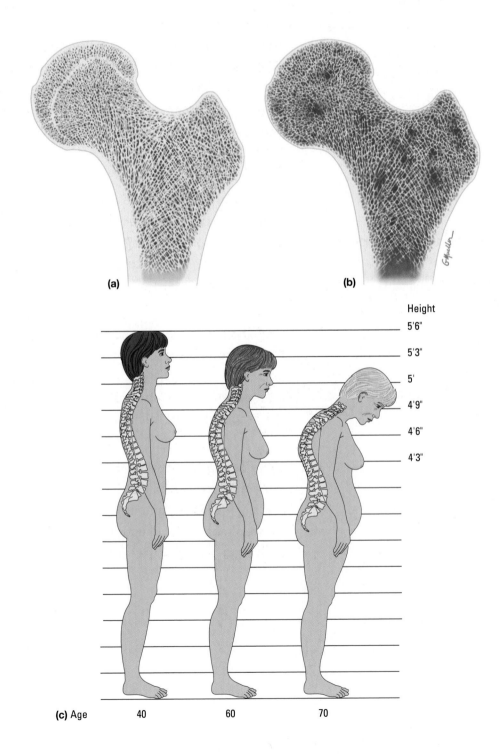

(a)

(b)

(c) Age 40 60 70

Height
5'6"
5'3"
5'
4'9"
4'6"
4'3"

paraplegia
PAIR ah PLEE jee ah

quadriplegia
KWAHD rih PLEE jee ah

6.47 The suffix *-plegia* means "paralysis." One form of paralysis is _____, in which there is a loss of sensation or voluntary movement of the area of the body below the hips, including both legs. In another form of paralysis, all four limbs are without sensation of voluntary movement. It utilizes the prefix that means "four" and is called _____.

polymyositis
PALL ee my oh SYE tiss

6.48 The term _____ means "inflammation of many muscles." It is a condition caused by bacterial infection in which a group of muscles become infected and react with inflammation. The constructed form of this term is written as poly/myos/itis, in which the prefix *poly-* means "many," *myos* means "muscle," and the suffix *-itis* means "inflammation."

rickets
RIHK ehts

6.49 In the disease **rickets**, the bones become softened due to the excessive removal of calcium for other body functions. _____ is caused by a lack of calcium and/or vitamin D in the diet. When it strikes a child, it often results in bowing of the legs and growth retardation.

rotator cuff injury

6.50 The rotator cuff is a combination of four muscles and their tendons that surround and stabilize the shoulder joint: teres minor, supraspinatus, infraspinatus, and subscapularis. A trauma to the shoulder can tear one or more tendons and muscles, resulting in a _____ _____ _____ that can cause local inflammation, pain, and joint dislocation.

spinal cord injury

6.51 A trauma to the vertebral column may result in _____ _____ _____, which is abbreviated **SCI**. If severe, the injury can cause paralysis of areas of the body below the vertebral level of the injury.

spondylarthritis
SPON dill ahr THRYE tiss

6.52 The clinical term that is formed by combining the suffix meaning "inflammation," the word root *arthr*, meaning "joint," and the word root *spondyl*, meaning "vertebra" is _____, which means "inflammation of joints of vertebrae." It is a relatively uncommon condition of intervertebral joints that leads to a gradual inability to flex and bend the back. The constructed form of this term is written spondyl/arthr/itis.

sprain

6.53 A _____ is a tear of collagen fibers within a ligament. See Figure 6.11 ■. It usually is caused by stretching the ligament beyond its normal range without warming or slow stretching.

Figure 6.11 ■
Sprain. A sprain involves damage to one or more ligaments, and is categorized into three degrees of injury as shown.

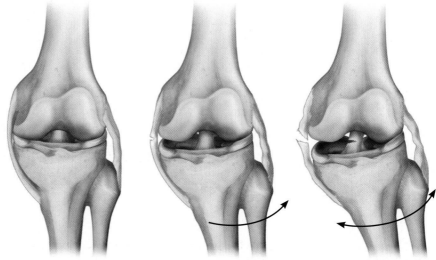

1st-degree sprain
Localized joint pain and tenderness, but no joint laxity.

2nd-degree sprain
Detectable joint laxity, plus localized pain and tenderness.

3rd-degree sprain
Complete disruption of ligaments and gross joint instability.

strain

6.54 Similar to a sprain but involving a muscle, a _____ usually is caused by stretching a muscle beyond its normal range. It often causes a bruise due to the tearing of muscle tissue and capillary damage.

temporomandibular joint disease
TEMP or oh man DIH byoo lahr *
JOYNT * DIS eez

6.55 The temporomandibular joint is the junction of the mandible and the temporal bone, which allows the lower jaw to move when speaking and chewing. A disease of this joint is known as _____ _____ _____, or **TMJ**, and results in frequent dislocations that make it difficult and painful to move the jaw during speaking and chewing.

tendonitis
TEN dunn EYE tiss

6.56 Inflammation of a tendon is a common sports injury and is known as _____. An example occurs when damage is caused by throwing a ball without warming up, which is known as **rotator cuff tendonitis**. Tendonitis is a constructed term, written as tendon/itis.

tenosynovitis
TEN oh sin oh VYE tiss

6.57 A form of tendonitis that also involves inflammation of the synovial membrane surrounding the joint is known as _____. This term has four word parts and is written as ten/o/synov/itis, in which ten/o means "tendon," synov means "synovial," and -itis means "inflammation."

PRACTICE: Diseases and Disorders of the Skeletal and Muscular Systems

The Right Match

Match the term on the left with the correct definition on the right.

_____ 1. Pott's

_____ 2. gout

_____ 3. bunion

_____ 4. Duchenne's muscular dystrophy

_____ 5. cramps

_____ 6. sprain

_____ 7. fracture

_____ 8. strain

_____ 9. comminuted

_____ 10. rotator cuff injury

a. an abnormal enlargement of the joint at the base of the big toe

b. a condition that causes skeletal muscle degeneration, which results in progressive muscle weakness and deterioration; abbreviated DMD

c. prolonged, involuntary muscular contractions

d. a trauma that causes tearing of tendons and/or muscles of the shoulder

e. caused by an abnormal accumulation of uric acid crystals in the joints; usually affects the big toe joints

f. an injury that results from stretching a muscle beyond its normal range

g. a type of fracture that involves a break resulting in fragmentation of the bone

h. a tear of collagen fibers within a ligament

i. a type of fracture that involves a break at the ankle that affects both bones of the leg

j. clinical term for a break in the bone

Linkup

Link the word parts in the list to create the terms that match the definitions. You may use word parts more than once. Remember to add combining vowels when needed—and that some terms do not use any combining vowel. The first one is completed as an example.

Prefix	Combining Form	Suffix
epi-	arthr/o	-asthenia
poly-	burs/o	-itis
	condyl/o	-malacia
	lith/o	-osis
	lord/o	
	menisci/o	
	my/o, myos/o	
	oste/o	
	synov/o	
	ten/o	

Definition   Term

1.   weakness in the muscles   *myasthenia*

2.   inflammation of many muscles simultaneously   _____

3.   a spine deformity with an anterior curve of the spine   _____

4.   inflammation of bony elevations (epicondyles) near the elbow joint   _____

5.   inflammation and degeneration of a joint   _____

6.   a gradual and painful softening of bones   _____

7.   inflammation of a bursa   _____

8.   inflammation of bone tissue   _____

9.   a calcium deposit or stone within a bursa   _____

10. inflammation of a meniscus   _____

11. form of tendonitis that also involves inflammation of the synovial membrane   _____

Treatments, Procedures, and Devices of the Skeletal and Muscular Systems

Following are the word parts that specifically apply to the treatments, procedures, and devices associated with the skeletal and muscular systems that are covered in the following section. Note that the word parts are color-coded to help you identify them: combining forms are red, and suffixes are purple.

Combining Form	Definition
arthr/o	joint
burs/o	purse or sac, bursa
chondr/o	cartilage
cost/o	rib
crani/o	skull, cranium
electr/o	electricity
fasci/o	fascia
lamin/o	thin, lamina
orth/o	straight
ost/o, oste/o	bone
spondyl/o	vertebra
syn/o	connect
ten/o, tend/o	tendon
vertebr/o	vertebra

Suffix	Definition
-centesis	surgical puncture
-clasia, -clasis	break apart
-desis	surgical fixation or fusion
-ectomy	surgical removal or excision
-gram	a record or image
-graphy	recording process
-iatry	treatment or specialty
-ist	one who specializes
-lysis	loosen or dissolve
-pathy	disease
-plasty	surgical repair
-rrhaphy	suturing
-scope	instrument, used for viewing
-scopy	process of viewing
-tic	pertaining to
-tomy	incision or to cut

arthrocentesis

AHR throh sen TEE siss

6.58 The suffix *-centesis* means "surgical puncture," and the combining form *arthr/o* means "joint." Many joint injuries result in the condition of inflammation, which may slow healing and lead to additional complications. In the procedure known as _____, excess fluids are **aspirated**, or withdrawn by suction, through a surgical puncture into the synovial cavity of the joint. See Figure 6.12■. This constructed term is written as arthr/o/centesis.

Figure 6.12 ■
Arthrocentesis. The aspiration of fluid is a common treatment for joint injuries resulting in inflammation, such as carpal tunnel syndrome (CTS) in this illustration.

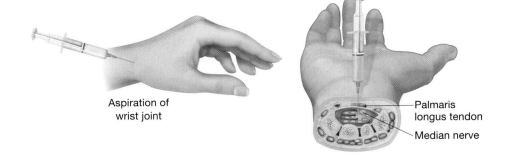

Aspiration of wrist joint

Palmaris longus tendon

Median nerve

arthroclasia
ahr throh KLAY see ah

6.59 Occasionally, an abnormally stiff joint must be broken during surgery to increase the **range of motion**, or **ROM**. This procedure is called _____, in which the suffix -clasia means "break apart." After surgery, it is common to undergo ROM exercises to increase muscle strength and joint mobility. Arthroclasia is a constructed term with three word parts that is written as arthr/o/clasia.

arthrodesis
ahr throh DEE siss

6.60 The suffix -desis means "surgical fixation." Thus, the term _____ means "surgical fixation of a joint." The constructed form of this term is written as arthr/o/desis.

arthrogram
AHR throh gram

6.61 Prior to joint surgery, it is common to obtain an X-ray of the joint after injection of contrast media, air, or both to highlight the synovial joint. The image is printed on a film and is called an _____ because the suffix -gram means "a record or image." The constructed form of this term is arthr/o/gram.

arthrolysis
ahr THROH loh siss

6.62 The suffix -lysis means "loosen." During an _____, a joint is loosened of abnormal restrictions, such as calcium deposits and bursoliths (see Frame 6.22). The constructed form of this term is arthr/o/lysis.

arthroplasty
AHR throh PLASS tee

6.63 The suffix -plasty means "surgical repair." The goal of an _____ procedure is to repair a joint. A complete arthroplasty refers to a joint replacement, the most common of which is a hip replacement. The constructed form of this term is arthr/o/plasty.

6.64 An endoscopic visual examination of a joint cavity uses an instrument that integrates fiber optics, live-action photography, and computer enhancement, known as an **arthroscope**. The viewing process is called _____. When arthroscopy is part of a surgery, the procedure is called **arthroscopic surgery**. See Figure 6.13■.

arthroscopy
ahr THROSS koh pee

Figure 6.13 ■
Arthroscopic surgery. In this illustration, the knee joint is undergoing surgery with a specialized endoscope called an arthroscope in the procedure known as arthroscopic surgery.

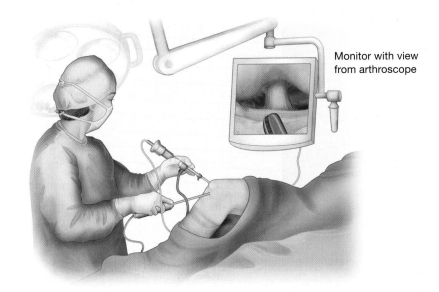

Monitor with view from arthroscope

arthrotomy
ahr THROTT oh mee

6.65 The suffix -*tomy* means "to cut" or "incision." A surgical incision into the synovial cavity of a joint is known as _____. The constructed form of the term is arthr/o/tomy.

bursectomy
ber SEK toh mee

6.66 A surgery involving the removal of a bursa from a joint is known as a _____. The constructed form of the term is burs/ectomy, in which *burs* means "sac" and -*ectomy* means "surgical removal" or "excision."

chiropractic
KIGH roh PRAK tik

6.67 The field of therapy that is centered on manipulation of bones and joints, most commonly the vertebral column, is known as _____. A practitioner of this therapy is called a **chiropractor** (KIGH roh prak tor).

chondrectomy
kon DREK toh mee

6.68 Surgical removal, or excision, of the cartilage associated with a joint is a common procedure known as _____. The surgery commonly uses arthroscopy to reduce the size of the incision and improve the surgeon's view. It is a constructed term that can be written as chondr/ectomy to reveal its two word parts: *chondr*, which means "cartilage," and -*ectomy*, which means "surgical removal" or "excision."

WORDS TO WATCH OUT FOR !

-ectomy or -tomy?

These two suffixes look very similar, but how do you tell them apart? One easy way is to remember that -ectomy means "excision" (see how they both start with an "e"?). The suffix -tomy means "incision" or "to cut," and this meaning does not start with an "e."

---

chondroplasty
KON droh plass tee

6.69 The suffix -plasty means "surgical repair." Surgical repair of cartilage associated with a joint is known as _____. The constructed form of the term is chondr/o/plasty.

---

costectomy
koss TEK toh mee

6.70 A surgery involving the removal of a rib (the combining form is cost/o) is known as a _____.

---

cranioplasty
KRAY nee oh plass tee

6.71 When one or more bones of the cranium (crani/o) undergo repair during surgery (-plasty), the procedure is called _____. The constructed term for this procedure is crani/o/plasty.

---

craniotomy
KRAY nee OTT oh mee

6.72 In order to perform surgery of the brain, a **craniotomy** is required, during which the surgeon enters the cranial cavity. The constructed form of _____ is written as crani/o/tomy, in which the combining form crani/o means "skull or cranium," and the suffix -tomy means "incision."

---

diskectomy
disk EK toh mee

6.73 A surgical procedure that is used frequently to reduce the pain of a herniated disk by surgically removing the intervertebral disk is a _____. It may also be called a **spinal fusion** when the adjacent vertebrae are fused together following the removal of the disk. An alternate term for spinal fusion is **spondylosyndesis** (SPON dih loh sin DEE siss), which literally means "surgical fixation to connect vertebrae." This constructed term is written as spondyl/o/syn/desis, in which the combining form spondyl/o means "vertebra," syn means "connect," and the suffix -desis means "surgical fixation." Also performed to treat a herniated disk is a **laminectomy** (lahm ih NEK toh mee), during which the part of a vertebra known as the lamina is surgically removed to relieve pressure on the spinal cord.

---

electromyography
ee LEK troh my OG rah fee

6.74 The strength of a muscle contraction can be measured and recorded by a procedure called **electromyography**. It utilizes an instrument that electrically stimulates a muscle, and the resulting contraction is recorded and analyzed on a computer. In this term, electr/o means "electricity," my/o means "muscle," and -graphy means "recording process." _____ includes five word parts and is written as electr/o/my/o/graphy.

fasciotomy
FASH ee OTT oh mee

6.75 A surgical incision into the connective tissue sheath surrounding a muscle, called fascia, is known as a _____. The constructed form of this term is fasci/o/tomy.

fracture reduction

6.76 Orthopedic surgeons, or orthopedists, treat fractures by aligning the broken bones to their normal positions in a procedure known as **reduction**. Manipulating the bone without surgery during reduction is known as **closed** _____ _____. If surgery intervention is needed to align the broken area, the procedure is called **open fracture reduction**. During this procedure, pins, screws, rods, or plates may be used to stabilize the alignment, known as **internal fixation**. In **external fixation**, metal rods and pins are attached from outside the skin surface. External fixation carries the advantage of avoiding the use of a plaster cast for immobilization. If the normal healing process is impeded, **bone grafting** or **electrical bone stimulation** may be applied to stimulate the healing process.

myoplasty
MY oh plass tee

myorrhaphy
my OR ah fee

6.77 The combining form *my/o* means "muscle." A muscle may become torn during a serious injury and require surgical intervention to promote healing. During a _____, a muscle undergoes surgical repair (*-plasty*). The constructed form of the term is written my/o/plasty. The repair often includes suturing the torn ends together in the procedure known as _____. The constructed form of the term is my/o/rrhaphy, in which the suffix *-rrhaphy* means "suturing."

NSAIDs

6.78 The most common pharmacological treatment for any condition, including inflammation or pain of muscle or bone tissue, is the use of **nonsteroidal anti-inflammatory drugs**, commonly abbreviated _____. Examples of NSAIDs are aspirin and ibuprofen.

orthotics
or THOTT iks

6.79 The field of medical support involving the construction and fitting of orthopedic appliances to assist a patient, such as lifts, artificial limbs, and retraction devices, is known as **orthotics**. Formed from the combining form *orth/o*, which means "straight," and the suffix *-tic*, which means "pertaining to," this constructed term is written as orth/o/tics. A specialist in _____ is called an **orthotist** (OR thott ist). The medical term for an artificial limb is **prosthesis** (pross THEE siss).

ostectomy
oss TEK toh mee

6.80 An _____ is the surgical removal, or excision, of bone tissue. It is performed to remove unwanted bony formations. The constructed form of this term is ost/ectomy, in which the suffix meaning "surgical removal or excision" is added to the word root for "bone" (ost).

osteoclasis
OSS tee oh KLAY siss

6.81 In some cases, it becomes necessary to break a bone purposely to correct a defect or an improperly healed fracture. Formed by adding the suffix -clasis, meaning "break apart," to the combining form for "bone," the name of the procedure is _____. It is a constructed term that is written oste/o/clasis.

osteopathy
OSS tee OPP ah thee

6.82 A medical field that emphasizes the relationship between the musculoskeletal system and overall health with an emphasis on body alignment and nutrition is called **osteopathy**. The constructed form is oste/o/pathy. A physician trained in _____ is known as an **osteopath** or **osteopathic surgeon**.

osteoplasty
OSS tee oh plass tee

6.83 The surgical repair of bone is a general procedure known as _____. This term is formed by adding the suffix -plasty (surgical repair) to the combining form oste/o (bone). The constructed form is oste/o/plasty.

WORDS TO WATCH OUT FOR !

-pathy or -plasty?

These two suffixes look very similar, but how do you tell them apart? The suffix -pathy means "disease," whereas the meaning of the suffix -plasty is "repair." One easy way to tell them apart is to think of the sound of -plasty: it sounds like "plaster," which is a home product that is used to repair walls.

podiatry
poh DYE ah tree

6.84 The Greek word for "foot" is podos. This word root, combined with the suffix -iatry, which means "treatment or specialty," is used to construct the term _____, which is the specialty that focuses on foot health. A healthcare professional trained in this field is called a **podiatrist** (poh DYE ah trist).

tenomyoplasty
TEN oh MY oh plass tee

6.85 Some injuries involve damage to both the muscle and its associated tendon. The surgical procedure involving the repair of both muscle and tendon is called a _____. This constructed term may be written as ten/o/my/o/plasty to reveal its word parts: the combining forms ten/o, meaning "tendon," and my/o, meaning "muscle"; and the suffix -plasty, meaning "surgical repair."

tenorrhaphy
ten OR ah fee

6.86 Stepping into a hole and falling can cause a serious injury to the calcaneal tendon of the ankle. This tendon, also known as the Achilles tendon, attaches the powerful calf muscles to the large heel bone (calcaneus). If it tears, mobility of the affected leg becomes impossible until surgical intervention corrects the injury. The surgery is called a _____ and involves the suturing of a tendon to close a tear. This constructed term is written as ten/o/rrhaphy to reveal its word parts. In this term, the suffix -rrhaphy, which means "suturing," is added to the combining form that means "tendon."

tenotomy
ten OTT oh mee

6.87 A tenorrhaphy often includes the _____ procedure, during which one or more incisions are made into a tendon. Also a constructed term, it is written as ten/o/tomy, using the combining form that means "tendon" and the suffix that means "incision."

vertebroplasty
VERT eh broh plass tee

6.88 A surgical procedure that repairs damaged or diseased vertebrae is called a _____. Adding the combining form that means "vertebra" with the suffix that means "surgical repair" creates this constructed term, which is written vertebr/o/plasty.

PRACTICE: Treatments, Procedures, and Devices of the Skeletal and Muscular Systems

The Right Match

Match the term on the left with the correct definition on the right.

_____ 1. reduction

_____ 2. aspiration

_____ 3. arthrocentesis

_____ 4. nonsteroidal anti-inflammatory drugs

_____ 5. spinal fusion

_____ 6. arthroscopy

_____ 7. chondroplasty

_____ 8. tenorrhaphy

_____ 9. podiatry

_____ 10. arthrogram

a. the most common pharmacological treatment for inflammation or pain of muscle or bone tissue

b. a procedure in which adjacent vertebrae are fused together following a diskectomy

c. withdrawing by suction

d. a procedure in which excess fluids are aspirated through a surgical puncture in the joint

e. a procedure that aligns broken bones to their normal positions

f. an X-ray image of a joint that is printed on a film

g. healthcare specialty that focuses on foot health

h. an endoscopic visual examination of a joint cavity

i. surgical repair of cartilage

j. a surgery that sutures a tear in a tendon

Break the Chain

Analyze these medical terms:

   a) Separate each term into its word parts; each word part is labeled for you (**p** = prefix, **r** = root, **cf** = combining form, and **s** = suffix).

   b) For the Bonus Question, write the requested word part or definition in the blank that follows.

1. a) arthrodesis   _____/__/_____
                                   cf   s

    b) *Bonus Question:* What is the definition of the suffix? _____

2. a) chondrectomy   ____/_____
                                 r   s

    b) *Bonus Question:* What is the definition of the word root? _____

3. a) craniotomy   _____/ __/ _____
                                   cf   s

    b) *Bonus Question:* Does this term contain a prefix? _____

4. a) laminectomy   _____ / _____
                                  r   s

    b) *Bonus Question:* What is the definition of the suffix? _____

5. a) electromyography   _____ / ___ / ____ / ___ / _____
                                   cf   cf   s

    b) *Bonus Question:* What is the definition of the second combining form? _____

6. a) orthotics   _____ / __ /____
                                   cf   s

    b) *Bonus Question:* What is the definition of the combining form? _____

7. a) osteoclasis   _____ / __ / _____
                                   cf   s

    b) *Bonus Question:* What is the definition of the suffix? _____

8. a) tenomyoplasty   _____ / __/___/__/ _____
                                   cf   cf   s

    b) *Bonus Question:* What is the definition of the suffix? _____

9. a) osteoplasty   _____ / __/ _____
                                   cf   s

    b) *Bonus Question:* What is the definition of the combining form? _____

Abbreviations of the Skeletal and Muscular Systems

The abbreviations that are associated with the skeletal and muscular systems are summarized here. Study these abbreviations, and review them in the exercise that follows.

Abbreviation	Definition
ACL	anterior cruciate ligament; a ligament that stabilizes the knee joint
CTS	carpal tunnel syndrome
DJD	degenerative joint disease
DMD	Duchenne's muscular dystrophy
DO	physician specializing in osteopathy
EMG	electromyography
HNP	herniated nucleus pulposus; a herniated intervertebral disk
MG	myasthenia gravis
NSAIDs	nonsteroidal anti-inflammatory drugs

Abbreviation	Definition
OA	osteoarthritis
ortho	orthopedics
RA	rheumatoid arthritis
ROM	range of motion
SCI	spinal cord injury
THR	total hip replacement
TKA	total knee arthroplasty
TKR	total knee replacement
TMJ	temporomandibular joint
Vertebrae	
C1 through C7	the seven cervical vertebrae
T1 through T12	the twelve thoracic vertebrae
L1 through L5	the five lumbar vertebrae

PRACTICE: Abbreviations

Fill in the blanks with the abbreviation or the complete medical term.

Abbreviation

1. _____
2. TKA
3. _____
4. DMD
5. _____
6. EMG
7. _____
8. THR
9. _____
10. CTS
11. _____
12. OA
13. _____
14. T1–T12
15. _____
16. TMJ
17. _____

Medical Term

spinal cord injury

_____

rheumatoid arthritis

_____

herniated nucleus pulposus

_____

anterior cruciate ligament

_____

the five lumbar vertebrae

_____

range of motion

_____

total knee replacement

_____

degenerative joint disease

_____

myasthenia gravis

▶▶▶▶▶ Chapter Review

Word Building _____

Construct medical terms from the following meanings. The first question has been completed for you as an example.

1. **a gradual and painful softening of bone**   osteo_malacia_____
2. abnormal loss of bone density   osteo_____
3. paralysis of lower body, including both legs   _____plegia
4. abnormal lateral curve of the spine   scoli_____
5. inflammation of a tendon and synovial membrane   teno_____
6. X-ray film of a joint   arthro_____
7. inflammation of a meniscus   _____itis
8. surgical incision into a joint   arthro_____
9. muscular weakness   my_____
10. protrusion of muscle through its fascia   myo_____
11. a repetitive stress injury of the wrist   _____tunnel syndrome
12. a therapy in which a joint is loosened of its restrictions   arthro_____
13. a viral infection of bone that accelerates bone loss   _____'s disease
14. a rupture of an intervertebral disk   _____ disk
15. surgical repair of a joint   arthro_____
16. pain in a tendon   teno_____
17. a calcium deposit within a bursa   burso_____
18. abnormal condition of joint stiffness   _____osis
19. abnormally slow movements   _____kinesia
20. an abnormal reduction of calcium in bone   _____ (do this one on your own!)
21. surgical stabilization of a joint   arthro_____
22. a progressive disease of the joints in which the   degenerative _____ _____
    cartilage degenerates; abbreviated DJD
23. an orthopedic procedure in which metal rods and pins are   external _____
    attached from outside the skin surface to align a bone fracture
24. a disease of unknown origin that produces widespread pain   _____myalgia
    of musculoskeletal structures of the limbs, face, and trunk
    (but not joints)
25. a tumor that forms in the red bone marrow   myel_____
26. lacking development, or wasting   _____trophy

Clinical Application Exercises

Medical Report

Read the following medical report, then answer the questions that follow.

University Hospital

5500 University Avenue
Metropolis, TX

Phone: (211) 594-4000
Fax: (211) 594-4001

Medical Consultation: Osteology

Date: 6/15/2007

Patient: Jorge Johnson

Patient Complaint: Severe pain of the right ankle with any movement of lower limb. Localized redness and inflammation. Open wound apparent.

History: 35-year-old male African-American with no prior histories of musculoskeletal challenges.

Family History: Father deceased at 82 years of age, Type II diabetic with COPD. Mother Type II diabetic with right amputation of lower limb at knee.

Allergies: None

Evidences: Broken skin at right ankle superior to tarsometatarsal joint to suggest compound Pott's fracture. Local inflammation and pain may also suggest damage to the Achilles tendon. X-rays required for confirmation prior to treatment.

Treatment: Evaluation to be performed following x-rays; possible surgery may be required to remove bone fragments and establish alignment. If surgery is not warranted, immobilize lower limb with casting.

Jonathan McIntyre, M.D.

---

1. What is the evidence supporting an initial diagnosis as a compound fracture? _____

_____

2. Why are x-rays required before treatment can begin? _____

_____

3. How might the family history influence the course of treatment? _____

_____

Medical Report Case Study

The following case study provides further discussion regarding the patient in the medical report. Fill in the blanks with the correct terms. Choose your answers from the list of terms that precedes the case study. (Note that some terms may be used more than once.)

compound	myositis	Pott's
myalgia	polymyositis	tendonitis

A 35-year-old patient named Jorge Johnson received injuries during a weekend touch football game in the park. Upon his arrival at emergency, he presented an open, or (a) _____ fracture of the tibia, pain and discoloration of the ankle that suggested damage to a tendon, or (b) _____, and muscle tenderness or (c) _____ that suggested damaged muscle fibers or (d) _____, and inflammation of all muscles of the right lower extremity, or (e) _____. An X-ray examination revealed a fracture at the ankle, called a (f) _____ fracture, with associated inflammation of the Achilles tendon, or generalized (g) _____.

Image Recall

Label each type of fracture in the following image.

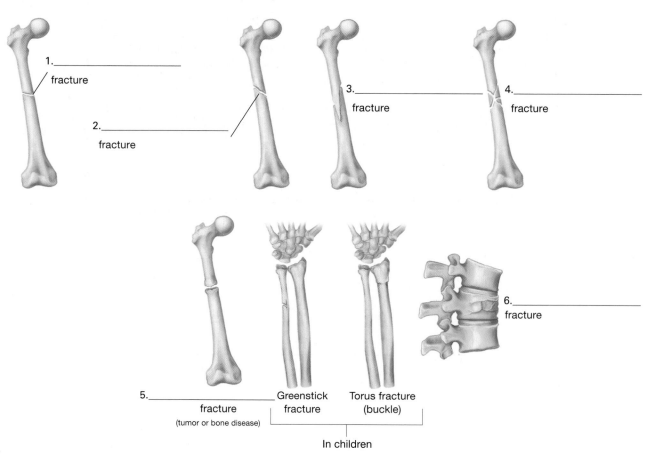

1. _____ fracture

2. _____ fracture

3. _____ fracture

4. _____ fracture

5. _____ fracture (tumor or bone disease)

Greenstick fracture

Torus fracture (buckle)

In children

6. _____ fracture

▶▶▶▶ Key Terms Double-Check

Remember that the chapter's key terms appeared alphabetically throughout this chapter. This exercise helps you check your knowledge AND review for tests.

1. First, fill in the missing word in the definitions for the chapter's key terms.
2. Then, check your answers using Appendix F.
3. If you got the answer right, put a check mark in the right column.
4. If your answer was incorrect, go back to the frame number provided and review the content.

Use the checklist to study the terms you don't know until you're confident you know them all.

Key Term	Frame	Definition	Know It?
1. achondroplasia	6.16	literally "without _____ formation"; causes dwarfism	☐
2. ankylosis	6.17	abnormal condition of _____ stiffness	☐
3. arthralgia	6.6	joint _____	☐
4. arthritis	6.18	_____ and degeneration of a joint	☐
5. arthrochondritis	6.19	inflammation of articular cartilage within synovial _____	☐
6. arthrocentesis	6.58	a procedure in which excess fluids are aspirated through a surgical _____ in the joint	☐
7. arthroclasia	6.59	procedure in which an abnormally stiff joint is _____ during surgery to increase range of motion	☐
8. arthrodesis	6.60	surgical _____ (stabilization) of a joint	☐
9. arthrogram	6.61	an X-ray (_____) image of a joint that is printed on a film	☐
10. arthrolysis	6.62	a therapy in which a joint is _____ of its restrictions	☐
11. arthroplasty	6.63	surgical _____ of a joint	☐
12. arthroscopy	6.64	an endoscopic visual examination of a(n) _____ cavity	☐
13. arthrotomy	6.65	surgical _____ into a joint	☐
14. ataxia	6.7	the inability to coordinate muscles during a voluntary activity or _____	☐
15. atrophy	6.8	lacking _____, or wasting	☐
16. bradykinesia	6.9	abnormally _____ movements	☐
17. bunion	6.20	abnormal enlargement of the joint at the base of the big _____	☐
18. bursectomy	6.66	a surgery involving the removal of a(n) _____ from a joint	☐
19. bursitis	6.21	_____ of a bursa	☐
20. bursolith	6.22	a calcium deposit or _____ within a bursa	☐
21. carpal tunnel syndrome	6.23	a repetitive stress injury of the _____	☐
22. carpoptosis	6.24	weakness of the wrist that results in difficulty supporting the _____	☐
23. chiropractic	6.67	the field of therapy that is centered on manipulation of bones and joints, most commonly the _____ column	☐

Key Term	Frame	Definition	Know It?
24. chondrectomy	6.68	surgical _____, or excision, of the cartilage associated with a joint	☐
25. chondroplasty	6.69	surgical repair of _____	☐
26. costectomy	6.70	a surgery involving the removal of a(n) _____	☐
27. cramps	6.25	prolonged, involuntary _____ contractions	☐
28. cranioplasty	6.71	a surgery that involves repair of one or more bones of the _____	☐
29. craniotomy	6.72	a(n) _____ into the cranial cavity during surgery	☐
30. decalcification	6.10	an abnormal reduction of _____ in bone	☐
31. degenerative joint disease	6.26	a progressive disease of the joints in which the cartilage degenerates; abbreviated _____	☐
32. diskectomy	6.73	a surgery that involves the removal of the intervertebral _____	☐
33. Duchenne's muscular dystrophy	6.27	a condition that causes skeletal muscle degeneration with progressive muscle _____ and deterioration; abbreviated DMD	☐
34. dyskinesia	6.11	difficulty in _____	☐
35. dystrophy	6.12	a deformity that arises during _____	☐
36. electromyography	6.74	a procedure that provides _____ stimulation of a muscle and records and analyzes the contractions	☐
37. epicondylitis	6.28	_____ of bony elevations (epicondyles) near the elbow joint	☐
38. fasciotomy	6.75	a surgical incision into the _____, the connective tissue sheath surrounding a muscle	☐
39. fibromyalgia	6.29	a disease of unknown origin that produces widespread _____ of musculoskeletal structures of the limbs, face, and trunk (but not joints)	☐
40. fracture	6.30	clinical term for a break in the _____	☐
41. fracture reduction	6.76	a procedure that involves aligning the broken bones to their _____ positions	☐
42. gout	6.31	caused by an abnormal accumulation of uric _____ crystals in the joints; usually affects the big toe joints	☐
43. herniated disk	6.32	a(n) _____ of an intervertebral disk	☐
44. hypertrophy	6.13	excessive muscle _____	☐
45. kyphosis	6.33	a spine deformity with a(n) _____ curve of the spine	☐
46. lordosis	6.33	a spine deformity with a(n) _____ curve of the spine	☐
47. Marfan's syndrome	6.34	congenital disease that results in excessive cartilage formation at the _____, or epiphyseal, plates	☐
48. meniscitis	6.35	inflammation of a(n) _____	☐
49. myalgia	6.14	_____ pain	☐
50. myasthenia gravis	6.36	literally "_____ muscle weakness"; a condition caused by a progressive failure of muscles to respond to nerve stimulation	☐

Key Term	Frame	Definition	Know It?
51. myeloma	6.37	a(n) _____ that forms in the red bone marrow	☐
52. myocele	6.38	_____ of muscle through its fascia	☐
53. myoplasty	6.77	surgical _____ of a muscle	☐
54. myorrhaphy	6.77	a surgical procedure that _____ the torn ends of a muscle	☐
55. myositis	6.39	_____ of a muscle	☐
56. nonsteroidal anti-inflammatory drugs (NSAIDs)	6.78	the most common _____ treatment for inflammation or pain of muscle or bone tissue	☐
57. orthotics	6.79	the field of medical support involving the construction and fitting of _____ appliances	☐
58. ostectomy	6.80	surgical removal (_____) of bone tissue	☐
59. osteitis	6.40	inflammation of _____ tissue	☐
60. osteitis deformans	6.41	a disease that results in bone deformities due to acceleration of bone loss; _____ disease	☐
61. osteocarcinoma	6.42	bone _____ arising from epithelial tissue that has invaded a bone	☐
62. osteoclasis	6.81	a surgical procedure that involves _____ a bone in order to correct a defect or an improperly healed fracture	☐
63. osteogenesis imperfecta	6.43	an inherited disease resulting in impaired bone _____ and fragile bones	☐
64. osteomalacia	6.44	a gradual and painful _____ of bones	☐
65. osteomyelitis	6.45	inflammation of the red bone _____	☐
66. osteopathy	6.82	a medical field that emphasizes the relationship between the _____ system and overall health with an emphasis on body alignment and nutrition	☐
67. osteoplasty	6.83	the _____ repair of bone	☐
68. osteoporosis	6.46	abnormal loss of bone _____	☐
69. osteosarcoma	6.42	_____ cancer arising from connective tissue, usually within the bone itself	☐
70. paraplegia	6.47	_____ of the lower body, including both legs	☐
71. podiatry	6.84	healthcare specialty that focuses on _____ health	☐
72. polymyositis	6.48	inflammation of _____ muscles simultaneously	☐
73. quadriplegia	6.47	a form of paralysis in which all _____ limbs are without sensation or voluntary movement	☐
74. rickets	6.49	a disease in which the bones become softened due to the excessive removal of _____ for other body functions	☐
75. rotator cuff injury	6.50	a trauma that causes tearing of tendons and/or muscles of the _____	☐
76. scoliosis	6.33	abnormal _____ curve of the spine	☐
77. spinal cord injury	6.51	trauma to the vertebral _____	☐

Key Term	Frame	Definition	Know It?
78. spondylarthritis	6.52	_____ of intervertebral joints	☐
79. sprain	6.53	a(n) _____ of collagen fibers within a ligament	☐
80. strain	6.54	an injury that results from _____ a muscle beyond its normal range	☐
81. temporomandibular joint disease	6.55	inflammation of the _____ joint that results in frequent, painful dislocations	☐
82. tendonitis	6.56	inflammation of a(n) _____	☐
83. tenodynia	6.15	_____ in a tendon	☐
84. tenomyoplasty	6.85	a surgical procedure involving the repair of both muscle and _____	☐
85. tenorrhaphy	6.86	a surgery that _____ a tear in a tendon	☐
86. tenosynovitis	6.57	form of tendonitis that also involves inflammation of the _____ membrane	☐
87. tenotomy	6.87	a procedure in which one or more _____ are made into a tendon	☐
88. vertebroplasty	6.88	a surgical procedure that repairs damaged or diseased _____	☐

Multimedia Preview ▶▶▶▶▶

Additional interactive resources and activities for this chapter can be found on the Companion Website. For videos, audio glossary, and review, access the accompanying DVD-ROM in this book.

DVD-ROM Highlights

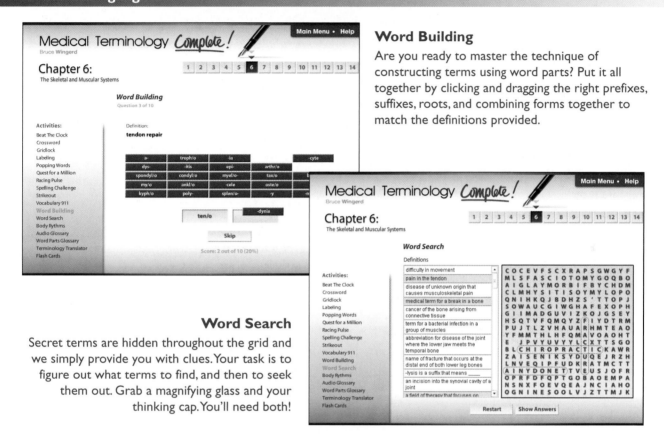

Word Building

Are you ready to master the technique of constructing terms using word parts? Put it all together by clicking and dragging the right prefixes, suffixes, roots, and combining forms together to match the definitions provided.

Word Search

Secret terms are hidden throughout the grid and we simply provide you with clues. Your task is to figure out what terms to find, and then to seek them out. Grab a magnifying glass and your thinking cap. You'll need both!

Website Highlights—www.prenhall.com/wingerd

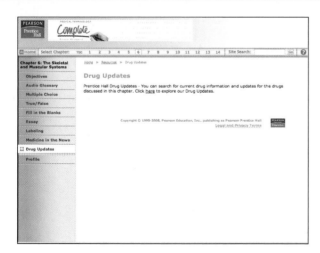

Drug Updates

Click here to take advantage of the free-access online study guide that accompanies your textbook. You'll find a feature that allows you to search for current information on the drugs discussed in this chatper. By clicking on this URL you'll also access links to download mp3 audio reviews, current news articles, and an audio glossary.

Blood and the Lymphatic System ▶▶▶▶▶

Learning Objectives

After completing this chapter, you will be able to:

- Define and spell the word parts used to create terms for the blood and the lymphatic system.

- Break down and define common medical terms used for symptoms, diseases, disorders, procedures, and treatments associated with the blood and the lymphatic system.

- Build medical terms from the word parts associated with the blood and the lymphatic system.

- Pronounce and spell common medical terms associated with the blood and the lymphatic system.

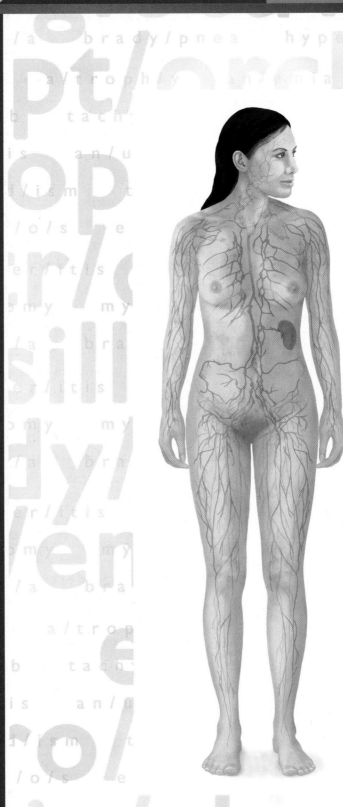

Anatomy and Physiology Terms ▶▶▶▶▶

The following table provides the combining forms that specifically apply to the anatomy and physiology of the blood and the lymphatic system. Note that the combining forms are colored red to help you identify them when you see them later in the chapter.

Combining Form	Definition	Combining Form	Definition
aden/o	gland	lymph/o	clear water or fluid
bacteri/o	bacteria	path/o	disease
blast/o	germ or bud, developing cell	splen/o	spleen
erythr/o	red	thromb/o	clot
hem/o, hemat/o	blood	thym/o	wartlike, thymus gland
immun/o	exempt or immunity	tox/o	poison
leuk/o	white		

blood

7.1 Although the blood is a tissue that is part of the cardiovascular system, the blood is also closely associated with another system, the lymphatic system. Therefore, the blood and lymphatic system are combined in this chapter. In the human body, blood is normally found only within the heart and blood vessels of the cardiovascular system. As _____ courses through these organs, it performs its primary function of transport. Its components include red blood cells, white blood cells, platelets, and plasma. Another type of body fluid, known as lymph, also transports substances throughout the body, but this fluid is found only within lymphatic vessels. Lymphatic vessels and lymph are important parts of the lymphatic system, along with the lymph nodes, spleen, and thymus gland. Lymph carries the components of immunity, such as white blood cells and the products they use to fight infection. Amazingly, blood and lymph are intertwined because lymph is formed from blood during capillary exchange and rejoins the bloodstream later. And, because both blood and lymph carry white blood cells, both fluids are involved in the fight against infection.

FUNCTION ▶▶▶▶

transport

7.2 The primary function of blood is the _____ of substances throughout the body. Vital substances carried by the blood include oxygen, carbon dioxide, hormones, enzymes, nutrients, and waste materials. The blood also protects against infectious disease and helps regulate body temperature. The primary function of the lymphatic system is protection from infectious disease. It also recycles fluids from the extracellular environment to the bloodstream.

7.3 Use the anatomy terms that appear in the left column to fill in the corresponding blanks in Figures 7.1■ and 7.2■.

1.   **neutrophil**
2.   **platelets**
3.   **red blood cells**

Figure 7.1 ■
A blood smear. The smear reveals representative cells from each formed element group: red blood cells, platelets, and two white blood cells (shown is a lymphocyte and a neutrophil).

4.   **lymphatic vessel**
5.   **thymus gland**
6.   **spleen**
7.   **lymph node**

Figure 7.2 ■
The lymphatic system. Lymphatic vessels, major lymph nodes, and lymphatic organs. The direction of lymph flow is toward the heart.

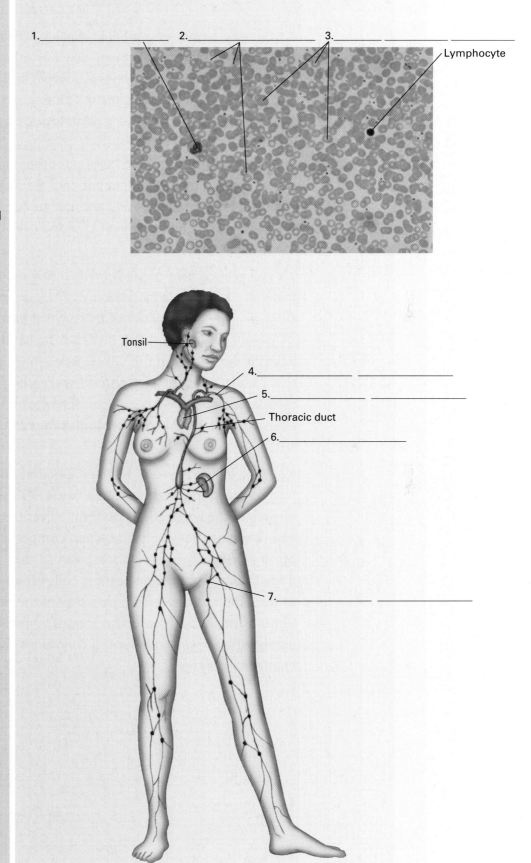

1._____ 2._____ 3._____ _____ _____

Lymphocyte

Tonsil

4._____ _____

5._____ _____

Thoracic duct

6._____

7._____ _____

Medical Terms of the Blood and the Lymphatic System ▶▶▶▶

transport

7.4 Because blood is a vital fluid, making sure it is healthy is an important part of healthcare management. Like any other tissue, blood can become diseased from any one of several sources, including inherited abnormalities, infection, or tumor development. The loss of blood itself can become a life-threatening situation if intervention is not provided in time, due to its important function as a _____ medium for gases, enzymes, nutrients, hormones, blood cells, and other substances. Fortunately, blood serves as an important diagnostic tool. Because blood can be conveniently removed from a blood vessel and analyzed, it is an important avenue for testing body chemistry as well as blood cells during a diagnostic evaluation.

hemat/o/logy

7.5 The general field of medicine focusing on blood-related disease is known as **hematology** (HEE mah TALL oh jee). You should recognize this term as being constructed of three word parts and shown as _____/____/_____. It includes the combining form *hemat/o*, which is derived from the Greek word for blood, *haima*, and the suffix *-logy* that means "study of." A physician specializing in the treatment of disease associated with blood is called a **hematologist** (HEE mah TALL oh jist), or alternatively a **hematopathologist** (hee MAH toh path ALL oh jist).

infection

7.6 The lymphatic system has dual functions: the filtering and recycling of fluid to the bloodstream and the battle against _____. A disease of the lymphatic system can affect either function, or perhaps both. Also, because the lymphatic system components are distributed throughout the body, a lymphatic disease can spread quickly to distant areas of the body. In fact, metastasizing cancer cells often use the low-pressure current of the lymph to travel from one area of the body to another. In addition to tumors, lymphatic disease also includes infections that may overwhelm the immune response and inherited conditions that result in deficiencies in immune protection.

immun/o/logy	**7.7** Our understanding of infectious disease has grown rapidly during the past 50 years, due mainly to new information coming from research labs. The field of medicine that treats this form of disease is generally called **immunology** (IM yoo NALL oh jee) or, at some hospitals, **infectious disease**. The term *immunology* refers to the body's ability to defend against infection and includes a variety of mechanisms. This is a constructed term, written as _____/____/_____, where *immun/o* is a combining form derived from the Latin word *immunis*, which means "exempt or immunity," and *-logy* is the often-used suffix that means "study of." Its subdisciplines include **virology** (vih RALL oh jee) (study of viruses), **bacteriology** (bak TEER ee ALL oh jee) (study of bacteria), and **toxicology** (TAHK sih KALL oh jee) (study of toxins).
bacteria	**7.8** The most important discovery in the field of immunology, and perhaps in any medical field, was made when Sir Alexander Fleming first reported the effects of the *Penicillium* mold on bacterial cultures. Fleming's work led to the discovery that bacterial infections could be treated with substances produced by some of their natural enemies, certain fungi. When this was understood, and **antibiotics** (AN tye bye OT tiks) became available to patients suffering from bacterial infections of many types, millions of lives were saved. Although some _____ have been able to develop resistance to antibiotics, antibiotic therapy remains our most effective weapon against bacterial infections.
lymphatic lim FAT ik	**7.9** In the following sections, we will review the prefixes, combining forms, and suffixes that combine to build the medical terms of the blood and the _____ system. Complete the frames and review exercises that follow. You are on your way to mastery of the medical terms related to the blood and the lymphatic system!

Signs and Symptoms of the Blood and the Lymphatic System

Following are the word parts that specifically apply to the signs and symptoms of the blood and the lymphatic system that are covered in the following section. Note that the word parts are color-coded to help you identify them: prefixes are blue, combining forms are red, and suffixes are purple.

Prefix	Definition
an-	without or absence of
iso-	equal
macro-	large
poly-	many

Combining Form	Definition
bacteri/o	bacteria
cyt/o	cell
erythr/o	red
hem/o	blood
leuk/o	white
poikil/o	irregular
splen/o	spleen
thromb/o	clot
tox/o	poison

Suffix	Definition
-emia	condition of blood
-ia	condition of
-lysis	loosen or dissolve
-megaly	abnormally large
-osis	condition of
-penia	abnormal reduction in number or deficiency
-rrhage	profuse bleeding, hemorrhage

KEY TERMS A-Z

anisocytosis
an EYE soh sigh TOH siss

7.10 The presence of red blood cells of unequal size in a sample of blood is an abnormal finding. It is a sign of a disease known as **anisocytosis**. The constructed form of this term is an/iso/cyt/osis, in which an- is a prefix that means "without or absence of," iso- is a prefix that means "equal," cyt/o is the combining form for "cell," and -osis means "condition of." Thus, _____ literally means "condition of without equal cells."

bacteremia
bak ter EE mee ah

7.11 The presence of bacteria in a sample of blood is a sign of an infection and is called **bacteremia**. The constructed form of this term reveals two word parts, bacter/emia. Because the suffix -emia means "condition of blood," _____ literally means "condition of bacteria in the blood."

erythropenia
ee RITH roh PEE nee ah

erythr/o/cyt/o/penia

7.12 The suffix -penia means "abnormal reduction in number." It is used in the term _____ to describe an abnormally reduced number of red blood cells in a sample of blood. This constructed term is written erythr/o/penia. It is also called **erythrocytopenia**, which is also a constructed term and is written _____/__/_____/__/_____.

hemolysis
hee MALL ih siss

7.13 The rupture of red blood cells may occur if a blood transfusion is not compatible with the recipient's blood. The rupture of the red blood cell membrane is called **hemolysis**. The constructed form of _____ is written hem/o/lysis, which literally means "dissolve blood."

hemorrhage HEM eh rihj	**7.14** The abnormal loss of blood from the circulation is a sign of trauma or illness. It is called _____, which is a constructed term written hem/o/rrhage.
leukopenia loo koh PEE nee ah leuk/o/cyt/o/penia	**7.15** An abnormally reduced number of white blood cells in a sample of blood is a sign of disease called _____. The constructed form of this term is leuk/o/penia. It is also called **leukocytopenia** (LOO koh SIGH toh PEE nee ah), which is also a constructed term and is written _____/__/_____/__/_____.
macrocytosis MAK roh sigh TOH siss	**7.16** The presence of abnormally large red blood cells in a sample of blood is a sign of disease and is called **macrocytosis**. The constructed form of _____ is written macro/cyt/osis, which literally means "condition of large cell."
poikilocytosis POY kih loh sigh TOH siss	**7.17** The combining form _poikil/o_ means "irregular." The presence of tear-shaped red blood cells in a sample of blood is called _____. The constructed form of this term is poikil/o/cyt/osis, which literally means "condition of irregular cell."
polycythemia pall ee sigh THEE mee ah	**7.18** The prefix _poly-_ means "many." When combined with the word root that means "cell" (_cyt_) and the suffix that means "condition of blood" (_-emia_), the term _____ is formed. This constructed term is written poly/cyt/hem/ia. Polycythemia, which is an abnormal increase in the number of red blood cells in the blood, may also be called **erythrocytosis** (eh RITH roh sigh TOH siss). This is also a constructed term, written erythr/o/cyt/osis, that literally means "condition of red cell."
splenomegaly splee noh MEG ah lee	**7.19** The suffix _-megaly_ means "abnormally large." Abnormal enlargement of the spleen is a symptom of injury or infection and is called _____. The constructed form is written splen/o/megaly, which literally means "abnormally large spleen."

thrombopenia

throm boh PEE nee ah

thromb/o/cyt/o/penia

7.20 An abnormally reduced number of platelets in a sample of blood is a symptom of disease called **thrombopenia.** The constructed form of _____ is thromb/o/penia. It is also called **thrombocytopenia** (THROM boh SIGH toh PEE nee ah), which is also a constructed term and is written _____/__/_____/__/_____.

toxemia

tahk SEE mee ah

7.21 The presence of toxins in the bloodstream is a symptom known as _____. The constructed form is tox/emia, which literally means "condition of blood poison."

PRACTICE: Signs and Symptoms of the Blood and the Lymphatic System

The Right Match

Match the term on the left with the correct definition on the right.

_____ 1. anisocytosis	a.	presence of bacteria in the blood
_____ 2. bacteremia	b.	abnormally reduced number of red blood cells
_____ 3. splenomegaly	c.	abnormally large red blood cells
_____ 4. toxemia	d.	presence of red blood cells of unequal size
_____ 5. erythropenia	e.	abnormal increase in number of red blood cells
_____ 6. macrocytosis	f.	irregularly shaped red blood cells
_____ 7. poikilocytosis	g.	presence of toxins in the bloodstream
_____ 8. polycythemia	h.	abnormal loss of blood from the circulation
_____ 9. hemorrhage	i.	abnormal enlargement of the spleen

Break the Chain

Analyze these medical terms:

    a) Separate each term into its word parts; each word part is labeled for you (**p** = prefix, **r** = root, **cf** = combining form, and **s** = suffix).

    b) For the Bonus Question, write the requested definition in the blank that follows.

The first set has been completed as an example.

1. a) polycythemia

         poly / cyt / hem / ia
           p   r   r   s

    b) *Bonus Question:* What is the definition of the suffix? _condition of_

2. a) thrombopenia

         _____ / _ / ____
             cf   s

    b) *Bonus Question:* What is the definition of the combining form? _____

3. a) leukopenia

         ____ / _ / _____
           cf   s

    b) *Bonus Question:* What is the definition of the suffix? _____

4. a) hemolysis

         _____ / _ / _____
           cf   s

    b) *Bonus Question:* What is the definition of the suffix? _____

5. a) leukocytopenia

         _____ / _ / _____ / _ / _____
           cf   cf   s

    b) *Bonus Question:* What is the definition of the first combining form? _____

Diseases and Disorders of the Blood and the Lymphatic System

Following are the word parts that specifically apply to the diseases and disorders of the blood and the lymphatic system that are covered in the following section. Note that the word parts are color-coded to help you identify them: prefixes are blue, combining forms are red, and suffixes are purple.

Prefix	Definition
ana-	up or toward
an-	without or absence of
mono-	one

Combining Form	Definition
aden/o	gland
aut/o	self
fung/o	fungus
globin/o	protein
hem/o, hemat/o	blood
hydr/o	water
iatr/o	physician
idi/o	individual
immun/o	exempt or immunity
leuk/o	white
lymph/o	clear water or fluid
necr/o	death
nosocom/o	hospital
nucle/o	kernel or nucleus
path/o	disease
sept/o	putrefying; wall or partition
staphylococc/o	Staphylococcus
streptococc/o	Streptococcus
thym/o	wartlike, thymus gland

Suffix	Definition
-emia	condition of blood
-genic	pertaining to producing
-ial	pertaining to
-ic	pertaining to
-ism	pertaining to
-itis	inflammation
-oma	tumor
-osis	condition
-pathy	disease
-philia	loving or affinity for
-phobia	fear
-rrhagic	pertaining to profuse bleeding

AIDS

7.22 The acronym for **acquired immunodeficiency syndrome** is _____. This devastating disease is caused by the human immunodeficiency virus (**HIV**), which disables the immune response by destroying important white blood cells known as helper T cells. The loss of immune function allows opportunistic diseases to proliferate, such as pneumonia caused by *Pneumocystis carinii*, dementia, Kaposi's sarcoma, and many others, which eventually cause death.

allergy
AL er jee

7.23 An **allergy** is the body's immune response to allergens, which are foreign substances that produce a reaction including immediate inflammation. An _____ may strike in different forms, the most common of which are **allergic rhinitis** (hay fever), which affects the mucous membranes of the nasal cavity and throat, and **allergic dermatitis**, which affects the skin where it has been in physical contact with the allergen (Figure 7.3■).

Figure 7.3 ■
Results from an allergy skin test. The patient's arm shows a reaction against the injected allergen, which has caused inflammation (swelling, redness, heat, and pain).
Source: SIU/Photo Researchers, Inc.

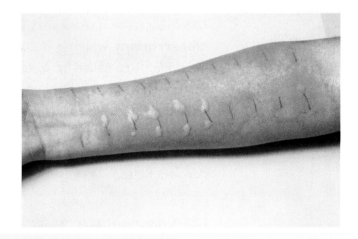

anaphylaxis
AN ah fih LAK siss

7.24 An immediate reaction to a foreign substance that includes rapid inflammation, vasodilation, bronchospasms, and spasms of the GI tract is called **anaphylaxis**. In severe cases it can become life threatening if medical intervention is not available. This term is constructed from the prefix *ana-* that means "up, toward" and the noun *phylaxis* that means "protection." Thus, the constructed form of _____ is written ana/phylaxis.

anemia
ah NEE mee ah

7.25 The prefix *an-* means "without," and the suffix *-emia* means "condition of blood." Combining these two word parts forms the term **anemia**, which literally means "without blood." The constructed form of this term is written an/emia. _____ is the reduced ability of red blood cells to deliver oxygen to tissues. It may be the result of a reduced number of normal circulating red blood cells or a reduction in the amount of the oxygen-binding protein in red blood cells called hemoglobin. Some common forms of anemia include **aplastic anemia**, in which the red bone marrow fails to produce sufficient numbers of normal blood cells; **iron deficiency anemia**, caused by a lack of available iron, resulting in the body's inability to make adequate amounts of hemoglobin; **sickle cell anemia**, in which the hemoglobin is defective within cells, resulting in misshaped red blood cells that cause obstructions in blood vessels; and **pernicious** (per NISH us) **anemia**, caused by an inadequate supply of folic acid usually obtained from a healthy diet.

anthrax
AN thraks

7.26 A bacterial disease that has been threatened to be used in **bioterrorism**, which is the application of disease-causing microorganisms (pathogens) to cause harm to a population, is **anthrax**. The spores of the bacteria can survive within a powder that can be distributed through the air, making it very dangerous. If inhaled, _____ can become fatal. The term is derived from the Greek word *anthrakos*, which means "coal," referring to the blackening effect the infection has on the skin and lungs.

autoimmune disease
au toe im YOON * dis EEZ

7.27 A disease that is caused by a person's own immune response attacking otherwise healthy tissues is called **autoimmune disease**. The term *autoimmune* is a constructed term, written aut/o/immune, and literally means "self-exempt" or "self-immunity." Examples of _____ _____ include rheumatoid arthritis, systemic lupus erythematosus, and multiple sclerosis. The triggering mechanism that results in autoimmune disease is not yet known.

botulism
BAHT yoo lizm

7.28 One lethal form of food-borne illness is called **botulism**. It is caused by the ingestion of food contaminated with the neurotoxin produced by the bacterium *Clostridium botulinum*. _____ usually occurs when canned food is not prepared properly and is often fatal due to the extreme toxic nature of the botulism neurotoxin.

communicable disease
co MYOON ik ah bul * dis EEZ

7.29 A disease that is capable of transmission from one person to another is called a _____ _____. Also known as a **contagious disease**, it may be transmitted by direct contact with an infected person, indirectly by way of contact with infected body fluids or other materials, or by way of vectors, usually insects such as mosquitoes, ticks, and fleas.

diphtheria
diff THEER ee ah

7.30 **Diphtheria** is an infectious disease resulting in acute inflammation of the mucous membranes, primarily in the mouth and throat. Derived from the Greek word for "leather," _____ is characterized by the formation of an obstructive, leatherlike membrane in the throat. It is illustrated in Figure 7.4■.

Figure 7.4 ■

Diphtheria. The bacteria that cause this disease, called *Corynebacterium diphtheriae*, proliferate in the mucous membranes of the throat to establish a leathery, white covering.

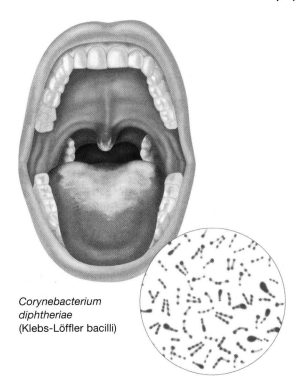

Corynebacterium diphtheriae (Klebs-Löffler bacilli)

DID YOU KNOW ?

Diphtheria

Before the availability of antibiotics, diphtheria was a life-threatening scourge among children, killing thousands each year within the United States. It is caused by the toxins produced by the bacterium *Corynebacterium diphtheriae,* which produces inflammation of the throat and the formation of a thick secretion. Because the infected throat becomes covered with a leathery membrane, it was named after the Greek word for leather, *diphthera.*

dyscrasia
diss KRAY zee ah

7.31 Derived from the Greek word *dyskrasia* that means "difficult temperament," the clinical term _____ is any abnormal condition of the blood. Apparently, the ones who named this condition observed a correlation between a difficult temperament and blood disease.

edema
eh DEE mah

7.32 The leakage of fluid from the bloodstream into the interstitial space between body cells causes swelling and is one aspect of inflammation. The swelling is called _____. The term is derived from the Greek word, *oidema,* which means "swelling."

fungemia
fun JEE mee ah

7.33 The combining form for fungus is *fung/o*, and the suffix *-emia* means "condition of blood." Putting these word parts together forms the term **fungemia**, which is a fungal infection that spreads throughout the body by way of the bloodstream. As a constructed term, _____ is written fung/emia and literally means "condition of blood fungus." Another common term for this infection is **fungal septicemia**.

gas gangrene
gas * GANG green

7.34 Infection of a wound may be caused by various anaerobic bacteria, which cause additional damage to local tissues when blood flow is reduced due to some reason, including frostbite or diabetes. The condition is called **gas gangrene**, which can become life threatening if it is allowed to spread. If antibiotics fail to control the _____ _____ infection, amputation may become a lifesaving option. The term *gangrene* is derived from the Greek word *gangraina*, which means "eating sore." The term *gas* is included in the term because of the fermentation gas that is a diagnostic of the disease.

hematoma
HEE mah TOH mah

7.35 When the word root for blood, *hemat/o*, is combined with the suffix that means "tumor" (*-oma*), the term _____ is formed. It is a mass of blood outside blood vessels and confined within an organ or space within the body, usually in a clotted form. It is commonly known as a bruise or a contusion. A hematoma is usually the result of injury or disease. The constructed form of this term is written hemat/oma.

hemoglobinopathy
HEE moh gloh bin AH path ee

7.36 A general term for a disease that affects hemoglobin within red blood cells is **hemoglobinopathy**. This constructed term contains five word parts, as shown when it is written as hem/o/globin/o/pathy. It literally means "disease of blood protein." Because sickle cell anemia is a disease affecting hemoglobin (Frame 7.25), it is a form of _____.

hemophilia
HEE moh FILL ee ah

7.37 An inherited bleeding disorder that results from defective or missing blood-clotting proteins that are necessary components in the coagulation process is known as **hemophilia**. Because the clotting proteins normally stop the loss of blood after minor injuries, a patient suffering from _____ experiences an abnormal loss of blood. The term is a constructed term, written hem/o/philia, which literally means "love for blood."

hemorrhagic fever
HEM or AJ ik

7.38 An infectious disease that causes internal bleeding, or internal hemor-rhage (Frame 7.14), and high fevers is generally known as _____ _____. The disease is often caused by viruses, such as Ebola, and exhibits a high rate of mortality.

Hodgkin's disease

7.39 In 1832, the British physician Thomas Hodgkin first described a malig-nant form of cancer of lymphatic tissue that is characterized by the pro-gressive enlargement of lymph nodes, fatigue, and deficiency of the immune response. Known as _____ _____ or **Hodgkin's lymphoma**, about 1,300 Americans die of the disease each year, usually from opportunistic infections. It is less common than **non-Hodgkin's lymphoma**, which had almost 55,000 new cases in 2004 compared to the 8,000 new cases of Hodgkin's disease.

iatrogenic disease
EYE a troh JEN ik * dis EEZ

7.40 A condition that is caused by a medical treatment is called an **iatrogenic disease**. This constructed term combines the combining form for physican, *iatr/o*, with the suffix that means "pertaining to producing," *-genic*. The resulting constructed form of _____ _____ is written iatr/o/genic.

idiopathic disease
id ee oh PATH ik * dis EEZ

7.41 A disease that develops without a known or apparent cause is called an _____ _____. The constructed form of this term is idi/o/path/ic, which literally means "pertaining to individual disease."

immunodeficiency
IM yoo noh dee FISH ehn see

7.42 A condition resulting from a defective immune response is called an **immunodeficiency**. It occurs when there are insufficient numbers of functional white blood cells, especially lymphocytes, available to defend the body from sources of infection. This constructed term is written immun/o/deficiency. A closely related term is **immunocompromised**, which is used to describe a patient suffering from an _____.

immunosuppression
IM yoo noh suh PREH shun

7.43 A reduction of an immune response may be caused by disease or by the use of chemical, pharmacological, or immunologic agents. The suppressed status of the immune response that results is called _____. The constructed form of this term is immun/o/suppression.

incompatibility
IN com PAT ih BILL ih tee

7.44 The combination of two blood types that result in the destruction of red blood cells is called _____. It may occur during a blood transfusion causing severe consequences, including the possibility of death if the donor blood antibodies attack the recipient's red blood cells.

infection
in FEK shun

7.45 A multiplication of disease-causing microorganisms, or pathogens, in the body is called an **infection**. The term is derived from the Latin word *infectus*, which means "to color, stain, or dye," referring to the discoloration of skin during an infection. A disease caused by _____ is called an **infectious disease**. The reaction of the body against an infection is illustrated in Figure 7.5■.

Figure 7.5 ■
Reaction against infection. Pathogens invade the body, in this example, by a pierce through the skin. The result of invasion is the proliferation of pathogens within body tissues, or infection. The body responds to the infection by mounting an attack that begins with inflammation, which promotes the movement of phagocytes to the site of the infection. Phagocytes localize the pathogens and destroy them by phagocytosis. Pus is released, which is composed of dead bacteria and phagocytes.

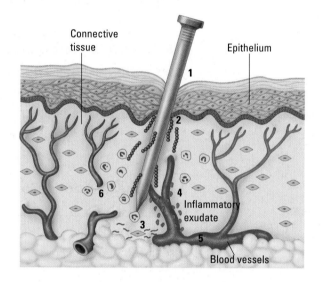

1. Dirty nail punctures skin.
2. Bacteria enter and multiply.
3. Injured cells release histamine.
4. Blood vessels dilate and become permeable, releasing inflammatory exudate.
5. Blood flow to the damaged site increases.
6. Neutrophils (polymorphs) move toward bacteria (chemotaxis) and destroy them (phagocytosis).

inflammation

in flah MAY shun

7.46 The physiological process that serves as the body's initial response to injury and many forms of illness involves the swelling of body tissue. Known as **inflammation**, the swelling results from the movement of plasma from capillaries into the extracellular space to produce **edema** (Frame 7.32), or fluid accumulation in tissue (Figure 7.6■). The common symptoms of _____ include swelling, redness, heat, and pain. The term _inflammation_ is derived from the Latin word _inflammatio_, which means "to ignite" or "to set ablaze."

Figure 7.6 ■
Inflammation. Inflammation is characterized by the presence of swelling, redness, heat, and pain. Swelling is caused by the accumulation of fluid in tissue spaces and is also known as edema. In this photograph, the patient exhibits severe edema of the leg.
Source: MSNB/Custom Medical Stock Photo, Inc.

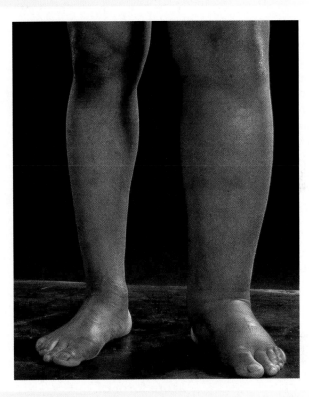

influenza

in floo EHN zah

7.47 A viral disease characterized by fever and an acute inflammation of respiratory mucous membranes is called **influenza**. Commonly called "the flu," _____ is highly contagious, and the virus is capable of mutating to escape detection by white blood cells.

leukemia
loo KEE mee ah

7.48 A form of cancer that literally means "condition of white blood cells" is _____. Leukemia originates from cells within the blood-forming tissue of the red marrow. The constructed form of the term is written leuk/emia. The primary tumor of leukemia spreads throughout the red marrow, transforming the blood-forming tissue into a dysfunctional mass that produces abnormal white blood cells (Figure 7.7■). As a result, common symptoms of leukemia include immunodeficiency and the development of opportunistic infections.

Figure 7.7 ■
Leukemia. A blood smear from a patient suffering from leukemia demonstrates the abundance of enlarged, nonfunctional leukocytes that serve as a diagnostic characteristic of this disease.
Source: Spike Walker/Getty Images, Inc.—Stone Allstock

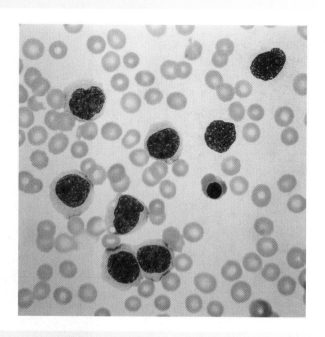

lymphadenitis
limm fad eh NYE tiss

7.49 Inflammation of the lymph nodes is a condition called **lymphadenitis**. The constructed form of this term is lymph/aden/itis. The acute form of _____ is common during infections. The chronic form indicates a more serious disorder may be the cause, such as lymphoma (Frame 7.50).

lymphoma
limm FOH mah

7.50 A malignant tumor originating in lymphatic tissue is called _____. The constructed form uses the suffix -oma, which means "tumor," and is written lymph/oma.

malaria
mah LAIR ee ah

7.51 A disease caused by a parasitic protozoan that infects red blood cells and the liver during different parts of its life cycle is called **malaria**. The vector, or carrier, of the protozoan is the *Anopheles* mosquito, and the symptoms of malaria include periodic flares of high fever. The term _____ literally means "bad air," referring to the swampy marshlands where the mosquitoes proliferate to cause higher incidences of the disease.

DID YOU KNOW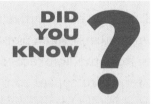

Malaria

The term *malaria* is derived from combining the Italian word for bad, *mal*, with that of air, *aria*. It was first used during the Middle Ages, when malaria was believed to have been caused by breathing bad air near swamplands. We now know that this dreaded disease is caused by the bite of an *Anopheles* mosquito carrying the protozoan known as *Plasmodium*. Approximately 200,000 people die of this disease each year, mainly in tropical regions where the mosquitoes flourish.

mononucleosis
MAHN oh nook lee OH siss

7.52 A viral disease characterized by enlarged lymph nodes and spleen, atypical lymphocytes, throat pain, pharyngitis, fever, and fatigue is called **mononucleosis**. Also called **infectious mononucleosis**, it is caused by the Epstein-Barr virus and is a communicable disease (Figure 7.8■). The term _____ is a constructed term made up of the prefix *mono-*, meaning "one," the word root *nucle*, meaning "kernel or nucleus," and the very common suffix *-osis*, meaning "condition of." It is written as mono/nucle/osis.

Figure 7.8 ■
Mononucleosis. Infectious mononucleosis is caused by the Epstein-Barr virus and produces the symptoms of swollen palatine tonsils (pharyngitis), swollen cervical lymph nodes (lymphadenopathy), high fever, and a blood sample that reveals atypical lymphocytes.

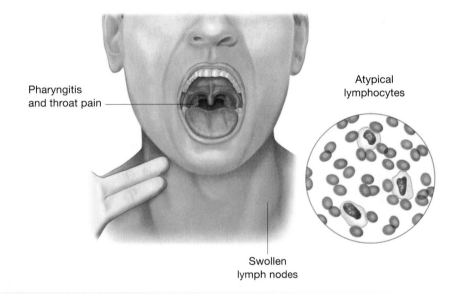

Pharyngitis and throat pain

Atypical lymphocytes

Swollen lymph nodes

necrosis
neh KROH siss

7.53 The death of one or more cells or a portion of a tissue or organ is called **necrosis**. The term _____ is derived from the Greek word *nekrosis*, which means "death." A cell or cells, tissue, or organ that is dead is often called **necrotic**.

nosocomial infection
noh soh KOH mee al * in FEK shun

7.54 An infectious disease that is contracted during a hospital stay is called a **nosocomial infection**. The term *nosocomial* is derived from the Greek word *nosokomeion*, which means "hospital." The most common cause of _____ _____ in recent years has been a lack of hand washing, made worse by the development of antibiotic-resistant strains of *Staphylococcus* (Frame 7.59).

plague
playg

7.55 Any infectious disease that is widespread and causes extensive mortality is called a **plague**. The term is derived from the Latin word *plago*, which means "to strike or beat." The term originated from the first recorded outbreak of bubonic plague in 542 AD. Today, the term also applies to the bubonic _____, which is caused by the bacterium *Yersinia pestis* and is characterized by high fever, skin eruptions (called buboes) and discoloration, internal hemorrhage, and pneumonia.

rabies
RAY beez

7.56 A viral infection that is spread from the saliva of an infected animal, usually by way of a bite, is known as **rabies**. In Latin, *rabies* means "savage, fierce," which refers to the ferocity of infected animals. The virus acts on the central nervous system to cause paranoia and paralysis and is usually fatal. _____ has also been called **hydrophobia** (HIGH droh FOH bee ah), which literally means "fear of water" and refers to the panic of infected animals unable to drink water due to the progressive paralysis. Hydrophobia is a constructed term, written as hydr/o/phobia.

septicemia
sep tih SEE mee ah

7.57 A systemwide disease caused by the presence of bacteria and their toxins in the circulating blood is called **septicemia**. This is a constructed term written sept/ic/emia and literally means "condition of putrefying blood." The word root, *sept*, is derived from the Latin word *sepsis*, which means "putrefying." Thus, _____ may also be called by its Latin origin, **sepsis**. A person suffering from this condition is referred to as **septic.**

smallpox

7.58 A viral disease caused by the *variola* virus that was the scourge of the human population prior to its eradication in 1975 is known as **smallpox**. The term was first used around 1400 AD to distinguish the disease from syphilis, the "great pox," which at the time was characterized by the formation of large pustules on the skin that exceeded the pustules of smallpox in size and number. The eradication of _____ was the crowning achievement of the World Health Organization, which battled the disease with an aggressive vaccination (Frame 7.88) campaign for about 8 years. Although it is eradicated from the population, reserves of *variola* remain in storage for research purposes.

staphylococcemia
STAFF ih loh kok SEE mee ah

7.59 The presence of the bacterium *Staphylococcus* in the blood is a condition known as staphylococcemia. Only two word parts, the word root *staphylococc* and the suffix meaning "condition of blood," *-emia*, are used to construct _____, which is written staphylococc/emia. *Staphylococcus* is a frequent cause of infections in wounds, a complication of normal healing. An infection caused by *Staphylococcus* is commonly called a **staph infection**. It is also the most common cause of foodborne illness, skin inflammation, osteomyelitis (infection of bone), and nosocomial infections (Frame 7.54). Varieties of *Staphylococcus* that are resistant to antibiotics are one of the greatest challenges to antiseptic medical procedures.

streptococcemia
STREP toh kok SEE mee ah

7.60 The presence of the bacterium *Streptococcus* in the blood is known as **streptococcemia**. The constructed term _____ is written streptococc/emia. An infection caused by *Streptococcus* is commonly called a **strep infection**. It frequently begins in the throat as a form of pharyngitis called **strep throat** and, if not managed, may spread to the bloodstream, which distributes the infection to vital organs. The heart valves in particular are a potential target of *Streptococcus* and are subject to permanent damage if infected.

tetanus
TETT ah nuss

7.61 A disease caused by a powerful neurotoxin released by the common bacterium *Clostridium tetani* is called **tetanus**. The toxin acts on the central nervous system to cause convulsions and spastic paralysis (in which muscles are unable to relax). The term _____ is derived from the Latin word *tetanos*, which means "convulsive tension." Infection can be obtained from a puncture wound that is not properly cleaned, but is easily prevented with periodic vaccination (Frame 7.88).

thymoma
thigh MOH mah

7.62 A tumor originating in the thymus gland is called a **thymoma**. The constructed form of _____ uses the word root *thym* and the suffix *-oma* and is written thym/oma.

PRACTICE: Diseases and Disorders of the Blood and the Lymphatic System

The Right Match

Match the term on the left with the correct definition on the right.

_____ 1. sickle cell anemia

_____ 2. rabies

_____ 3. botulism

_____ 4. Hodgkin's disease

_____ 5. tetanus

_____ 6. immunodeficiency

_____ 7. fungemia

_____ 8. plague

_____ 9. diphtheria

_____ 10. malaria

a. disease caused by a neurotoxin released by _Clostridium tetani_

b. anemia resulting from defective hemoglobin within cells, resulting in misshaped red blood cells

c. viral infection that is spread from the saliva of an infected animal

d. condition resulting from a defective immune response

e. any infectious disease that is widespread and causes extensive mortality

f. fungal infection that spreads throughout the body by way of the bloodstream

g. a cancer of lymph nodes

h. caused by a neurotoxin produced by _Clostridium botulinum_

i. disease caused by a parasitic protozoan that infects red blood cells and the liver

j. infectious disease resulting in acute inflammation with formation of a leathery membrane in the throat

Linkup

Link the word parts in the list to create the terms that match the definitions. You may use word parts more than once. Remember to add in combining vowels when needed—and that some terms do not use any combining vowel. The first one is completed for you as an example.

Prefix	Combining Form	Suffix
a-	aden/o	-emia
mono-	botul/o	-genic
	globin/o	-ia
	hemat/o	-ic
	hem/o	-ism
	hydr/o	-itis
	iatr/o	-oma
	leuk/o	-osis
	lymph/o	-pathy
	nucle/o	-philia
	sept/o	-phobia
	thym/o	

Definition

1. systemwide disease caused by the presence of bacteria and their toxins in the circulating blood

2. tumor originating in the thymus gland

3. reduced ability of red blood cells to deliver oxygen to tissues

4. poisoning caused by the ingestion of food contaminated with the toxin produced by the bacterium *Clostridium botulinum*

5. blood outside the blood vessels and confined within an organ or space within the body, usually in a clotted form

6. a condition that is caused by a medical treatment

7. an inherited bleeding disorder that results from missing or deficient blood-clotting proteins

8. general term for a disease that affects hemoglobin within red blood cells

9. inflammation of the lymph nodes

10. a viral disease characterized by enlarged lymph nodes, atypical lymphocytes, throat pain, pharyngitis, fever, and fatigue

11. another term for rabies that refers to infected animals' inability to drink water due to progressive paralysis

Term

septicemia

Treatments and Procedures of the Blood and the Lymphatic System

Following are the word parts that specifically apply to the treatments and procedures of the blood and the lymphatic system that are covered in the following section. Note that the word parts are color-coded to help you identify them: prefixes are blue, combining forms are red, and suffixes are purple.

Prefix	Definition	Combining Form	Definition	Suffix	Definition
anti-	against or opposite of	aden/o	gland	-crit	to separate
pro-	before	aut/o	self	-ectomy	surgical excision or removal
		bi/o	life	-ic	pertaining to
		globin/o	protein	-logous	pertaining to study
		hem/o, hemat/o	blood	-logy	study of
		hom/o	same	-lysis	loosen or dissolve
		immun/o	exempt or immunity	-stasis	standing still
		lymph/o	clear water or fluid	-therapy	treatment
		thromb/o	clot	-tic	pertaining to
				-phylaxis	protection

antibiotic therapy

AN tih bye AHT ik * THAIR ah pee

7.63 A therapeutic treatment involving the use of a substance with known toxicity to bacteria is called **antibiotic therapy**. The constructed form of the term *antibiotic* is written anti/bio/tic, which literally means "pertaining to against life." The antibiotic may be obtained from a fungus, usually a mold, or other bacteria. _____ _____ is effective only against bacteria, many types of which are capable of developing resistance, especially when antibiotics are not administered properly.

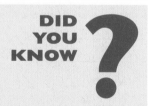
DID YOU KNOW ?

Discovery of Antibiotics

The first antibiotic was discovered in 1926 by Sir Alexander Fleming, who found that a common bread mold (a fungus) could produce toxins capable of killing bacterial colonies. The *Penicillium* mold produces an antibacterial toxin that is now known as penicillin. In time, the fungal toxins were proven to be effective against many strains of bacteria, and their use as antibiotics has been hailed as the single most important treatment against bacterial infections ever.

anticoagulant

AN tye koh AG yoo lant

7.64 A chemical agent that delays or prevents the clotting process in blood is called an **anticoagulant**. It is often administered to dissolve existing unwanted clots or to reduce the likelihood of clot formation after surgery. The constructed form of anticoagulant is written anti/coagulant. The most common _____ agent is **warfarin** (Coumadin).

7.65 A pharmacological therapy that is useful in battling a class of viruses that tend to mutate quickly, called retroviruses, is often called _____. It is used against the virus that causes AIDS (Frame 7.22), HIV. The drugs form a cocktail that includes nucleotide analog reverse transcriptase inhibitors and protease inhibitors, which block HIV replication by a variety of means.

antiretroviral therapy
AN tye REH troh VYE ral
* THAIR ah pee

7.66 The process in which pathogens are rendered less virulent, or infectious, prior to their incorporation into a vaccine preparation is called _____. The term is derived from the Latin word *attenuatus*, which means "to make thin."

attenuation
ah TEN yoo AY shun

7.67 A transfusion of blood donated by a patient for their personal use is called an **autologous transfusion**. The term includes a constructed term that is written aut/o/logous and means "pertaining to study of self." _____ _____ is a common procedure before a surgery to avoid potential incompatibility or contamination of blood. (See Figure 7.9■)

autologous transfusion
aw TALL oh guss * trans FYOO zhun

Figure 7.9 ■
Blood transfusion. A transfusion of one's own blood is called an autologous transfusion (see Frame 7.67). A transfusion of donated blood from another person is called a homologous transfusion (see Frame 7.78).
Source: Gaillard/Jerrican/Photo Researchers, Inc.

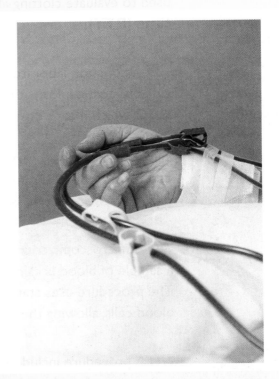

7.68 A test or series of tests on a sample of plasma to measure the levels of its composition, including glucose, albumin, triglycerides, pH, cholesterol, and electrolytes is called _____ _____.

blood chemistry

immunology IM yoo NALL oh jee	**7.80** The study concerned with immunity and allergy is called _____. The constructed form of this term is immun/o/logy.
immunotherapy IM yoo noh THAIR ah pee	**7.81** The treatment of infectious disease by the administration of pharmacological agents, such as serum, gamma globulin, treated antibodies, and suppressive drugs is called _____. This constructed term is written immun/o/therapy.
lymphadenectomy limm fad eh NEK toh mee	**7.82** The suffix -_ectomy_ means "surgical excision or removal." Placing this suffix at the end of a word root for an organ describes the procedure that surgically removes the organ. For example, the surgical removal of one or more lymph nodes is called _____. The constructed form of this term reveals three word parts, lymph/aden/ectomy.
platelet count	**7.83** A laboratory procedure that calculates the number of platelets in a known volume of blood is called a **platelet count**, or **PLT**. A reduced _____ _____ suggests a potential failure of hemostasis (Frame 7.77), since platelets play a major role in blood clot formation and coagulation.
prophylaxis proh fih LAK siss	**7.84** Any treatment that tends to prevent the onset of an infection or other type of disease is called **prophylaxis**. The constructed form of _____ is written as pro/phylaxis, which literally means "before protection."
red blood count	**7.85** A lab test included in a complete blood count that measures the number of red blood cells within a given volume of blood is called a _____ _____ _____, or **RBC**.
splenectomy splee NEK toh mee	**7.86** The surgical removal of the spleen is often necessary if it has ruptured, which may occur during a physical injury to the left side of the trunk. The procedure is called _____. The constructed form of this term is written splen/ectomy.
thrombolysis throm BALL ih siss	**7.87** A treatment that is performed to dissolve an unwanted blood clot, or **thrombus**, is called _____. The constructed form of this term is thromb/o/lysis, which literally means "dissolve clot."

vaccination
VAK sih NAY shun

7.88 The inoculation of a foreign substance that has reduced virulence, or a reduced ability to cause infection, as a means of providing a cure or prophylaxis (Frame 7.84), is called a _____.

vaccine
vak SEEN

7.89 A preparation that is used to activate an immune response to provide acquired immunity against an infectious agent is called a

_____.

DID YOU KNOW ?

Vaccines

Vaccines have been in use since the Middle Ages, when scrapings from smallpox sores were given to people as prophylaxis against this deadly disease. The use of the term *vaccine* (derived from the Latin word *vaccinus*, which means "relating to a cow") began in 1796, when Edward Jenner published his findings that scrapings of skin pustules from people infected with a similar virus that produced a different disease contracted from milking cows, known as cowpox, provided immunity against the *variola* virus that causes smallpox.

PRACTICE: Treatments and Procedures of the Blood and the Lymphatic System

The Right Match

Match the term on the left with the correct definition on the right.

_____ 1. attenuation

_____ 2. hematocrit

_____ 3. vaccine

_____ 4. immunization

_____ 5. red blood count

_____ 6. prothrombin time

_____ 7. blood chemistry

_____ 8. antiretroviral therapy

_____ 9. prophylaxis

_____ 10. antibiotic therapy

a. measures the number of red blood cells

b. procedure that establishes immunity against a particular antigen

c. process in which pathogens are rendered less virulent, or infectious, prior to their incorporation into a vaccine

d. tests on a sample of plasma to measure the levels of certain chemicals

e. a timed test for coagulation rate

f. measures the percentage of red blood cells in a volume of blood by centrifuging a sample

g. drugs used to battle retroviruses

h. a preventative treatment

i. a therapy against bacterial infections

j. a preparation used to activate an immune response

Break the Chain

Analyze these medical terms:

   a)   Separate each term into its word parts; each word part is labeled for you (**p** = prefix, **r** = root, **cf** = combining form, and **s** = suffix).

   b)   For the Bonus Question, write the requested definition in the blank that follows.

1.   a)   immunotherapy   _____/___/_____
                                        cf   s

     b)   *Bonus Question:* What is the definition of the suffix? _____

2.   a)   splenectomy   _____/_____
                                     r   s

     b)   *Bonus Question:* What is the definition of the word root? _____

3.   a)   lymphadenectomy   _____/_____/_____
                                     r   r   s

     b)   *Bonus Question:* What is the definition of the second word root? _____

4.   a)   immunology   _____/__/_____
                                        cf   s

     b)   *Bonus Question:* What is the definition of the combining form? _____

5.   a)   homologous   _____/__/_____
                                        cf   s

     b)   *Bonus Question:* What is the definition of the combining form? _____

6.   a)   hematology   _____/_/_____
                                        cf   s

     b)   *Bonus Question:* What is the definition of the suffix? _____

7.   a)   autologous   _____/__/____
                                      cf   s

     b)   *Bonus Question:* What is the definition of the combining form? _____

8.   a)   anticoagulant   _____/_____
                                        p   s

     b)   *Bonus Question:* What is the definition of the prefix? _____

9.   a)   hemostasis   _____/__/_____
                                        cf   s

     b)   *Bonus Question:* What is the definition of the suffix? _____

10. a)   thrombolysis   _____/__/_____
                                        cf   s

     b)   *Bonus Question:* What is the definition of the suffix? _____

Abbreviations of the Blood and the Lymphatic System

The abbreviations that are associated with the blood and the lymphatic system are summarized here. Study these abbreviations, and review them in the exercise that follows.

Abbreviation	Definition
AIDS	acquired immune deficiency syndrome
CBC	complete blood count
HCT, Hct	hematocrit
HGB, Hgb	hemoglobin
HIV	human immunodeficiency virus
PLT	platelet count

Abbreviation	Definition
PT	prothrombin time
PTT	partial thromboplastin time
RBC	red blood cell or red blood count
WBC	white blood cell or white blood count

PRACTICE: Abbreviations

Fill in the blanks with the abbreviation or the complete medical term.

Abbreviation

1. _____
2. CBC
3. _____
4. RBC
5. _____
6. PT
7. _____
8. WBC
9. _____
10. HIV

Medical Term

acquired immunodeficiency syndrome

_____

platelet count

_____

hemoglobin

_____

partial thromboplastin time

_____

hematocrit

_____

▶▶▶▶▶ Chapter Review

Word Building _____

Construct medical terms from the following meanings. (Some are built from word parts, some are not.) The first question has been completed as an example.

1. reduced ability of blood to deliver oxygen   an_emia_____

2. presence of red blood cells of unequal size   _____cytosis

3. any abnormal condition of the blood   dys_____

4. a serious protozoan infection of red blood cells   _____ia

5. abnormal reduction of red blood cells   erythro_____

6. inherited defect in blood coagulation   _____philia

7. cancer originating in red bone marrow   _____emia

8. abnormally large red blood cells   macro_____

9. a condition of staphylococci in the blood   staphylococc_____

10. disease caused by immune reaction against own tissues   _____ disease

11. abnormal increase in number of red blood cells   _____emia

12. red blood cells that are tear-shaped   _____cytosis

13. presence of bacteria and toxins in the blood   septic _____

14. a drug that reduces blood clotting   anti_____

15. transfusion of blood donated by another person   _____logous transfusion

16. measures percentage of red blood cells in a sample   hemato_____

17. stoppage of bleeding   _____stasis

18. calculation of the number of platelets in blood   _____ count

19. cancer of lymphatic tissue   _____ disease

20. inflammation of the lymph nodes   _____itis

21. bacterial disease that causes a membrane in the throat to form   _____ia

▶▶▶▶▶ Clinical Application Exercises

Medical Report

Read the following medical report, then answer the questions that follow.

University Hospital

5500 University Avenue   Phone: (211) 594-4000
Metropolis, TX   Fax: (211) 594-4001

Medical Consultation: Hematology

Date: 10/02/2007

Patient: Millie Nyugen

Patient Complaint: Persistent mild fever with general body aches; tenderness of the
armpit and groin regions to pressure that was first noticed more than one month previous.

History: 55-year-old female of Asian-American descent with no prior hospitalization or
serious complaints.

Family History: Father deceased at 62 years with primary hepatic cancer. Mother, 77
years, with complete hysterectomy following diagnosis of stage 1 cervical cancer; no reported
conditions otherwise.

Allergies: Dietary restrictions to sesame seeds and milk products.

Evidences: Upon physical examination, lymphadenitis noted in axillary and inguinal nodes;
mild fever of 99.8°C. Differential count: neutrophils, monocytes, lymphocytes elevated 25%.

Blood chemistry: positive for *Staphylococcus*.

Diagnosis: staphylococcemia

Treatment: Antibiotic treatment with streptomycin with follow-up in 6 days. If no recovery
is evident, administer antibiotic cocktail to target strep-resistant strain of *S. aureus*.

Sylvia S. Hernandez, M.D.

---

1. What complaints support the diagnosis?_____

   _____

2. Why do you think antibiotics might fail as a treatment?_____

   _____

3. Does the familial history provide any clues into the cause of the illness?

   _____

Key Term	Frame	Definition	Know It?
21. differential count	7.73	the number of each type of _____ blood cell	☐
22. diphtheria	7.30	infectious disease resulting in acute inflammation with formation of a leathery membrane in the _____	☐
23. dyscrasia	7.31	any _____ condition of the blood	☐
24. edema	7.32	swelling due to leakage of _____ from the bloodstream into the interstitial space between body cells	☐
25. erythropenia	7.12	abnormally _____ number of red blood cells	☐
26. fungemia	7.33	_____ infection that spreads throughout the body by way of the bloodstream	☐
27. gas gangrene	7.34	bacteria from a wound that enters the _____	☐
28. hematocrit	7.74	determination of _____ blood cells from centrifugation	☐
29. hematology	7.75	field that focuses on _____-related disease	☐
30. hematoma	7.35	_____ outside the vessels and confined within an organ or space within the body	☐
31. hemoglobin	7.76	procedure included in a complete blood count that measures the level of _____ in red blood cells	☐
32. hemoglobinopathy	7.36	disease that affects _____ within red blood cells	☐
33. hemolysis	7.13	_____ of the red blood cell membrane	☐
34. hemophilia	7.37	an inherited _____ disorder	☐
35. hemorrhage	7.14	abnormal loss of _____ from the circulation	☐
36. hemorrhagic fever	7.38	an infectious disease that causes internal _____	☐
37. hemostasis	7.77	the _____ of bleeding	☐
38. Hodgkin's disease	7.39	cancer of the _____ nodes	☐
39. homologous transfusion	7.78	transfusion of blood that is voluntarily _____ by another person	☐
40. iatrogenic disease	7.40	an unfavorable response to _____ treatment	☐
41. idiopathic disease	7.41	disease that develops without a known or apparent _____	☐
42. immunization	7.79	establishes _____ against a particular antigen	☐
43. immunodeficiency	7.42	condition resulting from a defective _____ response	☐
44. immunology	7.80	the _____ of immunity and allergy	☐
45. immunosuppression	7.43	a(n) _____ of the immune response	☐
46. immunotherapy	7.81	treatment of _____ disease by the administration of pharmacological agents	☐
47. incompatibility	7.44	the _____ of red blood cells that results from the combination of two blood types	☐
48. infection	7.45	a multiplication of _____-causing microorganisms	☐
49. inflammation	7.46	the _____ of body tissue	☐
50. influenza	7.47	viral disease characterized by fever and an acute inflammation of _____ mucous membranes	☐
51. leukemia	7.48	form of _____ that originates from cells within the blood-forming tissue of the red marrow	☐

Key Term	Frame	Definition	Know It?
52. leukopenia	7.15	abnormally reduced number of _____ blood cells	☐
53. lymphadenectomy	7.82	the _____ removal of one or more lymph nodes	☐
54. lymphadenitis	7.49	inflammation of the _____ nodes	☐
55. lymphoma	7.50	a malignant _____ that originates in lymphatic tissue	☐
56. macrocytosis	7.16	abnormally _____ red blood cells	☐
57. malaria	7.51	disease caused by a parasitic protozoan that infects red blood cells and the _____	☐
58. mononucleosis	7.52	viral disease characterized by _____ lymph nodes, atypical lymphocytes, throat pain, pharyngitis, fever, and fatigue	☐
59. necrosis	7.53	the _____ of one or more cells or a portion of a tissue or organ	☐
60. nosocomial infection	7.54	an infectious disease contracted during a(n) _____ stay	☐
61. plague	7.55	any _____ disease that is widespread and causes extensive mortality	☐
62. platelet count	7.83	laboratory procedure that calculates the number of _____ in a known volume of blood	☐
63. poikilocytosis	7.17	large, irregularly shaped red blood _____	☐
64. polycythemia	7.18	abnormal _____ in number of red blood cells	☐
65. prophylaxis	7.84	a preventative _____	☐
66. rabies	7.56	bacterial infection spread from the saliva of an infected _____	☐
67. red blood count	7.85	measures the _____ of red blood cells	☐
68. septicemia	7.57	systemwide disease caused by the presence of _____ and their toxins in the circulating blood	☐
69. smallpox	7.58	a(n) _____ disease that was eradicated in 1975 due to an aggressive vaccine campaign	☐
70. splenectomy	7.86	the surgical _____ of the spleen	☐
71. splenomegaly	7.19	abnormal enlargement of the _____	☐
72. staphylococcemia	7.59	the presence of the *Staphylococcus* bacterium in the _____	☐
73. streptococcemia	7.60	the presence of the *Streptococcus* _____ in the blood	☐
74. tetanus	7.61	disease caused by a(n) _____ released by *Clostridium tetani*	☐
75. thrombolysis	7.87	treatment that dissolves an unwanted blood _____	☐
76. thrombopenia	7.20	abnormally reduced number of _____	☐
77. thymoma	7.62	_____ originating in the thymus gland	☐
78. toxemia	7.21	presence of _____ in the bloodstream	☐
79. vaccination	7.88	_____ of a foreign substance to provide a cure or prophylaxis	☐
80. vaccine	7.89	a preparation used to activate an immune _____	☐

Multimedia Preview ▶▶▶▶▶

Additional interactive resources and activities for this chapter can be found on the Companion Website. For videos, audio glossary, and review, access the accompanying DVD-ROM in this book.

DVD-ROM Highlights

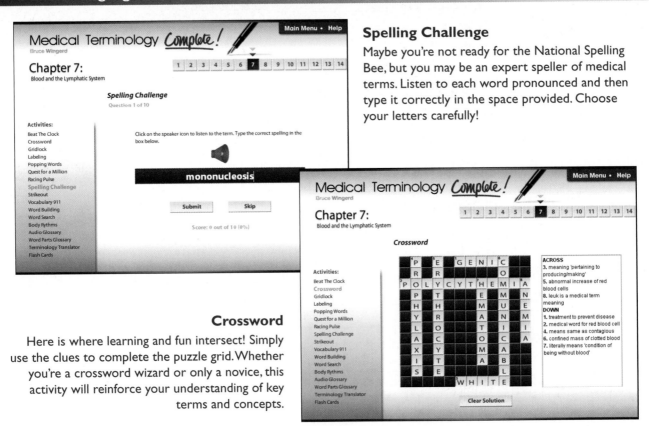

Spelling Challenge

Maybe you're not ready for the National Spelling Bee, but you may be an expert speller of medical terms. Listen to each word pronounced and then type it correctly in the space provided. Choose your letters carefully!

Crossword

Here is where learning and fun intersect! Simply use the clues to complete the puzzle grid. Whether you're a crossword wizard or only a novice, this activity will reinforce your understanding of key terms and concepts.

Website Highlights—www.prenhall.com/wingerd

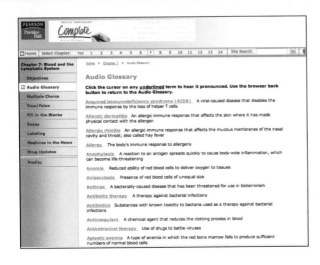

Audio Glossary

Take advantage of the free-access online study guide that accompanies your textbook. You'll find an audio glossary with definitions and audio pronunciations for every term in the book. By clicking on this URL you'll also access a variety of quizzes with instant feedback, links to download mp3 audio reviews, and current news articles.

The Cardiovascular System ▶▶▶▶

Learning Objectives

After completing this chapter, you will be able to:

- Define and spell the word parts used to create terms for the cardiovascular system.

- Break down and define common medical terms used for symptoms, diseases, disorders, procedures, treatments, and devices associated with the cardiovascular system.

- Build medical terms from the word parts associated with the cardiovascular system.

- Pronounce and spell common medical terms associated with the cardiovascular system.

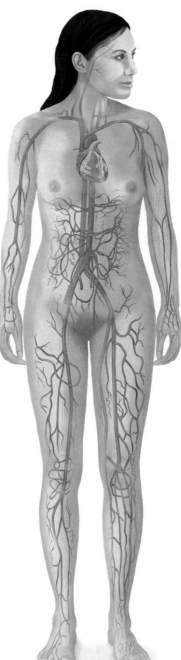
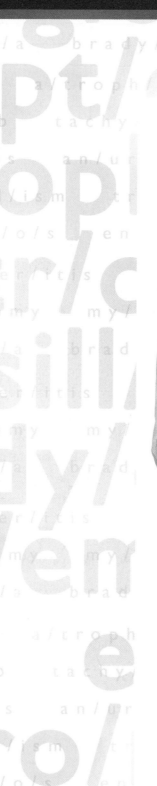

Anatomy and Physiology Terms ▶▶▶▶▶

The following table provides the combining forms that specifically apply to the anatomy and physiology of the cardiovascular system. Note that the combining forms are colored red to help you identify them when you see them again later in the chapter.

Combining Form	Definition	Combining Form	Definition
angi/o	blood vessel	valvul/o	little valve
aort/o	aorta	vas/o	blood vessel
arter/o, arteri/o	artery	vascul/o	little blood vessel
atri/o	atrium	ven/o	vein
cardi/o	heart	ventricul/o	little belly, ventricle
coron/o	crown or circle, heart		
my/o, myos/o	muscle		
pector/o	chest		

cardiovascular
kar dee oh VAS kyoo lar

blood

8.1 Every one of the 30 trillion or so cells in your body requires a continuous supply of oxygen and nutrients and an unending removal of waste materials. To meet these demands, the blood carries these materials in the body's circulation within a series of closed tubes, called blood vessels, pushed along mainly by the movements of the heart. The movement and transport of blood is thereby achieved by the _____ system, which consists of the heart and blood vessels, as the word parts that form the term *cardiovascular* suggest. The constructed form is written cardi/o/vascul/ar, in which *cardi/o* is a combining form that means "heart," and *vascul* is a word root that means "little blood vessel." The continuous flow of _____ to all tissues is vital to maintain normal body functions. If the supply of oxygen or nutrients or the removal of carbon dioxide is reduced or cut off, even for a few minutes, the affected cells may die. Thus, a disease of the cardiovascular system can pose life-threatening risks to health and survival.

FUNCTION ▶▶▶

8.2 The functions of the cardiovascular system may be summarized as:

- Propulsion of blood by the heart
- Transport of blood to all body tissues by the blood vessels
- Exchange of materials between the blood and body tissues

8.3 Use the anatomy terms that appear in the left column to fill in the corresponding blanks in Figures 8.1■ and 8.2■.

1. **alveoli**
2. **heart**
3. **artery**
4. **vein**

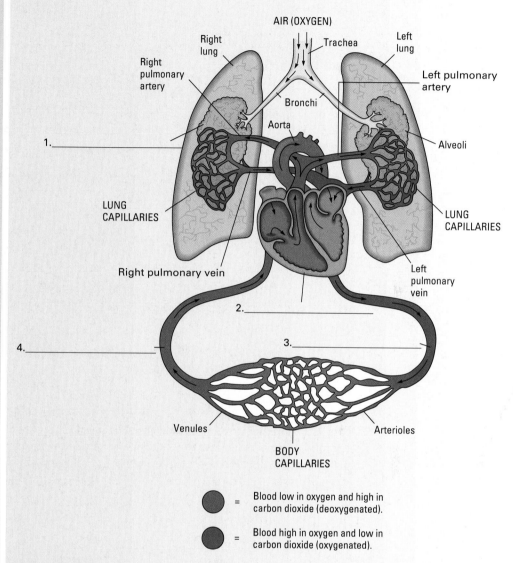

Figure 8.1 ■
The cardiovascular system. A schematic view of the closed circulation of blood. The heart is sectioned, and the capillaries are enlarged to enable you to see them.

5. **aorta**
6. **right**
7. **mitral**
8. **left**

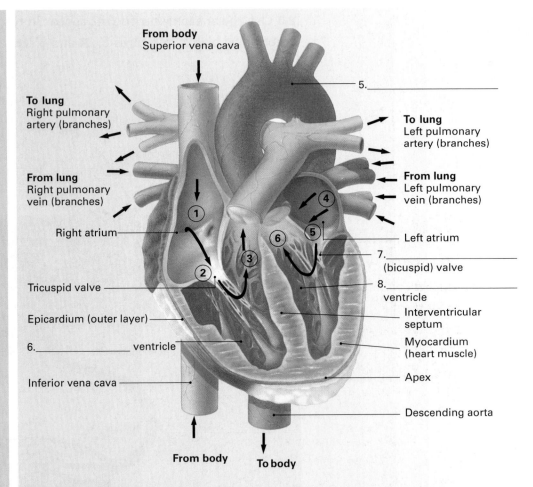

From body
Superior vena cava

To lung
Right pulmonary
artery (branches)

From lung
Right pulmonary
vein (branches)

Right atrium

Tricuspid valve

Epicardium (outer layer)

6._____ ventricle

Inferior vena cava

5._____

To lung
Left pulmonary
artery (branches)

From lung
Left pulmonary
vein (branches)

Left atrium

7._____
(bicuspid) valve

8._____
ventricle

Interventricular
septum

Myocardium
(heart muscle)

Apex

Descending aorta

From body   **To body**

Figure 8.2 ■
Internal anatomy of the heart. The heart is sectioned to reveal its internal features. The
numbers indicate the sequence of blood flow through the heart, and the arrows indicate
the direction of blood flow.

Medical Terms of the Cardiovascular System ▶▶▶▶▶

blood flow	**8.4** Many diseases of the cardiovascular system have a profound effect on the body's overall health. The result of cardiovascular disease is often the reduction or stoppage of blood flow to one or more parts of the body, which results in the death of cells. If _____ _____ reduction affects a large area or a critical organ like the brain, kidneys, or heart itself, the resulting cell death can produce a condition that quickly becomes life threatening.
cardi/o/logy **cardiologist** kar dee ALL oh jist	**8.5** The division of medicine known as **cardiology** (kar dee ALL oh jee) provides clinical treatment for heart disease. Cardiology is a constructed term, _____/__/_____, where the combining form *cardi/o* means "heart" and the suffix *-logy* means "study of." A physician specializing in this field is called a **cardiologist**. Generally, a _____ also treats conditions associated with blood vessels, due to the close functional relationship between blood vessels and the heart.
cardiovascular	**8.6** In the following sections, we will review the prefixes, combining forms, and suffixes that combine to build the medical terms of the cardiovascular system. Complete the frames and review exercises that follow. You are on your way to mastery of the medical terms related to the _____ system!

Signs and Symptoms of the Cardiovascular System

Following are the word parts that specifically apply to the signs and symptoms of the cardiovascular system that are covered in the following section. Note that the word parts are color-coded to help you identify them: prefixes are blue, combining forms are red, and suffixes are purple.

Prefix	Definition
a-	without or absence of
dys-	bad, abnormal, painful, or difficult
brady-	slow
tachy-	rapid

Combining Form	Definition
angi/o	blood vessel
cardi/o	heart
cyan/o	blue
pect/o, pector/o	chest
rhythm/o, rrhythm/o	rhythm
sten/o	narrow

Suffix	Definition
-a	singular
-algia, -dynia	condition of pain
-genic	pertaining to producing; formation
-ia	condition of
-osis	condition of
-plegia	paralysis
-sis	state of
-spasm	sudden involuntary muscle contraction

angina pectoris
an JYE nah * pek TOR iss

8.7 The primary symptom of an insufficient supply of oxygen to the heart is chest pain called _____ _____.This Latin term literally means "chest choke." The level of chest pain varies with the patient, varying from a very slight pressure to an overbearing pain that radiates to the shoulders, upper left arm, and back.

angiospasm
AN jee oh spazm

8.8 The common combining form of "blood vessel" is *angi/o*. Blood vessel disorders may include abnormal muscular contractions, or spasms, of the smooth muscles forming the vessel walls. This sign is called _____.The constructed form of this term is angi/o/spasm.

angiostenosis
an jee oh sten OH siss

8.9 Narrowing of a blood vessel is a sign of cardiovascular disease, causing a reduction of blood flow to the part of the body at the receiving end of the narrowed vessel.This sign is called **angiostenosis**.The constructed form of this term is written angi/o/sten/osis and includes one combining form: *angi/o*, which means "blood vessel"; and the word root *sten*, which means "narrow." Thus, the literal meaning of _____ is "condition of a narrow blood vessel."

arrhythmia
ah RITH mee ah

8.10 The prefix *a-* means "without or absence of," and the prefix *dys-* means "bad, abnormal, painful, or difficult." In some cases, they may be used interchangeably. For example, a loss of the normal rhythm of the heart is called _____, which means "condition of without rhythm" and is written a/rrhythm/ia. An alternate term for an abnormal heart rhythm is **dysrhythmia**.The constructed form of this term is written dys/rhythm/ia.

WORDS TO WATCH OUT FOR !

Arrhythmia and Dysrhythmia

These two medical terms relating to the abnormal rhythm of the heart appear and function similarly.As you have learned, the prefix *a-* means "without or absence of," and the prefix *dys-* means "bad, abnormal, painful, or difficult." Now look closer at the word roots.They are not identical. Both *rrhythm* and *rhythm* mean "rhythm." The term arrhythmia ("condition of without rhythm") has an extra **r** in front.To remember which term is spelled with two *r*'s, it might help to think of the expression "without rhyme or reason." A condition of arrhythmia is a heartbeat *"without rhyme or reason,"* while a condition of dysrhythmia is a heartbeat with an abnormal rhythm.

bradycardia brad ee KAR dee ah	**8.11** The common word root for heart is *cardi*. You will find it used in many terms in this chapter. In the term **bradycardia**, the prefix that means "slow" is used to form the meaning "slow heart." _____ is an abnormally slow heart rate, usually under 60 beats per minute. The normal resting heart rate ranges from 60 to 90 beats per minute.
cardiodynia kar dee oh DIN ee ah	**8.12** Two alternate suffixes are used for the condition of pain, *-algia* and *-dynia*. In the term commonly used for the symptom of pain associated with the heart, **cardiodynia**, the suffix *-dynia* is used for ease of speech. The constructed form of _____ is written cardi/o/dynia. The term **cardialgia** (kar dee AL gee ah) may also be used to identify heart pain, but it is less frequently used.
cardiogenic kar dee oh JENN ik	**8.13** The suffix *-genic* means "pertaining to producing." When combined with the word part for heart, the term _____ is formed. The constructed form of the term is written cardi/o/genic. It refers to a symptom or sign that originates from a condition of the heart. For example, the chest pain of angina pectoris (Frame 8.7) is a cardiogenic symptom because it is caused by insufficient blood flow to the heart.
cardioplegia kar dee oh PLEE jee ah	**8.14** The suffix *-plegia* means "paralysis." Therefore, a sign in which the heart has become paralyzed is called _____. The constructed form of this term is cardi/o/plegia.
cyanosis sigh ah NOH siss	**8.15** A symptom in which a blue tinge is seen in the skin and mucous membranes is called **cyanosis**, which literally means "condition of blue." It is written cyan/osis. _____ is caused by oxygen deficiency in tissues and is a common sign of respiratory failure often caused by cardiovascular disease.
palpitation pal pih TAY shun	**8.16** A symptom of pounding, racing, or skipping of the heartbeat is called _____. The term is derived from the Latin word *palpitatus*, which means "a throbbing."
tachycardia tack ee KAR dee ah	**8.17** The opposite of the prefix *brady-* is the prefix *tachy-*, which means "rapid." A rapid heart rate is called _____. It may be a symptom of heart disease if the heart exceeds 100 beats per minute at rest.

PRACTICE: Signs and Symptoms of the Cardiovascular System

The Right Match

Match the term on the left with the correct definition on the right.

_____ 1. cyanosis

_____ 2. angina pectoris

_____ 3. cardioplegia

_____ 4. cardiogenic

_____ 5. cardiodynia

_____ 6. arrhythmia

_____ 7. tachycardia

_____ 8. palpitation

a. sign or symptom that originates from a condition of the heart

b. pounding, racing, or skipping of the heartbeat

c. opposite of bradycardia; fast heartbeat

d. pain associated with the heart

e. chest pain or pressure

f. blue tinge in the skin and mucous membranes

g. paralyzed heart

h. term that literally means "condition of without rhythm"

Break the Chain

Analyze these medical terms:

a) Separate each term into its word parts; each word part is labeled for you (**p** = prefix, **r** = root, **cf** = combining form, and **s** = suffix).

b) For the Bonus Question, write the requested definition in the blank that follows.

The first set has been completed for you as an example.

1. a) angiostenosis   *angi / o / sten / osis*
                                 cf   r   s

   b) *Bonus Question:* What is the definition of the suffix? *condition of* _____

2. a) bradycardia   ____ / _____ / ___
                                p   r   s

   b) *Bonus Question:* What is the definition of the word root? _____

3. a) cardiodynia   _____ / __ / _____
                               cf   s

   b) *Bonus Question:* What is the definition of the suffix? _____

4. a) cardiogenic   _____ / __ / _____
                               cf   s

   b) *Bonus Question:* What is the definition of the suffix? _____

5. a) cyanosis   _____ / _____
                          r   s

   b) *Bonus Question:* What is the definition of the word root? _____

6. a) angiospasm   _____ / __ / _____
                             cf   s

   b) *Bonus Question:* What is the definition of the suffix? _____

Diseases and Disorders of the Cardiovascular System

Following are the word parts that specifically apply to the diseases and disorders of the cardiovascular system that are covered in the following section. Note that the word parts are color-coded to help you identify them: prefixes are blue, combining forms are red, and suffixes are purple.

Prefix	Definition
endo-	within
epi-	upon, over, above, or on top
hyper-	excessive, abnormally high, above
hypo-	deficient, abnormally low, below
peri-	around
poly-	many

Combining Form	Definition
angi/o	blood vessel
aort/o	aorta
arter/o, arteri/o	artery
ather/o	fatty
atri/o	atrium
cardi/o	heart
coron/o	crown or circle, heart
hem/o	blood
isch/o	hold back
my/o	muscle
phleb/o	vein
scler/o	thick or hard; sclera
sept/o	wall or partition; putrefying
sten/o	narrow
tampon/o	plug
tens/o	pressure
thromb/o	clot
valvul/o	little valve
varic/o	dilated vein
ventricul/o	little belly, ventricle

Suffix	Definition
-ac	pertaining to
-ade	process
-al	pertaining to
-ar	pertaining to
-emia	condition of blood
-ic	pertaining to
-ion	process
-itis	inflammation
-megaly	abnormally large
-oma	tumor
-osis	condition of
-pathy	disease

aneurysm
AN yoo rism

8.18 An abnormal bulging of an arterial wall is called an **aneurysm** and is illustrated in Figure 8.3■. The term is derived from the Greek word *aneurysma*, which means "a widening." An _____ is usually caused by a congenital defect or an acquired weakness of the arterial wall, which worsens in time as blood is pushed against it. The bursting of a large aneurysm is usually life threatening, resulting in massive hemorrhage.

Figure 8.3 ■
Aneurysm. In this illustration of the ventral side of the brain, three large aneurysms are clearly present.

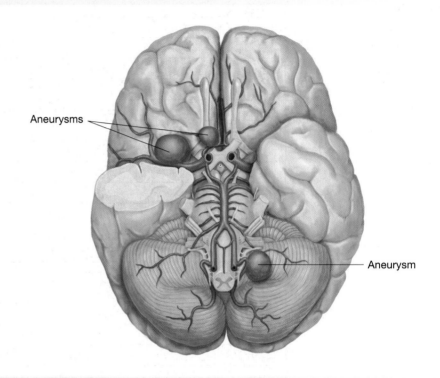

Aneurysms

Aneurysm

angiocarditis
AN jee oh kar DYE tiss

8.19 Inflammation of the heart and blood vessels is a disease called **angiocarditis**. It is usually caused by a widespread bacterial infection of the blood, or septicemia (Frame 8.55). The four word parts of _____ are shown when it is written angi/o/card/itis.

angioma
an jee OH mah

8.20 A term describing a tumor arising from a blood vessel combines the word root for blood vessel, *angi*, with the suffix for mass or tumor, *-oma*, to form _____. This constructed term is written angi/oma. Also known as **hemangioma** (heh MAN gee OH mah), it is a benign clump of endothelium forming a mass. In some cases the mass can obstruct the flow of blood through the vessel, although it is often a red or purple birthmark on the skin that does not obstruct blood flow.

aortic insufficiency
a OR tik * in suf FISH un see

8.21 The aortic valve is the semilunar valve located at the base of the aorta, which normally prevents blood from returning to the left ventricle. If it fails to close completely during ventricular diastole, blood may return to the left ventricle, causing the left ventricle to work harder. This condition is called **aortic insufficiency**. The long-term result of _____ _____, abbreviated **AI**, is a chronic condition of the heart known as **congestive heart failure**, which is described in Frame 8.36. An alternate term for AI is **aortic regurgitation**.

aortic stenosis
a OR tik * sten OH siss

8.22 The word root *sten* means "narrow." An **aortic stenosis** is a narrowing of the aorta that reduces the flow of blood through this large vessel, which causes the left ventricle to work harder than normal. It is usually a more serious condition than aortic insufficiency, although the long-term effect is similar by leading to **congestive heart failure** (Frame 8.36). The constructed form of _____ _____ is written aort/ic sten/osis.

aortitis
ay or TYE tiss

8.23 Inflammation of the aorta is called _____. The constructed form of this term is aort/itis. Often caused by a bacterial infection, it can lead to acute aortic insufficiency (Frame 8.21).

arteriopathy
ahr tee ree AH path ee

8.24 A general term for a disease of an artery is _____. This constructed term uses the suffix *-pathy* (meaning "disease") and is written arteri/o/pathy.

arteriosclerosis
ahr TEE ree oh skleh ROH siss

8.25 One common form of arteriopathy occurs when an artery wall becomes thickened and loses its elasticity, resulting in a reduced flow of blood to tissues. The risk of developing this disease, known as **arteriosclerosis**, increases with advanced age. The constructed form of _____ is written arteri/o/scler/osis, which literally means "condition of hard artery." If coronary arteries supplying the heart are damaged by this disease, the condition is called **arteriosclerotic heart disease (ASHD)**.

atherosclerosis
ATH er oh skleh ROH siss

8.26 A term describing a specific form of arteriosclerosis (Frame 8.25), in which one or more fatty plaques form along the inner walls of arteries, uses the combining form that means "fatty" to form the term **atherosclerosis**. The plaques thicken with time, which reduces the flow of blood through the affected vessel (Figure 8.4■). The constructed form of this term is written ather/o/scler/osis, which literally means "condition of hard fat." A major cause of coronary artery disease (Frame 8.38), _____ poses an immediate threat to life if a plaque disrupts blood flow and releases blood clots, which may trigger an acute myocardial infarction (Frame 8.49).

Figure 8.4 ■
Atherosclerosis. (a) A sectioned coronary artery that exhibits an accumulation of fatty plaque, which reduces the internal diameter of the vessel.
(b) In this close-up, you can see that the plaque consists of cholesterol, triglycerides, phospholipids, collagen, and smooth muscle cells.
(c) Two types and degrees of atherosclerotic narrowing, or stenosis.

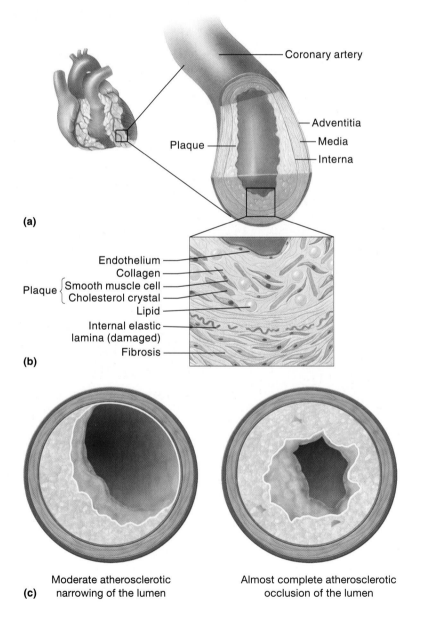

(a)

Coronary artery
Adventitia
Media
Interna
Plaque

Endothelium
Collagen
Smooth muscle cell
Plaque {
Cholesterol crystal
Lipid
Internal elastic lamina (damaged)
Fibrosis

(b)

Moderate atherosclerotic narrowing of the lumen

Almost complete atherosclerotic occlusion of the lumen

(c)

atrial septal defect
AY tree al * SEP tal * DEE fekt

8.27 A congenital condition characterized by a failure of the foramen ovale to close at birth, producing an opening in the septum that separates the right and left atria, is called _____ _____ _____. It allows blood to pass between the two atria, which bypasses the pulmonary circulation. Atrial and septal are constructed terms, as you can see when they are written as atri/al and sept/al.

atriomegaly
AY tree oh MEG ah lee

atri/o/megaly

8.28 The suffix -megaly means "abnormally large." In the condition **atriomegaly**, the atria have become abnormally enlarged or dilated, reducing their ability to push blood into the ventricles. The constructed form of _____ reveals three word parts when written _____/__/_____. It is a form of **cardiomegaly** (Frame 8.32).

atrioventricular block
AY tree oh ven TRIK yoo lar

8.29 An injury to the atrioventricular node (AV node), which normally receives impulses from the sinoatrial node (SA node) and transmits them to the ventricles to stimulate ventricular systole, is called an _____ _____, or **AV block**. The injury is usually caused by a myocardial infarction (Frame 8.49), during which the cells of the AV node die due to a loss of blood flow. The term atrioventricular is a constructed term, written atri/o/ventricul/ar.

cardiac arrest
KAR dee ak * ah REST

8.30 The cessation of heart activity is called _____ _____. As you should know, cardiac is a constructed term written cardi/ac. Arrest means "stop."

cardiac tamponade
KAR dee ak * tamp oh NAHD

8.31 Acute compression of the heart due to the accumulation of fluid within the pericardial cavity is known as **cardiac tamponade**. The term is constructed from word parts and is shown as cardi/ac tampon/ade. It literally means "pertaining to heart plug process." _____ _____ is a complication of an inflammatory disease of the pericardium known as pericarditis (Frame 8.52).

cardiomegaly
KAR dee oh MEG ah lee

8.32 Recall that the suffix -megaly means "abnormally large." The abnormal enlargement of the heart is called _____, which occurs when the heart must work harder than normal to meet the oxygen demands of body cells. The constructed form of this term is cardi/o/megaly.

cardiomyopathy
kar dee oh my OPP ah thee

8.33 A general term for a disease of the myocardium of the heart is **cardiomyopathy**. The constructed form of _____ reveals five word parts and is written cardi/o/my/o/pathy. The most common causes of cardiomyopathy include hypertension (Frame 8.46), chronic alcoholism, bacterial infection, and congenital defects of the myocardial cells.

cardiovalvulitis
KAR dee oh val vyoo LYE tiss

8.34 An inflammation of the valves of the heart is called **cardiovalvulitis**. The constructed form of this term is cardi/o/valvul/itis. The most common causes of this disease are bacterial infection, which leads to the deposition of calcium deposits on heart valves, and congenital defects, which results in abnormally shaped valves. _____ is usually diagnosed from the presence of a **heart murmur**, which is a gurgling sound detected during auscultation (Frame 8.68).

coarctation
ko ark TAY shun

8.35 A congenital defect characterized by aortic stenosis (Frame 8.22) that is present at birth is known as **coarctation of the aorta**. The term _coarctation_ is derived from the Latin word _coarcto_, which means "to press together." _____ of the **aorta** (ay OR tah) causes reduced systemic circulation of blood and accumulation of fluid in the lungs and requires surgical repair.

congestive heart failure

8.36 A chronic form of heart disease characterized by the failure of the left ventricle to pump enough blood to supply systemic tissues and lungs is called **congestive heart failure (CHF)**. Also known as **left ventricular failure**, the reduced function of the left ventricle characteristic of

_____ _____ _____

makes the heart work harder, resulting in cardiomegaly (Frame 8.32), pulmonary congestion, and reduced stroke volume that eventually leads to cardiac arrest (Frame 8.30).

cor pulmonale
kor * pull moh NAY lee

8.37 A chronic enlargement of the right ventricle resulting from congestion of the pulmonary circulation is called **cor pulmonale**. A French word that literally means "heart lung," _____ _____ is also known as **right ventricular failure**.

coronary artery disease

8.38 A general term for a disease that afflicts the coronary arteries supplying the heart is _____ _____ _____ **(CAD)**. The most common form of CAD is atherosclerosis (Frame 8.26).

coronary occlusion	**8.39** *Occlusion* is a general term that means "blockage." A **coronary occlusion** is a blockage within a coronary artery, resulting in a reduced blood flow to an area of the heart muscle. The most common single cause of a _____ _____ is atherosclerosis (Frame 8.26). Atherosclerosis or other diseases may also lead to emboli (drifting blood clots), and a congenital stenosis may also contribute to coronary occlusion.
embolism EM boh lizm	**8.40** A blockage or occlusion that forms when a blood clot or other foreign particle (including air or fat) moves through the circulation is called an **embolism**. The term is derived from the Greek word *embolisma*, which means "piece or patch." An _____ can produce a severe circulatory restriction when the blood clot or particle, called an **embolus** (plural form is emboli), lodges in an artery.
endocarditis EHN doh kar DYE tiss	**8.41** Inflammation of the endocardium, the thin membrane lining the inside walls of the heart chambers, is an acute disease called _____. The constructed form of this term is endo/card/itis. Because the endocardium also covers the heart valves, endocarditis often results in cardiovalvulitis (Frame 8.34). It is usually caused by a bacterial infection.
fibrillation fih bril AY shun	**8.42** A condition of uncoordinated, rapid contractions of the muscle forming the ventricles or atria is called _____. It is a severe form of arrhythmia (Frame 8.10). **Atrial fibrillation** leads to a reduction of blood expelled from the atria and is usually not fatal. However, **ventricular fibrillation** results in circulatory collapse due to the failure of the ventricles to expel blood.
heart block	**8.43** A block or delay of the normal electrical conduction of the heart is called _____. It is often the result of a myocardial infarction that damages the SA node or AV node.
heart murmur	**8.44** An abnormal soft, gurgling or blowing sound heard on auscultation (Frame 8.68) of the heart is called **heart murmur**. It indicates the regurgitation of blood through one or more heart valves. The most common source of _____ _____ occurs when the mitral valve leaks during ventricular contraction, called **mitral valve prolapse**.

tetralogy of Fallot
teh TRALL oh jee * of * fah LOH

8.56 A severe congenital disease in which four defects associated with the heart are present at birth is called **tetralogy of Fallot**. The four defects are pulmonary stenosis (narrowing of the pulmonary artery), ventricular septal defect (Frame 8.59), incorrect position of the aorta, and right ventricular hypertrophy. As a result of _____ _____ _____, the pulmonary circulation is partially bypassed.

thrombosis
throm BOH siss

8.57 The presence of stationary blood clots within one or more blood vessels is called **thrombosis**. The term is the Greek word for clotting, *thrombosis*. A coronary _____ is often caused by atherosclerosis (Frame 8.26), and its rupture can result in sudden death due to an acute myocardial infarction (Frame 8.49).

varicosis
vair ih KOH siss

8.58 An abnormally dilated vein is called _____, or varicose vein. Varicosis is a constructed term, written varic/osis, which literally means "condition of dilated vein." It results when valves within a superficial vein of the leg or elsewhere fail, allowing blood to pool in response to gravitational forces (Figure 8.6■).

Figure 8.6 ■
Varicosis. (a) Varicose veins develop due to the failure of valves in the superficial veins of the leg, which leads to blood accumulation in response to gravity and vein dilation.
(b) Photograph of spider veins of the leg.
Courtesy of Jason L. Smith, MD.

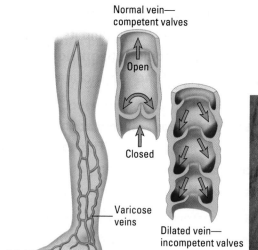

Normal vein—
competent valves

Open

Closed

Varicose
veins

Dilated vein—
incompetent valves

(a)

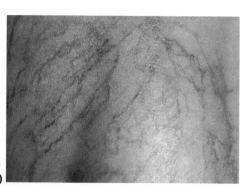

(b)

ventricular septal defect
vehn TRIK yoo lar * SEPP tal *
DEE fekt

8.59 A congenital disease in which an opening in the septum separating the right and left ventricles is present at birth is called _____ _____ _____. The opening allows some blood to flow from the right ventricle to the left ventricle, reducing blood flow to the lungs and the pulmonary circulation.

PRACTICE: Diseases and Disorders of the Cardiovascular System

The Right Match

Match the term on the left with the correct definition on the right.

_____ 1. aneurysm

_____ 2. cardiac tamponade

_____ 3. cor pulmonale

_____ 4. heart murmur

_____ 5. cardiac arrest

_____ 6. coronary artery disease

_____ 7. coronary occlusion

_____ 8. atrial septal defect

_____ 9. congestive heart failure

_____ 10. heart block

_____ 11. fibrillation

a. a disease of the coronary vessels

b. a congenital heart defect

c. a block of the heart conduction system

d. a blockage in a coronary vessel

e. abnormal bulging of an arterial wall

f. soft, gurgling, or blowing sound heard through auscultation

g. cessation of heartbeat

h. uncoordinated, rapid heartbeat

i. literally, "heart lung"

j. left ventricular failure

k. caused by fluid within pericardial cavity

Linkup

Link the word parts in the list to create the terms that match the definitions. You may use word parts more than once. Remember to add in combining vowels when needed—and that some terms do not use any combining vowel. The first one is completed as an example.

Prefix	Combining Form	Suffix
hyper-	angi/o	-ion
peri-	ather/o	-ism
	card/o, cardi/o	-itis
	embol/o	-oma
	my/o	-osis
	scler/o	-pathy
	tens/o	
	thromb/o	
	varic/o	

Definition

1. **An occlusion of blood flow**

2. A general term for a disease of the myocardium of the heart

3. A specific form of arteriosclerosis in which one or more fatty plaques form along the inner walls of arteries

4. A tumor arising from a blood vessel

5. Inflammation of the membrane surrounding the heart

6. Inflammation of the heart and blood vessels

7. An abnormally dilated vein

8. The presence of a stationary blood clot within a blood vessel

9. Persistently high blood pressure

Term

embolism

_____

_____

_____

_____

_____

_____

_____

_____

auscultation
oss kull TAY shun

8.68 A part of a physical examination that involves listening to internal sounds using a **stethoscope** (STETH oh skope) is called _____. Certain sounds suggest abnormalities of heart function, especially arrhythmias and valve disorders.

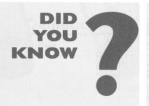
DID YOU KNOW ?

Auscultation

Auscultation is derived from the Latin word *ausculto,* which means "to listen." During the ancient times of Aristotle, early physicians practiced this form of evaluation by pressing an ear against the patient's chest. The stethoscope, which literally means "to view the chest," is a device that made this procedure much more efficient after its first use around 1725.

cardiac catheterization
KAR dee ak * kath eh ter ih ZAY shun

8.69 Insertion of a narrow flexible tube, called a **catheter**, through a blood vessel leading into the heart is called _____ _____. The procedure is performed to withdraw blood samples from heart chambers, measure pressures, and inject contrast medium for imaging purposes. The term *catheter* is derived from the Greek word *katheter,* which means "to send down."

cardiac pacemaker
KAR dee ak * PAYS maker

8.70 A **cardiac pacemaker** is a battery-powered device that is implanted under the skin and wired to the SA node in the heart (Figure 8.8■). It produces timed electric pulses that replace the function of the SA node as a treatment for a heart block and certain other arrhythmias. Recently, the _____ _____ has been improved to adjust to the patient's physical activity and SA node function. This is called an "on demand" pacemaker.

Figure 8.8 ■
Cardiac pacemaker. (a) The pacemaker device is implanted beneath the skin near the heart, and the electrode is surgically connected to the heart wall. (b) Photograph of a pacemaker in a patient's chest.
Source: Photo Researchers, Inc./Science Photo Library.

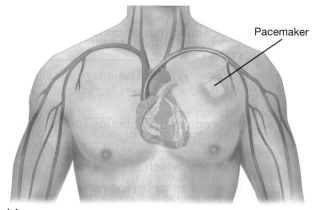

Pacemaker

(a)

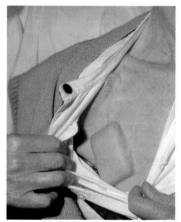

(b)

**cardiopulmonary
resuscitation**

KAR dee oh PULL mon air ee *
ree SUSS ih TAY shun

8.71 Artificial respiration that is used to restore breathing by applying a combination of chest compression and artificial ventilation at intervals is commonly abbreviated **CPR**, which means _____ _____. The constructed form of this term is written cardi/o/pulmon/ary resuscitation. The term *resuscitation* is derived from the Latin word *resuscitatio*, which means "to revive."

**coronary artery
bypass graft**

8.72 A surgical procedure that involves removing a blood vessel from another part of the body and inserting it into the coronary circulation is called _____ _____ _____ _____, or **CABG**. The grafted vessel restores blood flow to an oxygen-deprived area of the heart by carrying blood around an occluded (blocked) coronary artery (Figure 8.9■).

Figure 8.9 ■
Coronary artery bypass graft (CABG). The grafts are often obtained from the patient's saphenous veins in the legs and are inserted to carry blood around the blockage (occlusion).

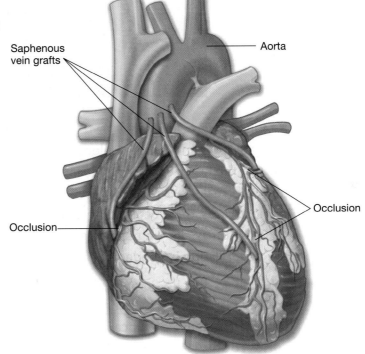

Saphenous vein grafts

Aorta

Occlusion

Occlusion

Holter monitor

8.80 A portable electrocardiograph may be worn by the patient to monitor electrical activity of the heart over 24-hour periods. The device is called a _____ _____ and is useful to detect periodic or transient cardiac abnormalities.

nitroglycerin
NIGH troh GLIH ser ihn

8.81 A drug that is commonly used as an emergency vasodilator as a treatment for severe angina pectoris (Frame 8.7) or myocardial infarction (Frame 8.49) is the compound **nitroglycerin**. The vasodilation that results from _____ temporarily improves blood flow to the heart and other vital organs.

phlebectomy
fleh BEK toh mee

8.82 **Phlebectomy** is constructed from the word root meaning "vein" (*phleb*) and the suffix meaning "surgical excision or removal" (-*ectomy*). From its word parts, we know that a _____ is a procedure involving the surgical removal of a vein. The constructed form of this term is phleb/ectomy.

phlebotomy
fleh BOT oh mee

8.83 A puncture into a vein to remove blood for sampling or donation is called **phlebotomy**. This constructed term combines the word root for vein, the combining vowel o, and the suffix meaning "incision or to cut" to create the term _____, which is written phleb/o/tomy. Although the word part for incision is included, a small puncture is made rather than an incision when withdrawing blood (called a **venipuncture**). A healthcare professional who performs this procedure is called a **phlebotomist** (fleh BOT oh mist).

positron emission tomography scan
PAHZ ih tron * ee MISH uhn * toh MOG rah fee

8.84 A noninvasive procedure that provides blood flow images using positron emission tomography (PET) techniques combined with radioactive isotope labeling may be used to produce images of the heart to reveal functional defects. The procedure is called _____ _____ _____ _____, or **PET scan.**

sphygmomanometry
SFIG moh mah NOM eh tree

8.85 A common procedure that measures arterial blood pressure is called _____. This constructed term is written sphygm/o/man/o/metry, which literally means "the process of measuring pulse." It utilizes a device called a **sphygmomanometer** (sfig moh mah NOM eh ter), which consists of an arm cuff and air pressure pump with a mercury pressure gauge (Figure 8.11 ■). In recent years, the mercury pressure gauge has been replaced by aneroid dials and digital technology.

Figure 8.11 ■
Sphygmomanometry. Photograph of a nurse taking blood pressure readings with the use of a sphygmomanometer, which includes an arm cuff and pressure gauge. A stethoscope is used to listen for sounds within the brachial artery.

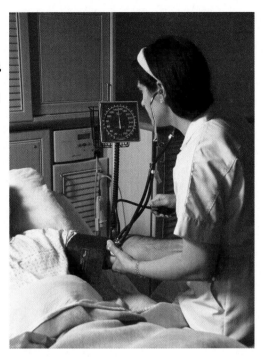

thrombolytic therapy
throm boh LITT ik * THAIR ah pee

8.86 Treatments to dissolve unwanted blood clots are often necessary after surgery to prevent the development of emboli (Frame 8.40). It is also performed soon after a myocardial infarction (Frame 8.49) to minimize damage to the heart and is credited with saving many lives. Known as _____ _____, it includes the use of drugs such as streptokinase and tissue plasminogen activator (TPA). The constructed term *thrombolytic* is made up of the combining form that means "clot" (*thrombo*) and the suffix that means "pertaining to loosen or dissolve" (*-lytic*).

treadmill stress test

8.87 If a heart condition is suspected, a cardiologist will often require the patient to undergo exercise during echocardiography or electrocardiography (or both) in an effort to examine heart function under stress. The most common term for this procedure is _____ _____ _____.

valvuloplasty
VAL vyoo loh plass tee

8.88 The surgical repair of a heart valve is called _____. The constructed form of this term is written valvul/o/plasty. If repair is not possible due to the extent of the damage or defect, valve replacement may be required using an artificial valve or a porcine (pig) valve.

PRACTICE: Treatments, Procedures, and Devices of the Cardiovascular System

The Right Match _____

Match the term on the left with the correct definition on the right.

_____ 1. cardiac pacemaker

_____ 2. defibrillation

_____ 3. phlebotomy

_____ 4. Holter monitor

_____ 5. coronary stent

_____ 6. PET scan

_____ 7. treadmill stress test

_____ 8. nitroglycerin

_____ 9. auscultation

_____ 10. Doppler sonography

a. an artificial, usually plastic, scaffold that is used to anchor a surgical implant, or graft

b. a drug that is commonly used as an emergency vasodilator

c. patient undergoes exercise during echocardiography or electrocardiography to examine heart function under stress

d. a battery-powered device that is implanted under the skin and wired to the SA node in the heart

e. puncture into a vein, usually to remove blood for sampling or donation

f. a portable electrocardiograph worn by the patient

g. an electric charge applied to the chest wall to stop the heart conduction system momentarily, then restart it with a more normal heart rhythm

h. a noninvasive procedure that provides blood flow images using positron emission tomography (PET) techniques combined with radioactive isotope labeling

i. an ultrasound procedure that evaluates blood flow to determine the cause of a localized reduction in circulation

j. a physical examination that involves listening to internal sounds

Break the Chain

Analyze these medical terms:

    a)   Separate each term into its word parts; each word part is labeled for you (**p** = prefix, **r** = root, **cf** = combining form, and **s** = suffix).

    b)   For the Bonus Question, write the requested definition in the blank that follows.

1. a) arteriogram   _____/__/_____
                                      cf   s

    b) *Bonus Question:* What is the definition of the suffix? _____

2. a) echocardiography   _____/__/___/__/_____
                                     cf   cf   s

    b) *Bonus Question:* What is the definition of the first combining form? _____

3. a) embolectomy   _____/_____
                                    r   s

    b) *Bonus Question:* What is the definition of the word root? _____

4. a) sphygmomanometry   _____/__/_____/__/_____
                                     cf   cf   s

    b) *Bonus Question:* What is the definition of the suffix? _____

5. a) phlebotomist   _____/__/_____/_____
                                    cf   r   s

    b) *Bonus Question:* What is the definition of the combining form? _____

6. a) electrocardiography   _____/__/_____/__/_____
                                     cf   cf   s

    b) *Bonus Question:* What is the definition of the suffix? _____

7. a) cardiopulmonary resuscitation _____/__/_____/_____
                                          cf   r   s

    b) *Bonus Question:* What is the definition of the word root in the first word? _____

8. a) endarterectomy   ___/____/_____
                                  p   r   s

    b) *Bonus Question:* What is the definition of the prefix? _____

9. a) valvuloplasty   _____/__/_____
                                    cf   s

    b) *Bonus Question:* What is the definition of the suffix? _____

Abbreviations of the Cardiovascular System

The abbreviations that are associated with the cardiovascular system are summarized here. Study these abbreviations, and review them in the exercise that follows.

Abbreviation	Definition		Abbreviation	Definition
ASHD	atherosclerotic heart disease		CHF	congestive heart failure
ASD	atrial septal defect		CPR	cardiopulmonary resuscitation
AV	atrioventricular		ECG, EKG	electrocardiogram
CABG	coronary artery bypass graft		MI	myocardial infarction
CAD	coronary artery disease		PET	positron emission tomography

PRACTICE: Abbreviations

Fill in the blanks with the abbreviation or the complete medical term.

Abbreviation

Medical Term

1. _____   congestive heart failure

2. ASD

3. _____   coronary artery bypass graft

4. MI

5. _____   positron emission tomography

6. CPR

7. _____   atherosclerotic heart disease

8. AV

9. _____   electrocardiogram

10. CAD

▶▶▶▶ Chapter Review

Word Building _____

Construct medical terms from the following meanings. (Some are built from word parts, some are not.) The first question has been completed as an example.

1. generalized disease of the heart muscle — *cardiomyo*pathy

2. inflammation of the heart and blood vessels — angio_____

3. narrowing of a blood vessel — angio_____

4. tumor arising from a blood vessel — angi_____

5. hardening of the arteries — _____sclerosis

6. abnormally slow heart rate — _____cardia

7. a sensation of pain in the heart — cardio_____

8. incision into an artery to remove plaque — end_____ectomy

9. abnormal hypertrophy of the heart — cardio_____

10. inflammation of the inner heart membrane — endo_____

11. an abnormal heart rhythm — dys_____

12. high blood pressure that is persistent — _____tension

13. death of a portion of the myocardium — _____cardial in_____

14. inflammation of the myocardium — myo_____

15. a process of recording heart electrical activity — _____cardiography

16. inflammation of a vein — _____itis

17. a recording of an X-ray of an artery — angio_____

18. general surgical repair of a blood vessel — _____plasty

19. use of an endoscope to evaluate a blood vessel — angio_____

20. an incision into an artery — arterio_____

21. listening to heart sounds with a stethoscope — aus_____

22. use of sound waves to diagnose a heart condition — _____cardiography

Clinical Application Exercises

Medical Report

Read the following medical report, then answer the questions that follow.

University Hospital

5500 University Avenue
Metropolis, TX

Phone: (211) 594-4000
Fax: (211) 594-4001

Medical Consultation: Cardiology

Date: 11/16/2007

Patient: Robert Gorman

Patient Complaint: Chest pain uncharacteristic of angina pectoris, which intensifies with deep breathing.

History: 62-year-old Caucasian male with a recent history of mild chest pain, shortness of breath, and malaise. Dental tooth extractions were performed recently and no follow-up treatment with antibiotics was reported.

Family History: Father deceased at 79 years with HF following bypass surgery. Mother, 89 years, with complete hysterectomy following diagnosis of stage 1 cervical cancer; no reported conditions otherwise.

Allergies: Penicillin

Evidences: Mild chest pain that worsens with inspiration; ECG and stress ECHO normal; recent history of dental extractions without AT.

Treatment: Effuse the pericardial cavity with inpatient antibiotic treatment using nonpenicillin antibiotic therapy on IV drip.

Donald Freeman, M.D.

---

1. What complaints support the diagnosis? _____

_____

2. Why is the patient history an important part of this diagnosis? _____

_____

3. Why is the reported allergy to penicillin an important factor in deciding a course of treatment? _____

_____

Medical Report Case Study

The following Case Study provides further discussion regarding the patient in the medical report. Fill in the blanks with the correct terms. Choose your answers from the following list of terms. (Note that some terms may be used more than once.)

angina pectoris	cardiologist	myocardial infarction
angiostenosis	cardiology	pericarditis
atherosclerosis	electrocardiography	stress ECHO
block	endocarditis	

A patient named Robert Gorman complained of pain in the heart area of the chest, or (a) _____

_____, and was subsequently referred to (b) _____ for immediate diagnosis and

treatment. The specialist, a (c) _____, diagnosed the pain as having a cause from insufficient blood supply

to the heart. The patient was given medication and educated about heart disease management. Several weeks later, the

patient was readmitted due to continued complaints of chest pain. After evaluating heart electrical events with

(d) _____, the physician performed a technique using sound waves to evaluate heart activity during

physical exercise, known as a(n) (e) _____ _____. The ECG showed a normal con-

duction system, thereby ruling out damage to the conduction system, or a heart (f) _____. The stress

ECHO also showed mostly normal results, ruling out damage to the heart muscle, or a(n) (g) _____

_____ because the heart muscle was receiving sufficient levels of oxygen. Because blood flow was nor-

mal, the narrowing of a coronary artery, generally called a(n) (h) _____, was eliminated as a cause,

which also eliminated the common plaque-forming disease that causes a stenosis, known as (i) _____.

However, the stress ECHO did reveal an abnormal contact with the pericardial sac with each heartbeat, suggesting in-

flammation of the membrane or (j) _____. Inflammation of the inner heart membrane, a condition

known as (k) _____, was also suspected. A blood analysis was ordered and found to be positive for

bacterial infection. A course of treatment was ordered that began with a surgical technique to create an opening in the

pericardial sac and followed with antibiotic therapy to destroy the infectious microorganisms and counter the

inflammation.

Key Terms Double-Check

Remember that the chapter's key terms appeared alphabetically throughout this chapter. This exercise helps you check your knowledge AND review for tests.

1. First, fill in the missing word in the definitions for the chapter's key terms.

2. Then, check your answers using Appendix F.

3. If you got the answer right, put a check mark in the right column.

4. If your answer was incorrect, go back to the frame number provided and review the content.

Use the checklist to study the terms you don't know until you're confident you know them all.

Key Term	Frame	Definition	Know It?
1. aneurysm	8.18	abnormal _____ of an arterial wall usually caused by a congenital defect or an acquired weakness of the arterial wall	☐
2. angina pectoris	8.7	chest pain that is a primary symptom of an insufficient supply of _____ to the heart	☐
3. angiocarditis	8.19	inflammation of the _____ and blood vessels	☐
4. angiography	8.60	diagnostic procedure that includes x-ray photography, MRI, or _____ _____ images of a blood vessel after injection of a contrast medium	☐
5. angioma	8.20	tumor arising from a blood vessel, also known as a(n) _____	☐
6. angioplasty	8.61	surgical repair of a blood vessel, including _____ angioplasty and laser angioplasty	☐
7. angioscopy	8.62	use of a flexible fiber-optic instrument, or _____, to observe a diseased blood vessel and to assess any lesions	☐
8. angiospasm	8.8	abnormal _____ contractions, or spasms, of the smooth muscles forming the vessel walls	☐
9. angiostenosis	8.9	narrowing of a blood _____ causing the reduction of blood flow to a part of the body	☐
10. angiostomy	8.63	creation of an opening into a blood vessel, usually for the insertion of a(n) _____	☐
11. angiotomy	8.64	surgical _____ into a blood vessel	☐
12. aortic insufficiency	8.21	condition in which the semilunar valve fails to close completely during ventricular _____ causing blood to return to the left ventricle, which makes the left ventricle work harder	☐
13. aortic stenosis	8.22	narrowing of the _____ that reduces the flow of blood through this large vessel, which causes the left ventricle to work harder than normal	☐
14. aortitis	8.23	_____ of the aorta often caused by a bacterial infection	☐
15. aortography	8.65	procedure that obtains an X-ray photograph, MRI, or CAT scan image of the aorta; image is called a(n) _____	☐
16. arrhythmia	8.10	loss of the normal rhythm of the heart; _____	☐
17. arteriography	8.66	procedure that obtains an image of an artery that is called a(n) _____	☐

Key Term	Frame	Definition	Know It?
18. arteriopathy	8.24	general term for a disease of a(n) _____	☐
19. arteriosclerosis	8.25	disease in which an artery wall becomes thickened and loses its _____, resulting in a reduced flow of blood to tissues	☐
20. arteriotomy	8.67	an incision into a(n) _____	☐
21. atherosclerosis	8.26	form of arteriosclerosis in which one or more fatty _____ form along the inner walls of arteries	☐
22. atrial septal defect	8.27	congenital condition characterized by a failure of the foramen ovale to close at birth, producing an opening in the septum that separates the right and left _____	☐
23. atriomegaly	8.28	abnormally enlarged or dilated atria with reduced ability to push blood into the _____	☐
24. atrioventricular block	8.29	an injury to the _____ node (AV node), which normally receives impulses from the sinoatrial node (SA node) and transmits them to the ventricles to stimulate ventricular systole	☐
25. auscultation	8.68	listening to internal sounds using a(n) _____	☐
26. bradycardia	8.11	abnormally _____ heart rate	☐
27. cardiac arrest	8.30	_____ of heart activity	☐
28. cardiac catheterization	8.69	insertion of a narrow flexible tube, called a(n) _____, through a blood vessel leading into the heart	☐
29. cardiac pacemaker	8.70	a battery-powered device that is implanted under the skin and wired to the _____ _____ in the heart to produce timed electric pulses that replace the function of the SA node	☐
30. cardiac tamponade	8.31	acute compression of the heart due to the accumulation of _____ within the pericardial cavity	☐
31. cardiodynia	8.12	heart pain, less frequently called_____	☐
32. cardiogenic	8.13	symptom or sign that _____ from a condition of the heart	☐
33. cardiomegaly	8.32	a(n) _____ heart, which occurs when the heart must work harder than normal to meet the oxygen demands of body cells	☐
34. cardiomyopathy	8.33	general term for a disease of the _____ of the heart	☐
35. cardioplegia	8.14	sign in which the heart has become _____	☐
36. cardiopulmonary resuscitation	8.71	artificial _____ that is used to restore breathing by applying a combination of chest compression and artificial ventilation at intervals	☐
37. cardiovalvulitis	8.34	inflammation of the valves of the heart that is usually diagnosed from the presence of a(n) _____ _____, which is a gurgling sound detected during auscultation	☐
38. coarctation of the aorta	8.35	congenital defect characterized by aortic _____ that is present at birth; it causes reduced systemic circulation of blood and accumulation of fluid in the lungs	☐

Key Term	Frame	Definition	Know It?
39. congestive heart failure	8.36	chronic form of heart disease characterized by the failure of the left ventricle to pump enough blood to supply systemic tissues and lungs, abbreviated _____	☐
40. cor pulmonale	8.37	chronic enlargement of the right ventricle resulting from congestion of the _____ circulation	☐
41. coronary artery bypass graft	8.72	surgical procedure that involves removing a blood vessel from another part of the body and inserting it into the coronary circulation, abbreviated _____	☐
42. coronary artery disease	8.38	disease that afflicts the _____ arteries supplying the heart	☐
43. coronary occlusion	8.39	a(n) _____ within a coronary artery, resulting in a reduced blood flow to an area of the heart muscle	☐
44. coronary stent	8.73	an artificial, usually plastic, scaffold that is used to anchor a surgical implant, or _____	☐
45. cyanosis	8.15	blue tinge seen in the skin and mucous membranes caused by oxygen _____ in tissues	☐
46. defibrillation	8.74	an electric charge applied to the chest wall to stop the heart conduction system _____, then restart it with a more normal heart rhythm	☐
47. Doppler sonography	8.75	_____ procedure that evaluates blood flow to determine the cause of a localized reduction in circulation	☐
48. echocardiography	8.76	ultrasound procedure that directs sound waves through the heart to evaluate heart function; recorded data is typically called a(n) _____	☐
49. electrocardiography	8.77	electrodes are pasted to the skin of the chest to detect and record the electrical events of the heart conduction system; the record or image of the data is called an electrocardiogram, and abbreviated _____ or EKG	☐
50. embolectomy	8.78	surgical removal of a floating blood clot, or _____	☐
51. embolism	8.40	a blood _____ or foreign particle (including air or fat) that moves through the circulation	☐
52. endarterectomy	8.79	surgical removal of the inner lining of an artery to remove a(n) _____ plaque	☐
53. endocarditis	8.41	inflammation of the _____	☐
54. fibrillation	8.42	condition of _____, rapid contractions of the ventricles or atria	☐
55. heart block	8.43	an interference with the normal _____ conduction of the heart	☐
56. heart murmur	8.44	abnormal soft, gurgling or blowing sound heard on _____ of the heart	☐
57. hemorrhoids	8.45	dilated, or _____, veins in the anal region	☐

Key Term	Frame	Definition	Know It?
58. Holter monitor	8.80	portable _____ worn by the patient to monitor electrical activity of the heart over 24-hour periods	☐
59. hypertension	8.46	abnormally high blood pressure; includes _____ hypertension and secondary hypertension	☐
60. hypotension	8.47	abnormally _____ blood pressure	☐
61. ischemia	8.48	abnormally low flow of _____ to tissues	☐
62. myocardial infarction	8.49	_____ of a portion of the myocardium, abbreviated MI	☐
63. myocarditis	8.50	inflammation of the _____ of the heart	☐
64. nitroglycerin	8.81	a drug commonly used as an emergency _____ as a treatment for severe angina pectoris or myocardial infarction	☐
65. palpitation	8.16	symptom of pounding, racing, or skipping of the _____	☐
66. patent ductus arteriosus	8.51	congenital condition characterized by a(n) _____ between the pulmonary artery and the aorta due to a failure of the fetal vessel to close	☐
67. pericarditis	8.52	inflammation of the membrane _____ the heart, the pericardium	☐
68. phlebectomy	8.82	_____ removal of a vein	☐
69. phlebitis	8.53	inflammation of a(n) _____	☐
70. phlebotomy	8.83	puncture into a vein to remove blood for sampling or donation by a(n) _____	☐
71. polyarteritis	8.54	simultaneous inflammation of _____ arteries	☐
72. positron emission tomography scan	8.84	noninvasive procedure that provides blood flow images using positron emission tomography techniques combined with radioactive isotope labeling known as a(n) _____ _____	☐
73. septicemia	8.55	bacterial infection of the _____	☐
74. sphygmomanometry	8.85	procedure that measures arterial blood pressure with a device called a(n) _____	☐
75. tachycardia	8.17	a(n) _____ heart rate	☐
76. tetralogy of Fallot	8.56	a severe congenital disease in which four defects associated with the heart are present at _____	☐
77. thrombolytic therapy	8.86	treatments to _____ unwanted blood clots to prevent the development of emboli	☐
78. thrombosis	8.57	presence of stationary _____ _____ within one or more blood vessels	☐
79. treadmill stress test	8.87	_____ during echocardiography or electrocardiography (or both) to examine heart function under stress	☐
80. valvuloplasty	8.88	surgical repair of a heart _____	☐
81. varicosis	8.58	an abnormally dilated vein that results when valves within a superficial vein of the leg or elsewhere fail, allowing blood to _____	☐
82. ventricular septal defect	8.59	congenital disease in which an opening in the septum separating the right and left ventricles is present at _____	☐

Multimedia Preview ▶▶▶▶▶

Additional interactive resources and activities for this chapter can be found on the Companion Website. For videos, audio glossary, and review, access the accompanying DVD-ROM in this book.

DVD-ROM Highlights

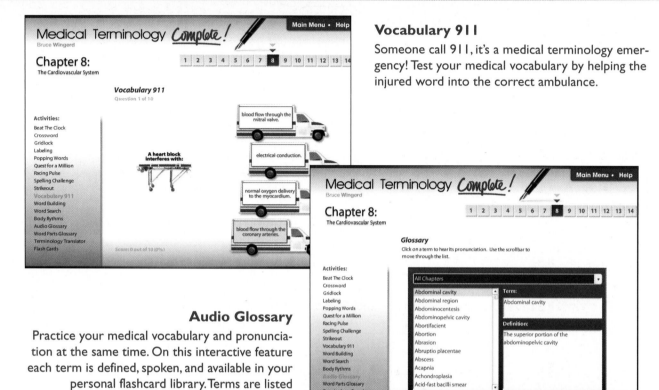

Vocabulary 911

Someone call 911, it's a medical terminology emergency! Test your medical vocabulary by helping the injured word into the correct ambulance.

Audio Glossary

Practice your medical vocabulary and pronunciation at the same time. On this interactive feature each term is defined, spoken, and available in your personal flashcard library. Terms are listed alphabetically and by chapter.

Website Highlights—www.prenhall.com/wingerd

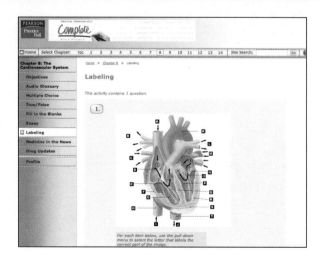

Labeling Exercise

Click here to take advantage of the free-access online study guide that accompanies your textbook. You'll find a figure labeling quiz that corresponds to the chapter. By clicking on this URL you'll also access links to download mp3 audio reviews, current news articles, and an audio glossary.

The Respiratory System ▶▶▶▶▶

Learning Objectives

After completing this chapter, you will be able to:

- Define and spell the word parts used to create terms for the respiratory system.

- Break down and define common medical terms used for symptoms, diseases, disorders, procedures, treatments, and devices associated with the respiratory system.

- Build medical terms from the word parts associated with the respiratory system.

- Pronounce and spell common medical terms associated with the respiratory system.

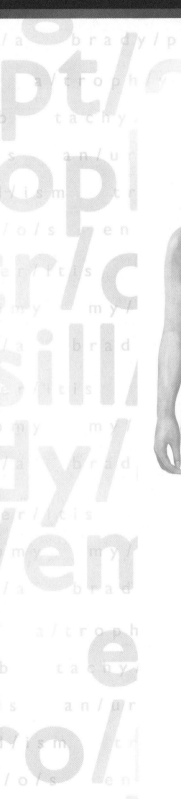
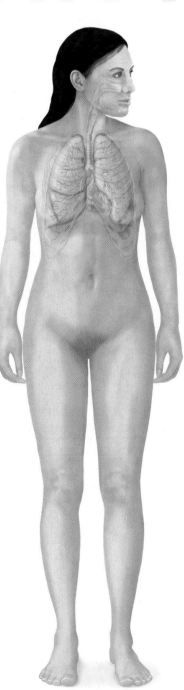

Anatomy and Physiology Terms ▶▶▶▶

The following table provides the combining forms that specifically apply to the anatomy and physiology of the respiratory system. Note that the combining forms are colored red to help you identify them when you see them again later in the chapter.

Combining Form	Definition	Combining Form	Definition
alveol/o	air sac, alveolus	phragm/o, phragmat/o	partition
bronch/o	airway, bronchus	pleur/o	pleura, rib
hem/o, hemat/o	blood	pneum/o, pneumon/o, pneumat/o	air, lung
laryng/o	voice box, larynx		
lob/o	a rounded part, lobe	pulmon/o	lung
muc/o	mucus	rhin/o	nose
nas/o	nose	sept/o	wall, partition; putrefying
ox/o	oxygen	sinus/o	cavity
pharyng/o	throat, pharynx	thorac/o	chest, thorax
		trache/o	windpipe, trachea

respiratory system	**9.1** The **respiratory** (RESS pih rah tor ee) **system** brings oxygen into the bloodstream, through which it is transported to all body cells. The system gets its name from its function: The process of providing cells with oxygen is commonly known as **respiration**. This term is derived from the word *respiratio*, which means "to breathe again." In addition to bringing oxygen into the bloodstream, the _____ _____ also removes the waste product, carbon dioxide, from the blood and channels it outside the body.
lower respiratory tract	**9.2** When you inhale, oxygen flows into the lungs after traveling through a series of chambers and tubes, known as the upper respiratory tract. It includes the nasal cavity, pharynx, and larynx. The lower portion of the respiratory system, known as the _____ _____ _____, consists of the trachea in the chest, the bronchial tree, which branches extensively throughout the lungs, the tiny air sacs within the lungs known as alveoli, and the lungs themselves. Gas exchange occurs across the walls of alveoli and adjacent capillaries. When you exhale, carbon dioxide flows out of the lungs through the same route but in the opposite direction.

FUNCTION ▶▶▶

carbon dioxide

1. **pharynx**
2. **trachea**
3. **bronchiole**
4. **lung**

9.3 The functions of the respiratory system may be summarized as follows:

- Provide a stream of oxygen into the blood through the process of inspiration, followed by diffusion.
- Remove _____ _____ from the blood through the process of diffusion, followed by expiration.

9.4 Use the anatomy terms that appear in the left column to fill in the corresponding blanks in Figures 9.1■ and 9.2■.

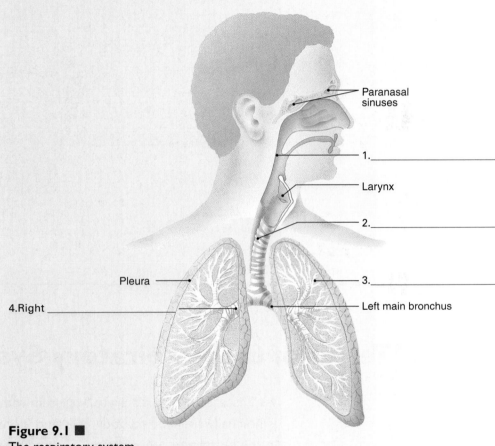

Paranasal sinuses

1._____

Larynx

2._____

3._____

Pleura

Left main bronchus

4. Right _____

Figure 9.1 ■
The respiratory system.

5. palate
6. tonsil
7. epiglottis
8. thyroid

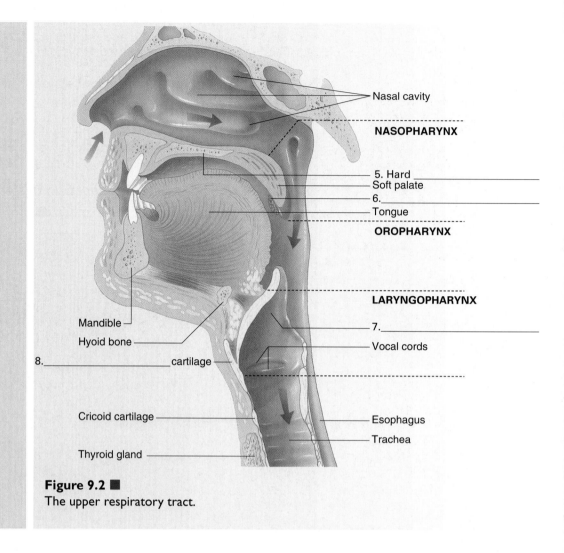

Nasal cavity

NASOPHARYNX

5. Hard _____
Soft palate
6. _____
Tongue

OROPHARYNX

LARYNGOPHARYNX

7. _____

Vocal cords

Mandible

Hyoid bone

8. _____ cartilage

Cricoid cartilage

Esophagus

Trachea

Thyroid gland

Figure 9.2 ■
The upper respiratory tract.

Medical Terms of the Respiratory System ▶▶▶▶

respiratory

9.5 Diseases of the respiratory system reduce the amount of oxygen that is normally supplied to body cells and increase the levels of carbon dioxide in the blood and other tissues. Severe respiratory disease can lead to a failure of oxygen delivery and may result in death. The most common symptoms of respiratory disease are breathing problems. If these problems are not identified and treated early, additional complications may arise. In general, _____ disease may be caused by congenital conditions, infections, allergies, tumors, heart disease, or injury.

9.6 The clinical treatment of a respiratory disease is performed by a physician with a specialization in treating the body region, the particular disorder, or a set of similar disorders. For example, lung disease is treated by a pulmonary specialist, or **pulmonologist**, disease of the pharynx is treated by a nose and throat specialist, or **otolaryngologist** (**ENT**), and lung cancer is treated by a _____ specialist, or **oncologist**. Often assisting the physician is a **respiratory therapist** who has received special training in the operation of equipment used to diagnose or treat breathing problems.

cancer

9.7 In the following sections, you will study the prefixes, combining forms, and suffixes that combine to build the medical terms of the respiratory system. Complete the frames and review exercises that follow. You are on your way to mastery of the medical terms related to the respiratory system!

Signs and Symptoms of the Respiratory System

Following are the word parts that specifically apply to the signs and symptoms of the respiratory system that are covered in the following section. Note that the word parts are color-coded to help you identify them: prefixes are blue, combining forms are red, and suffixes are purple.

Prefix	Definition
a-, an-	without or absence of
brady-	slow
dys-	bad, abnormal, painful, or difficult
epi-	upon, over, above, on top
eu-	normal or good
hyper-	excessive, abnormally high, or above
hypo-	deficient, abnormally low, or below
tachy-	rapid or fast

Combining Form	Definition
bronch/o	airway
hem/o	blood
laryng/o	voice box, larynx
orth/o	straight
rhin/o	nose
thorac/o	chest, thorax

Suffix	Definition
-algia	condition of pain
-capnia	condition of carbon dioxide
-dynia	pain
-emia	condition of blood
-oxia	condition of oxygen
-phonia	condition of sound or voice
-pnea	breath
-ptysis	to cough up
-rrhagia	condition of profuse bleeding, hemorrhage
-spasm	sudden involuntary muscle contraction
-staxis	dripping

acapnia
ah KAP nee ah

9.8 The suffix -capnia means "condition of carbon dioxide." When the prefix that means "without or absence of" is added, the term _____ is constructed, which is the absence of carbon dioxide. The constructed form of this term is a/capnia. A sign of reduced carbon dioxide in an expiration (exhaled air) sample indicates hyperventilation has been occurring, and an absence of this waste product of metabolism indicates metabolic failure.

DID YOU KNOW ?

-capnia

The suffix -capnia is derived from the Greek word kapnos, which means "smoke," referring to exhaled air. It refers specifically to the gas, carbon dioxide.

anoxia
ah NOK see ah

9.9 The suffix for "condition of oxygen" is -oxia. When the prefix that means "without or absence of" is added, the term _____ is made, which is the absence of oxygen. The constructed form of anoxia is written an/oxia.

aphonia
ah FOH nee ah

9.10 The suffix -phonia means "condition of sound or voice." Adding the prefix that means "without or absence of" forms the term _____, which is the absence of voice. The constructed form of this term is written a/phonia.

apnea
AP nee ah
a/pnea

9.11 The suffix -pnea means "breath." Adding the prefix that means "without or absence of" forms the term _____, which is the inability to breathe or inhale. This constructed term is written _____/_____.

bradypnea
brad ip NEE ah

9.12 Adding the prefix brady-, which means "slow," to the suffix for "breath" produces the term for an abnormal slowing of the breathing rhythm, _____. The constructed form of bradypnea is written brady/pnea.

bronchospasm
BRONG koh spazm

9.13 A narrowing of the airway caused by the contraction of smooth muscles in the walls of the tiny tubes known as bronchioles within the lungs is called **bronchospasm**. The constructed form of this term is bronch/o/spasm. A _____ is a common sign of the respiratory disease asthma (Frame 9.32), and may lead to the additional symptom of apnea (Frame 9.11).

Cheyne-Stokes respiration
chain stohks * ress pih RAY shun

9.14 The sign known as **Cheyne-Stokes respiration** is a repeated pattern of distressed breathing marked by a gradual increase of deep breathing, followed by shallow breathing, and apnea. _____-_____ _____ is a sign of nervous dysfunction or congestive heart failure.

dysphonia
diss FOH nee ah

9.15 The prefix *dys-* means "bad, abnormal, painful, or difficult." When used with the suffix that means "condition of sound or voice," the term _____ is formed. It is the symptom of a hoarse voice. The constructed form of dysphonia is written dys/phonia.

dyspnea
DISP nee ah

9.16 Adding the prefix *dys-* to the suffix that means "breath" forms the term _____. It is the symptom of difficult breathing, usually caused by a respiratory disease or cardiac disorder. In contrast, a normal breathing rhythm is called **eupnea** (yoop NEE ah). The constructed form of dyspnea is written dys/pnea, and eupnea is eu/pnea.

WORDS TO WATCH OUT FOR !

Terms with No Word Roots

There are many terms related to the respiratory system that contain no word root (or combining form), such as *dysphonia, dyspnea, epistaxis, hyperpnea,* and *hypopnea*. Don't let those terms confuse you when you're interpreting their meanings.

epistaxis
ep ih STAK siss

9.17 A nosebleed is clinically called **epistaxis**. It is a constructed term that literally means "dripping upon" and is written epi/staxis. An _____ can be a sign of high blood pressure, a nasal sinus infection, inhalation of a toxic irritant or particle, or a blow to the face. It is also called **rhinorrhagia** (rye noh RAH jee ah), another constructed term. The constructed form is written rhin/o/rrhagia and literally means "condition of profusely bleeding nose."

hemoptysis
hee MOP tih siss

9.18 The symptom of coughing up and spitting out blood is called _____, which combines the word root *hem* that means "blood" and the suffix *-ptysis* that means "to cough up." The constructed form of this term is written hem/o/ptysis.

hemothorax
hee moh THOH raks

9.19 A term composed of two word parts, which literally means "chest blood" is _____. It is the pooling of blood within the pleural cavity surrounding the lungs. The term is written hem/o/thorax Note that this term has no prefix or suffix; it is comprised of a combining form and a word root.

hypercapnia
HIGH per KAP nee ah

9.20 The prefixes *hyper-* and *hypo-* have opposite meanings. For example, excessive levels of carbon dioxide in the blood is a sign called _____. The opposite sign, in which carbon dioxide blood levels are deficient, or abnormally low, is **hypocapnia** (HIGH poh KAP nee ah).

hyperpnea
HIGH perp NEE ah

9.21 The sign of abnormally deep breathing or an abnormally high rate of breathing is called _____ and is common among patients suffering from the respiratory disease emphysema (Frame 9.43). Hyperpnea is also a common symptom of heart failure and anxiety (panic) attacks. By contrast, the sign of abnormally rapid breathing is more common among patients experiencing asthma (Frame 9.32), and is called **hyperventilation** (HIGH per vent ih LAY shun). The constructed form of hyperpnea is written hyper/pnea, and that of hyperventilation is hyper/ventilation.

WORDS TO WATCH OUT FOR !

-pnea and *-capnia*

Two suffixes pertaining to the respiratory system sound similar but have very different meanings: *-pnea* means "breath" and is found in numerous medical terms such as apnea, tachypnea, and orthopnea. The suffix *-capnia*, meaning "condition of carbon dioxide" and appearing in terms such as *hypocapnia* and *hypercapnia*, sounds similar but is spelled with an *i* instead of an *e*.

hypopnea
high POPP nee ah

9.22 The opposite sign of hyperpnea is abnormally shallow breathing and is called _____. This constructed term is written hypo/pnea.

hypoventilation
HIGH poh vent ih LAY shun

9.23 A reduced breathing rhythm that fails to meet the body's gas exchange demands is called _____. The constructed form of this term is hypo/ventilation.

hypoxemia
high pahk SEE mee ah

hypoxia
high PAHK see ah

9.24 Abnormally low levels of oxygen in the blood is a sign of a respiratory deficiency called **hypoxemia**. This constructed term is written hyp/ox/emia. Notice that the letter "o" in *hypo-* is dropped to make _____ easier to pronounce. This technique is also used to form the term **hypoxia**, which is written as hyp/oxia. _____ is the sign of abnormally low levels of oxygen throughout the body.

laryngospasm
lair ING goh spazm

9.25 A **laryngospasm** is the closure of the glottis, the opening into the larynx, due to muscular contractions of the throat. _____ is a constructed term written laryng/o/spasm.

orthopnea or THAHP nee ah	**9.26** The combining form *orth/o* means "straight." When the suffix for "breath" is added, the term **orthopnea** is formed. _____ is the limited ability to breathe when lying down, which becomes relieved when sitting upright. The constructed form of this term is *orth/o/pnea*.
paroxysm PAIR ahk sizm	**9.27** The term **paroxysm** refers to a sudden, sharp reoccurrence of symptoms or a convulsion. _____ is derived from the Greek word *paroxysmos*, which means "to sharpen or to irritate."
sputum SPYOO tum	**9.28** Respiratory diseases often include the symptom of **sputum**, which is an expectorated (coughed out from the lungs) matter. _____ contains mucus, inhaled particulates, and sometimes pus or blood.
tachypnea tak ihp NEE ah	**9.29** The prefix *tachy-* means "rapid or fast." When combined with the suffix that means "breath," it forms the term _____. The constructed form of this term for rapid breathing is written *tachy/pnea*.
thoracalgia thor ah KAL jee ah	**9.30** The symptom of pain in the chest region is called _____. The constructed form of this term is written *thorac/algia*. An alternate term with the same meaning is **thoracodynia** (thor AH koh DIN ee ah).

PRACTICE: Signs and Symptoms of the Respiratory System

The Right Match _____

Match the term on the left with the correct definition on the right.

_____ 1. thoracalgia

_____ 2. apnea

_____ 3. eupnea

_____ 4. bradypnea

_____ 5. paroxysm

_____ 6. hemoptysis

_____ 7. sputum

_____ 8. hemothorax

_____ 9. hypercapnia

_____ 10. hypoxemia

_____ 11. Cheyne-Stokes respiration

a. reoccurrence of a symptom or a convulsion

b. coughing up and spitting out blood

c. expectorated (spit out) matter that contains mucus, inhaled particulates, and sometimes pus and blood

d. normal breathing

e slow breathing

f. inability to breathe

g. excessive carbon dioxide blood levels

h. deficient levels of oxygen in the blood

i. pain in the chest region

j. blood in the pleural cavity

k. pattern of repeated distressed breathing marked by a gradual increase of deep breathing, followed by shallow breathing, and apnea

Break the Chain

Analyze these medical terms:

a) Separate each term into its word parts; each word part is labeled for you (**p** = prefix, **r** = root, **cf** = combining form, and **s** = suffix).

b) For the Bonus Question, write the requested definition in the blank that follows.

The first set has been completed for you as an example.

1. a) bronchospasm

   bronch/o/spasm
   cf   s

   b) *Bonus Question:* What is the definition of the suffix? *sudden involuntary muscle contraction*

2. a) dysphonia

   _____/_____
   p   s

   b) *Bonus Question:* What is the definition of the suffix? _____

3. a) dyspnea

   _____/_____
   p   s

   b) *Bonus Question:* What is the definition of the prefix? _____

4. a) epistaxis

   _____/_____
   p   s

   b) *Bonus Question:* What is the definition of the suffix? _____

5. a) hyperpnea

   _____/_____
   p   s

   b) *Bonus Question:* What is the definition of the suffix? _____

6. a) laryngospasm

   _____/__/_____
   cf   s

   b) *Bonus Question:* What is the definition of the combining form? _____

Diseases and Disorders of the Respiratory System

Following are the word parts that specifically apply to the diseases and disorders of the respiratory system that are covered in the following section. Note that the word parts are color-coded to help you identify them: prefixes are blue, combining forms are red, and suffixes are purple.

Prefix	Definition
a-	without or absence of
epi-	upon, over, above, or on top

Combining Form	Definition
atel/o	incomplete
bronch/o, bronchi/o	airway
carcin/o	cancer
coccidioid/o	Coccidioides immitis organism
coni/o	dust
cyst/o	bladder
embol/o	a plug
fibr/o	fiber
glott/o	opening into the windpipe
laryng/o	voice box, larynx
myc/o	fungus
nas/o	nose
pharyng/o	throat, pharynx
pleur/o	pleura, rib
pneum/o, pneumon/o	lung or air
pulmon/o	lung
py/o	pus
rhin/o	nose
sinus/o	cavity
sphyx/o	pulse
sten/o	narrow
thorac/o	chest, thorax
tonsill/o	almond, tonsil
trache/o	windpipe, trachea
tubercul/o	little swelling

Suffix	Definition
-al, -ic	pertaining to
-ectasis	expansion or dilation
-genic	pertaining to producing, formation, or causing
-ia, -ism, -osis	condition of
-itis	inflammation
-oma	tumor

KEY TERMS A-Z

asphyxia
ass FIK see ah

9.31 The word root meaning "pulse" is *sphyx*. It is included in the term **asphyxia**, which is the absence of respiratory ventilation, or suffocation. The constructed form of _____ is written a/sphyx/ia and literally means "condition of without pulse."

asthma
AZ mah

9.32 A condition of the lungs that is characterized by widespread narrowing of the bronchioles and formation of mucous plugs is known as **asthma**. Illustrated in Figure 9.3■, _____ produces the symptoms of wheezing, shortness of breath, chest pain, and frequent coughing during an episode, the frequency of which varies with every patient. It is regarded as an inflammatory response to an allergic substance by the lungs. According to the American Academy of Allergy, roughly 20 million Americans suffer from this chronic disease, nine million of whom are under the age of 18 years. When asthma is complicated with bronchitis (see Frame 9.35), it is referred to as **asthmatic bronchitis** (az MAHT ik * brong KYE tiss).

Figure 9.3 ■
Asthma. (a) A normal bronchiole. (b) An asthmatic bronchiole. During an asthma "attack," the bronchioles constrict to reduce the airway. Thickened mucous secretions form plugs that further reduce the airway.

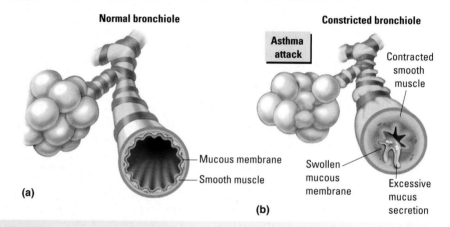

Normal bronchiole

Constricted bronchiole

Asthma attack

Contracted smooth muscle

Mucous membrane

Smooth muscle

(a)

Swollen mucous membrane

Excessive mucus secretion

(b)

DID YOU KNOW ?

Asthma

The term _asthma_ is derived from the Greek word _astma,_ which means "to pant." This panting disease is on the rise in the United States for unknown reasons. There is no cure, and the most common treatment is the use of inhalers that dilate the bronchioles.

atelectasis
at eh LEK tah siss

9.33 The alveoli in the lungs normally retain a small amount of air even during a forced expiration, which prevents them from collapsing. In the condition called **atelectasis**, trauma or disease has disabled this protective mechanism and caused the alveoli to collapse, preventing air from entering (see Frame 9.60). _____ is a constructed term composed of two word parts, _atel,_ which means "incomplete," and _-ectasis,_ which means "expansion or dilation." Its constructed form is written atel/ectasis. The common term for this condition is **collapsed lung**.

bronchiectasis
BRONG kee EK tah siss

9.34 Another term that uses the suffix -*ectasis* is _____, which is an abnormal dilation of the bronchi. The constructed form of this term is written bronchi/ectasis. It is most commonly seen in infants and young children and is relatively rare among adults.

bronchitis
brong KYE tiss

9.35 Recall that the suffix that means "inflammation" is -*itis*. This will be used in many terms in this section. Inflammation of the bronchi is called _____. The constructed form of this term is bronch/itis. Acute bronchitis is usually associated with a respiratory tract infection, with the symptoms of coughing, chest pain, and sputum. Chronic bronchitis is usually caused by smoking, although allergies may cause this condition in some people. Symptoms of chronic bronchitis include chest pain, difficult breathing, and a hoarse cough with sputum.

bronchogenic carcinoma
brong koh JENN ik *
kar sih NOH mah

9.36 An aggressive form of cancer arising from cells within the bronchi is known as **bronchogenic carcinoma** (Figure 9.4■). The constructed form of this term is written bronch/o/genic carcin/oma. In 2005, there were approximately 92,000 cases of _____ _____ in men and 80,000 cases in women in the United States. Although it is commonly referred to as lung cancer, it is different because the cells arise from the bronchi rather than the soft tissues of the lung. Cancer arising from the soft tissues of the lung is more aggressive and life threatening (Frame 9.47). However, bronchogenic carcinoma can also become fatal by spreading into the soft lung tissues and by blocking the major airways.

Figure 9.4 ■
Bronchogenic carcinoma. (a) An illustration of a sectioned lung that contains two tumors associated with a bronchial wall.
(b) A chest X-ray that reveals the tumor location.
Source: Phototake NYC.

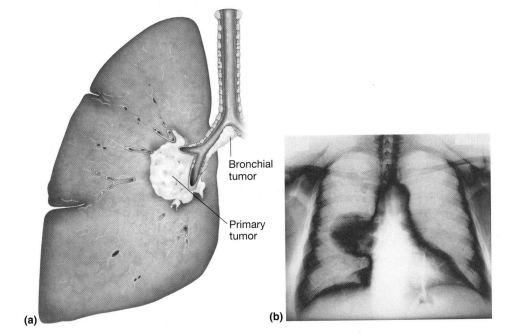

Bronchial tumor

Primary tumor

(a)   (b)

bronchopneumonia
BRONG koh noo MOH nee ah

9.37 An acute inflammatory disease involving the bronchioles and the alveoli is called **bronchopneumonia**. This constructed term is written bronch/o/pneumon/ia. It is usually caused by a bacterial infection that involves the bronchi and the soft tissue of the lungs, causing the alveoli to fill with fluid (called exudate) that leads to the loss of air space. _____ often occurs in a lobe of a lung, lending it the alternate name of **lobar pneumonia**.

chronic obstructive pulmonary disease

9.38 An obstruction of air flow to and from the lungs is a consequence of several forms of pulmonary disease, including chronic bronchitis (Frame 9.35), bronchospasm (Frame 9.13), cystic fibrosis (Frame 9.42), and emphysema (Frame 9.43). The general term for these forms of pulmonary obstruction is **chronic obstructive pulmonary disease**, abbreviated **COPD**. _____ _____ _____ _____ is usually persistent until death.

coccidioidomycosis
kok SIDD ee oy doh mye KOH siss

9.39 The combining form *myc/o* means "fungus." A fungal infection of the upper respiratory tract, which often spreads to the lungs and other organs, is called **coccidioidomycosis**. This constructed term is written coccidioid/o/myc/osis and is based on the name of the causative organism, *Coccidioides immitis*. Also called **valley fever** due to its place of origin in the San Joaquin Valley of California, _____ is caused by inhaling spores of the fungal pathogen.

coryza
koh RYE zah

9.40 The common cold is caused by a virus that infects the upper respiratory tract causing local inflammation. It is clinically called **coryza**, which is derived from the Greek word for runny nose, *koryza*. Because a cold is an acute illness, it is often called acute _____. It is also called **rhinitis** (rye NYE tiss), due to the inflammation. This constructed term is written rhin/itis.

croup
kroop

9.41 A viral infectious disease that is relatively common among infants and young children produces a characteristic hoarse cough with a sound resembling the bark of a dog. Commonly known as **croup**, the cough results from the acute obstruction of the larynx. The clinical term for _____ is **laryngotracheobronchitis** (lair RING goh TRAY kee oh brong KYE tiss), abbreviated **LTB**. The constructed form of this term reveals six word parts and is written laryng/o/trache/o/bronch/itis.

cystic fibrosis
SISS tik * fye BROH siss

9.42 A hereditary disease characterized by excess mucus production in the respiratory tract, digestive tract, and elsewhere is called **cystic fibrosis** and is abbreviated **CF**. This constructed term is written cyst/ic fibr/osis. _____ _____ literally means "condition of fibrous cysts (bladders)," which were early observations by 19th-century physicians who examined postmortem lungs and observed pockets of trapped mucus. CF causes difficulty breathing because of the dense mucus that obstructs the airways. It strikes roughly 1 in 2,500 children and is commonly fatal before the age of 30 years due to lung destruction.

emphysema
em fih SEE mah

9.43 A chronic lung disease characterized by the symptoms of dyspnea (Frame 9.16), a chronic cough, formation of a barrel chest due to labored breathing, and a gradual deterioration caused by chronic hypoxemia (Frame 9.24) and hypercapnia (Frame 9.20) is called **emphysema**. It is a Greek word that means "to inflate." The symptoms arise when the alveolar walls deteriorate, resulting in a loss of elasticity that causes an inability to breathe. Smoking is the leading cause of _____. It is illustrated in Figure 9.5■.

Figure 9.5 ■
Emphysema. (a) Illustration comparing normal lungs and emphysemic lungs. The inserts illustrate how alveolar walls deteriorate in emphysema, reducing their surface area by convergence.
(b) Typical appearance of a patient with emphysema. Characteristic signs include reduced weight, a barrel chest, and a drawn facial appearance.

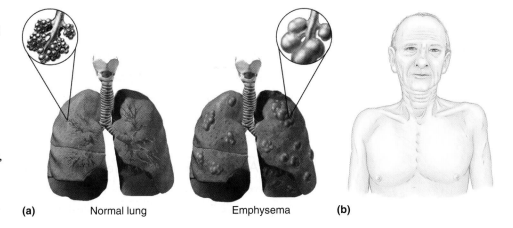

(a)   Normal lung   Emphysema   (b)

epiglottitis
ep ih glah TYE tiss

9.44 Inflammation of the epiglottis is called **epiglottitis**. This constructed term is written epi/glott/itis. _____ is usually caused by a bacterial infection that spreads from the throat to the epiglottis and can be very serious in children due to the danger of airway obstruction.

laryngitis
LAIR in JYE tiss

9.45 Inflammation of the larynx is called _____. The constructed form of this term is written laryng/itis. It is characterized by the symptom of dysphonia (Frame 9.15).

pneumothorax
NOO moh THOH raks

9.56 A **pneumothorax** is the abnormal presence of air or gas within the pleural cavity (Figure 9.6■). It is caused by a penetrating injury to the chest or severe coughing and leads to atelectasis (Frame 9.33). _____ is a constructed term that is written pneum/o/thorax. *Thorax* is a noun that is used as a suffix in this term.

Figure 9.6 ■
Pneumothorax, caused by a penetrating chest wound.

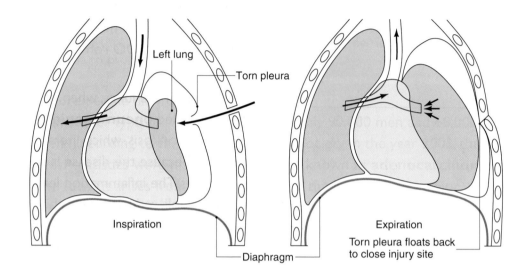

Left lung

Torn pleura

Inspiration

Diaphragm

Expiration

Torn pleura floats back to close injury site

pulmonary edema
PULL mon air ee * eh DEE mah

9.57 The accumulation of fluid within the tiny air sacs within the lungs (the alveoli) is a response to infection or injury and is called **pulmonary edema.** The most common cause of _____ _____ is cardiovascular disease, including congestive heart failure. It is often associated with pneumonitis (Frame 9.55). Pulmonary is a constructed term that is written as pulmon/ary.

pulmonary embolism
PULL mon air ee * EM boh lizm

9.58 A blood clot that moves along with the bloodstream is called an **embolus** (EM boh lus). It is derived from the Greek word *embolos,* which means "a plug." An embolus can become dangerous if it lodges in a blood vessel, causing an occlusion that blocks the flow of blood to form an **embolism.** A blockage in the pulmonary circulation by a blood clot is called a _____ _____. Abbreviated **PE**, it is a complication to an injury or surgery elsewhere in the body. Pulmonary embolism is a constructed term that is written as pulmon/ary embol/ism.

pyothorax pye oh THOH raks	**9.59** The presence of pus in the pleural cavity is called **pyothorax**. This constructed term is written py/o/thorax. _____ is also known as **empyema** (em pye EE mah).
respiratory distress syndrome	**9.60** A respiratory disease that is characterized by atelectasis (Frame 9.33) is known as **respiratory distress syndrome (RDS)**. It occurs in two different forms. One form affects newborns and is called **neonatal** _____ _____ _____ (**NRDS**), or **hyaline membrane disease (HMD)**. It is caused by insufficient surfactant, a substance produced by alveolar cells that prevents atelectasis. The second form affects adults and is called **adult** (or **acute**) **respiratory distress syndrome (ARDS)**. It is caused by severe lung infections or injury.
rhinitis rye NYE tiss	**9.61** Inflammation of the mucous membrane lining the nasal cavity is called **rhinitis**. The constructed form of this term is written rhin/itis. Acute _____ is one of the clinical terms for the common cold (see Frame 9.40).
severe acute respiratory syndrome	**9.62** A severe, rapid-onset viral infection resulting in respiratory distress that includes acute lung inflammation, alveolar damage, and atelectasis (Frame 9.33) is often referred to by its abbreviation, **SARS**. The long form is _____ _____ _____ _____. It is usually caused by the influenza virus and can become fatal.
sinusitis sigh nuss EYE tiss	**9.63** Similar to rhinitis, the condition known as _____ is an inflammation of the mucous membranes. It affects the nasal cavity and also the paranasal sinuses that are located within the frontal, sphenoid, ethmoid, and maxillary bones of the skull. The constructed form of this term is written sinus/itis.
tonsillitis TAHN sill EYE tiss	**9.64** Inflammation of one or more tonsils is called _____. This constructed term is written tonsill/itis.

tracheitis
tray kee EYE tiss

tracheostenosis
TRAY kee oh steh NOH siss

9.65 Inflammation of the trachea is called _____. The constructed form of this term is written trache/itis. It is usually caused by a bacterial infection that travels downward from the larynx. The combining form that means "narrow" is sten/o. Inflammation leads to a narrowing of the trachea, known as _____. Also constructed of word parts, it can be written trache/o/sten/osis.

tuberculosis
too BER kyoo LOH siss

9.66 Infection of the lungs by the bacterium _Mycobacterium tuberculosis_ causes the disease _____, abbreviated **TB.** This term is constructed of two word parts, tubercul/osis, and literally means "condition of a little swelling." The little swelling, or tubercle, is a colony of bacteria within the soft tissue of the lung that forms a hardened barrier, preventing white blood cells from entering and destroying the bacteria. In time, the bacterial colonies multiply throughout the lung until necrosis and inflammation overwhelm the function of gas exchange.

upper respiratory infection

9.67 A generalized infection of the upper respiratory tract (nasal cavity, pharynx, and larynx) is called an _____ _____ _____, or **URI.**

PRACTICE: Diseases and Disorders of the Respiratory System

The Right Match

Match the term on the left with the correct definition on the right.

_____ 1. emphysema

_____ 2. pertussis

_____ 3. asthma

_____ 4. severe acute respiratory syndrome

_____ 5. croup

_____ 6. atelectasis

_____ 7. tracheitis

_____ 8. tuberculosis

_____ 9. coryza

_____ 10. pyothorax

a. severe viral infection resulting in respiratory distress that includes lung inflammation, alveolar damage, and atelectasis

b. condition of pus in the chest

c. inflammation of the trachea

d. collapsed lung

e. also known as whooping cough

f. clinical term for the common cold

g. condition of the lungs that is characterized by widespread narrowing of the bronchioles and formation of mucous plugs

h. chronic lung disease named by a Greek word that means "to inflate"

i. a barking cough caused by an acute obstruction in the larynx among children

j. a highly contagious bacterial disease

Linkup

Link the word parts in the list to create the terms that match the definitions. You may use word parts more than once. Remember to add combining vowels when needed—and that some terms do not use any combining vowel. The first one is completed as an example.

Prefix	Combining Form	Suffix
a-	bronch/o	-ary
dia-	coni/o	-cele
neo-	embol/o	-ectasis
	legionell/o	-ia
	phragmat/o	-ism
	pleur/o	-itis
	pneum/o	-osis
	pulmon/o	-plasm
	py/o	
	sinus/o	
	sphyx/o	
	sten/o	
	thorac/o	
	tonsill/o	
	trache/o	
	tubercul/o	

Definition

Term

1. **inflammation of the pleurae; also called pleurisy**   *pleuritis*

2. inflammation of the mucous membranes of the nasal cavity and also the paranasal sinuses   _____

3. dilation of the bronchi   _____

4. narrowing of the trachea   _____

5. the absence of respiratory ventilation, or suffocation   _____

6. inflammation of a tonsil   _____

7. tumor of the lung   _____

8. inflammation of the lungs caused by the chronic inhalation of fine particles, which leads to the formation of a fibrotic tissue around the alveoli   _____

9. infection of the lungs by the bacterium *Mycobacterium tuberculosis*   _____

10. pneumonia caused by the bacterium *Legionella pneumophilia*   _____

11. blockage in the pulmonary circulation by a mobile blood clot   _____

Treatments, Procedures, and Devices of the Respiratory System

Following are the word parts that specifically apply to the treatments, procedures, and devices of the respiratory system that are covered in the following section. Note that the word parts are color-coded to help you identify them: prefixes are blue, combining forms are red, and suffixes are purple.

Prefix	Definition
anti-	against or opposite of
endo-	within

Combining Form	Definition
aden/o	gland
angi/o	blood vessel
bronch/o	airway
dilat/o	to widen
laryng/o	voice box, larynx
lob/o	round part, lobe
ox/i	oxygen
pleur/o	pleura, rib
pneum/o, pneumon/o	lung, airway
pulmon/o	lung
rhin/o	nose
spir/o	breathe
thorac/o	chest, thorax
trache/o	windpipe, trachea

Suffix	Definition
-al	pertaining to
-ary	pertaining to
-centesis	surgical puncture
-ectomy	surgical removal or excision
-gram	a record or image
-graphy	recording process
-ion	process
-meter	measuring device
-metry	measurement
-oid	resembling
-plasty	surgical repair
-scopy	process of viewing
-stomy	surgical creation of an opening
-tomy	incision or to cut

KEY TERMS A-Z

acid-fast bacilli smear

9.68 A clinical test performed on sputum to identify the presence of bacteria that react to acid is called **acid-fast bacilli smear**, abbreviated **AFB**. An _____-_____ _____ _____ is frequently used with chest X-rays to confirm a diagnosis of tuberculosis.

adenoidectomy
ADD eh noyd EK toh mee

9.69 A pharyngeal tonsil is called an **adenoid** (ADD eh noyd). This constructed term, written aden/oid, means "resembling a gland." In some cases, a chronically inflamed adenoid must be surgically removed to avoid complications including obstruction of the nasopharynx. Remember that the suffix -ectomy means "surgical removal." So, combine that with the term adenoid, and it creates the name for this procedure, _____. The constructed form of this term reveals three word parts and is written aden/oid/ectomy.

antihistamine an tih HISS tah meen	**9.70** A histamine is a compound released by certain cells in response to allergens that cause bronchial constriction and blood vessel dilation. The dilation of blood vessels increases the movement of plasma out of capillaries and into the interstitial space, resulting in the swelling of tissues with fluid, or **edema**. A therapeutic drug that inhibits the effects of histamines is called an _____.
arterial blood gases	**9.71** A clinical test on arterial blood to identify the levels of oxygen and carbon dioxide is called _____ _____ _____. It is abbreviated **ABGs**.
aspiration ass pih RAY shun	**9.72** The removal of fluid, air, or foreign bodies with suction is a procedure called **aspiration**. _____ is derived from the Latin word *aspiratus*, which means "to breathe on."
auscultation aw skull TAY shun	**9.73** A procedure that involves listening to sounds within the body as part of a physical examination, often with the aid of a stethoscope, is called **auscultation**. The term _____ is derived from the Latin word *ausculto*, which means "to listen to." As part of a physical examination that addresses the respiratory system, auscultation involves listening to chest sounds during inhalation and exhalation (Figure 9.7■). Abnormal sounds include wheezing, a sign of asthma (Frame 9.32); rales, a sign of pulmonary edema (Frame 9.57) or atelectasis (Frame 9.33); and gurgles, a sign of pneumonia (Frame 9.54).

Figure 9.7 ■
Auscultation. The stethoscope is pressed against the chest wall to listen for sound waves associated with breathing.

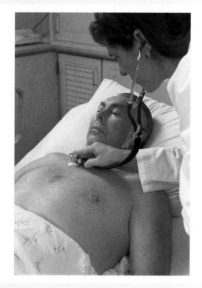

bronchodilation BRONG koh dye LAY shun	**9.74** A procedure that uses a bronchodilating agent in an inhaler to reduce bronchial constriction in an effort to open the airway and improve breathing is called _____. The constructed form of this term is written bronch/o/dilat/ion, which means "process of widening the airway."

bronchography
brong KOG rah fee

9.75 The suffix *-graphy* means "recording process." The X-ray imaging of the bronchi is called _____. This procedure produces an X-ray image of the bronchi called a **bronchogram** (BRONG koh gram) and uses a contrast medium to highlight the bronchial tree. In many respiratory clinics, bronchography is being replaced by bronchoscopy (Frame 9.76) and CAT scans.

bronchoscopy
brong KOSS koh pee

9.76 Remember that the suffix *-scopy* means "process of viewing." The evaluation of the bronchi using a flexible fiber-optic tube mounted with a small lens at one end and attached to an eyepiece and computer monitor at the other end is called _____. This constructed term is written bronch/o/scopy. The instrument is a modified endoscope, known as a **bronchoscope** (BRONG koh skope), which is inserted through the nose to observe the trachea and bronchi (Figure 9.8■).

Figure 9.8 ■
Bronchoscopy.

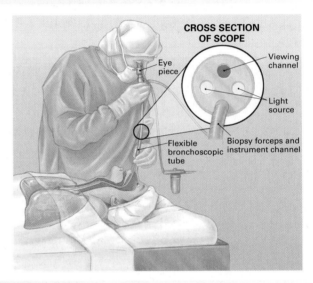

chest CT scan

9.77 Diagnostic imaging of the chest by a computed tomography (CT) instrument is called _____ _____ _____ (Figure 9.9■). The procedure is used to diagnose respiratory tumors, pleural effusion, pleuritis, and other diseases by providing 3-D images of the thoracic cavity.

Figure 9.9 ■
Chest CT scan.
Source: Getty Images, Inc.—Stone Allstock.

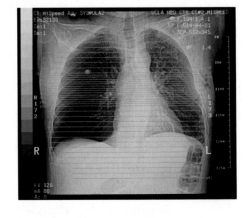

9.78 An X-ray image of the thoracic cavity that is used to diagnose tuberculosis, tumors, and other conditions of the lungs is called a

chest X-ray

_____ _____ (Figure 9.10■). Abbreviated **CXR**, it is also called a **chest radiograph**.

Figure 9.10 ■
Chest X-ray. (a) A patient undergoing the chest X-ray procedure.
Source: Bachman/Photo Researchers, Inc.
(b) An example of a normal chest X-ray.
Source: © Dorling Kindersley.

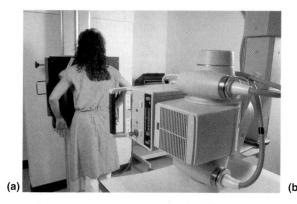
(a)

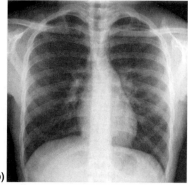
(b)

ears, nose, and throat specialist

9.79 A physician specializing in the treatment of upper respiratory tract disease is called an **ENT**, which is the abbreviation of _____

_____ _____ _____ _____.

Alternate terms include **otolaryngologist** (OH toh LAIR in GAHL oh jist), **otonasolaryngologist** (OH toh NAY so LAIR in GAHL oh jist), and **otorhinolaryngologist** (oh toh RYE no LAIR in GAHL oh jist).

endotracheal

9.80 Insertion of a noncollapsible breathing tube into the trachea through the nose or mouth is called **endotracheal intubation** (EHN doh TRAY kee al * in too BAY shun). It is performed to open the airway or, if the patient is comatose, to keep the airway open. _____ is a constructed term written endo/trache/al, which means "pertaining to within the trachea."

expectorant
ek SPEK toh rant

9.81 A drug that breaks up mucus and promotes the coughing reflex to expel the mucus is called an **expectorant**. The term _____ is derived from the Latin word, *expectoro* which means "spit out of the chest."

incentive spirometry
in SEHN tiv * spy RAH meh tree

9.82 A valuable postoperative breathing therapy is called **incentive spirometry**. It involves the use of a portable **spirometer** (Frame 9.93) to promote deeper breathing to improve lung expansion after an operation. Usually self-administered, _____ _____ reduces pulmonary complications and helps to correct atelectasis.

laryngectomy
lair in JEK toh mee

9.83 Surgical removal of the larynx is performed during a _____. The constructed form of this term is written laryng/ectomy. It is often required as a treatment for laryngeal cancer and is usually followed by training or insertion of a device to enable the patient to communicate orally. Laryngectomy patients have a permanent **tracheostomy** (Frame 9.102).

laryngoscopy
lair ring GOSS koh pee

9.84 A diagnostic procedure that uses a modified endoscope, called a **laryngoscope** (lair RING goh skope), to visually examine the larynx is called _____.

laryngotracheotomy
lair ring goh TRAY kee OTT oh mee

9.85 A surgical incision into the larynx and trachea is usually performed to provide a secondary opening for inspiration and expiration, allowing air to bypass the upper respiratory tract. Remember that the suffix -tomy means "incision or to cut." Combine that with the combining forms for larynx and trachea, and you form the term for this procedure, _____. The constructed form of this term reveals five word parts, and is written laryng/o/trache/o/tomy.

lobectomy
loh BEK toh mee

9.86 Surgical removal of a single lobe of a lung is sometimes required as a treatment for lung cancer, if the tumor is isolated in one lobe. The procedure is called _____. It may involve the removal of more than one lobe if required. Lobectomy is a constructed term, written lob/ectomy.

mechanical ventilation

9.87 A medical treatment to provide supplemental oxygen to patients in respiratory distress is called **mechanical ventilation.** It provides assisted breathing using a **ventilator**, which pushes air into the patient's airway (Figure 9.11■). _____ _____ is often used by a respiratory therapist in a clinical setting or by an emergency medical technician at the site of injury and in transit to a hospital.

Figure 9.11 ■
Mechanical ventilation. The ventilator is an instrument that pushes air through a tube that is connected to the airway, providing an artificial means of ventilation. (a) A positive pressure ventilator.
(b) A patient fitted with a face mask, which is connected to a positive pressure ventilator.

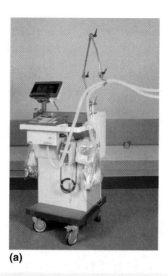
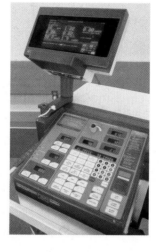

(a)

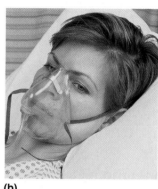

(b)

nebulizer
NEBB yoo lye zer

9.88 A device used to convert a liquid medication to a mist and deliver it to the lungs with the aid of deep inhalation is called a **nebulizer**. The term _____ is derived from the Latin word *nebula*, which means "fog."

oximetry
ok SIM eh tree

9.89 The suffix *-metry* means "measurement," and the combining form that means "oxygen" is *ox/i*. Therefore, the procedure that measures oxygen levels in the blood using an instrument called an **oximeter** (ok SIM eh ter) is called _____. The constructed form of this term is ox/i/metry. A small, handheld oximeter that provides a digital readout of oxygen levels by noninvasive physical contact with a finger is called a **pulse oximeter** (Figure 9.12■).

Figure 9.12 ■
Pulse oximetry. The small device provides a digital readout of oxygen levels in the blood.

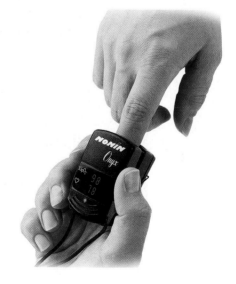

pleurocentesis
ploor oh sehn TEE siss

9.90 The suffix -*centesis* means "surgical puncture." The surgical puncture and aspiration of fluid from the pleural cavity is a diagnostic procedure called _____. After aspiration, the fluid is analyzed for the presence of bacteria and white blood cells, the presence of which indicates pleuritis (Frame 9.52). Pleurocentesis is a constructed term, written pleur/o/centesis. It is also called **thoracentesis** (Frame 9.98) or **thoracocentesis**.

pneumonectomy
NOO moh NEK toh mee

9.91 Many terms in this section have used the suffix that means "surgical removal or excision," -*ectomy*. A word root that means "lung" is *pneumon*. Therefore, surgical removal of a lung is called _____, or **pneumectomy** (noo MEK toh mee). It is performed as a radical treatment for lung cancer, in which tumors have progressed throughout one lung. Pneumonectomy is a constructed term, written pneumon/ectomy. The constructed form of pneumectomy is written pneum/ectomy. If the surgery is limited to the removal of a single lobe, recall that the procedure is called a **lobectomy** (Frame 9.86).

pulmonary angiography
PULL mon air ee * AN jee OG rah fee

9.92 A diagnostic procedure that evaluates the blood circulation of the lungs is called **pulmonary angiography**. In this procedure, X-ray images are taken of the lungs following the injection of a contrast medium into the pulmonary circulation. _____ _____ is a constructed term represented as pulmon/ary angi/o/graphy, which literally means "recording of blood vessel pertaining to lung."

pulmonary function tests

9.93 A series of diagnostic tests performed to determine the cause of lung disease by evaluating lung capacity through the use of **spirometry** (Frame 9.82) is called _____ _____ _____. Spirometry involves breathing into a tube connected to an instrument, called a **spirometer**. Both are terms that use the combining form that means "breathe," *spir/o*. The spirometer measures the amount of air inhaled and exhaled after a normal breathing cycle, called tidal volume (TV), the amount of air inhaled and exhaled during a forced expiration, called vital capacity (VC), and other values shown in Figure 9.13■.

Figure 9.13 ■

Pulmonary function test: spirometry. (a) Normal respiratory volumes, as measured during spirometry. A patient's spirometry data is compared to this chart to identify breathing deficiencies.
(b) Illustration of a patient expiring into a spirometer, which measures air volume.

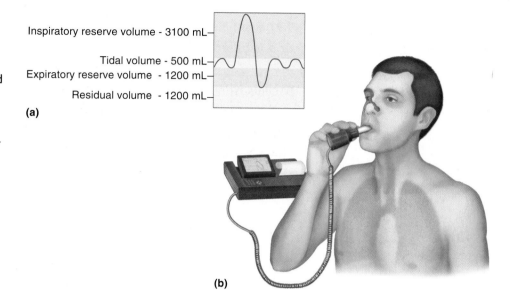

Inspiratory reserve volume - 3100 mL
Tidal volume - 500 mL
Expiratory reserve volume - 1200 mL
Residual volume - 1200 mL

(a)

(b)

pulmonologist
PUL moh NAHL oh jist

9.94 A physician specializing in the treatment of diseases affecting the lower respiratory tract, particularly the lungs, is called a pulmonary specialist or _____.

resuscitation
ree SUSS ih TAY shun

9.95 Artificial respiration that is used to restore breathing is known as pulmonary **resuscitation**. The most common form is cardiopulmonary _____, or **CPR**, which combines chest compression with artificial breathing.

DID YOU KNOW?

Resuscitation

The term *resuscitation* is derived from the Latin word *resuscito*, which means "to rise up again" or "revive." Its present meaning refers to any procedure that involves a restoration of breathing and includes the popular technique of compressing the chest and heart called cardiopulmonary resuscitation (CPR). It also includes mouth-to-mouth resuscitation, in which air is blown into the patient's mouth while holding the nose, and the Heimlich maneuver, during which an obstruction (usually food) may be dislodged by reaching around a standing patient and pushing upward on the diaphragm to force an expulsion of air.

rhinoplasty
RYE noh plass tee

9.96 Add the combining form that means "nose" (*rhin/o*) to the suffix that means "surgical repair" to form the term _____, which is the surgical repair of the nose. This constructed term is written rhin/o/plasty. Although this procedure is commonly used to modify the external appearance of the nose during cosmetic surgery, it may include **septoplasty** (SEP toh plass tee), during which deviation of the nasal septum is corrected to improve breathing.

TB skin test

9.97 A simple skin test to determine the presence of a tuberculosis infection is called a **TB skin test**. During a _____ _____ _____, a purified protein derivative (PPD) sample of the TB bacillus is injected beneath the epidermis of the skin (intradermal injection). A reddened, swollen skin lesion at the injection site a few days later indicates a previous exposure (Figure 9.14■) and requires follow-up with a chest X-ray. It is also called **PPD skin test** and **Mantoux skin test** (after the French physician Charles Mantoux).

Figure 9.14 ■
TB skin test.

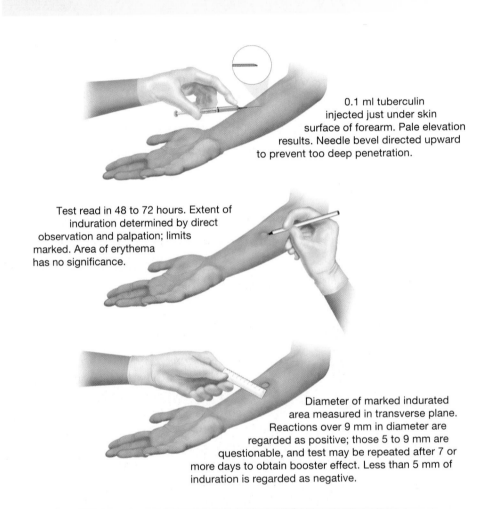

0.1 ml tuberculin injected just under skin surface of forearm. Pale elevation results. Needle bevel directed upward to prevent too deep penetration.

Test read in 48 to 72 hours. Extent of induration determined by direct observation and palpation; limits marked. Area of erythema has no significance.

Diameter of marked indurated area measured in transverse plane. Reactions over 9 mm in diameter are regarded as positive; those 5 to 9 mm are questionable, and test may be repeated after 7 or more days to obtain booster effect. Less than 5 mm of induration is regarded as negative.

thoracentesis
THOR ah sehn TEE siss

9.98 The suffix that means "surgical puncture" is -*centesis*. Surgical puncture using a needle and syringe into the thoracic cavity to aspirate pleural fluid for diagnosis or treatment is called a _____. It is also called **thoracocentesis** (THOR ah koh sehn TEE siss) or **pleurocentesis** (Frame 9.90). Thoracentesis is a constructed term written thora/centesis; note that, in this term, the *co* is removed from the combining form *thorac/o* for ease of pronunciation.

thoracostomy
THOR ah KOSS toh mee

9.99 The suffix *-stomy* means "surgical creation of an opening." Surgical puncture into the chest cavity, usually for the insertion of a drainage or air tube, is called a _____. The constructed form of this term is written thorac/o/stomy. The procedure is often termed "placing a chest tube."

thoracotomy
THOR ah KOTT oh mee

9.100 Recall the suffix that means "incision." Add this to the combining form that means "chest, thorax," and you form the term _____, which is a surgical incision into the chest wall. The constructed form of this term is thorac/o/tomy. The procedure is often used to treat pleural effusion (Frame 9.51) by draining the excess fluid from the pleural cavity.

tracheoplasty
TRAY kee oh PLASS tee

9.101 The suffix *-plasty* means "surgical repair." Surgical repair of the trachea is called _____. The constructed form of this term reveals three word parts and is written trache/o/plasty.

tracheostomy
TRAY kee OSS toh mee

9.102 Recall the suffix that means "surgical creation of an opening." Surgical creation of an opening into the trachea, usually for the insertion of a breathing tube, is called _____. This constructed term is written trache/o/stomy. The procedure is shown in Figure 9.15■.

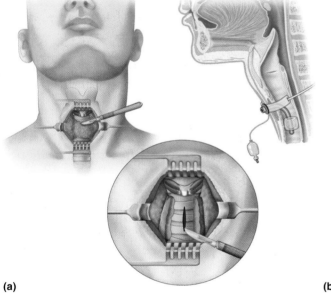
(a)

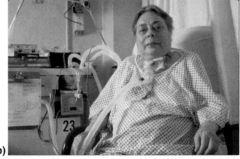
(b)

Figure 9.15 ■

Tracheostomy. (a) A tracheotomy, or incision into the trachea, is performed to create an opening into the trachea as shown in this series of illustrations. (b) A patient with a tracheostomy uses a breathing tube connected to a mechanical ventilator in this photograph.
Source: Phototake NYC.

tracheotomy TRAY kee OTT oh mee	**9.103** Surgical incision into the trachea is a required part of a tracheostomy (Frame 9.102). The incision is called a _____. The constructed form of this term is written trache/o/tomy.
ventilation-perfusion scanning	**9.104** A diagnostic tool that uses nuclear medicine, or the use of radioactive material, to evaluate pulmonary function is called **ventilation-perfusion scanning**. Abbreviated **VPS**, it can identify pulmonary embolism (Frame 9.58) and pulmonary edema (Frame 9.57). _____ - _____ _____ is also called **lung scan** and **V/Q scan**.

PRACTICE: Treatments, Procedures, and Devices of the Respiratory System

The Right Match

Match the term on the left with the correct definition on the right.

_____ 1. pulmonary function tests

_____ 2. pulse oximeter

_____ 3. bronchodilation

_____ 4. arterial blood gases

_____ 5. TB skin test

_____ 6. auscultation

_____ 7. ventilation-perfusion scanning

_____ 8. nebulizer

_____ 9. pulmonary angiography

_____ 10. expectorant

a. breaks up mucus and promotes coughing

b. also called PPD skin test and Mantoux skin test

c. oxygen and carbon dioxide blood levels

d. device used to convert a liquid medication to a mist and deliver it to the lungs

e. physical examination that includes listening to sounds within the body

f. a blood oxygen measuring device that reads oxygen levels by noninvasive physical contact with a finger

g. procedure that uses a bronchodilating agent in an inhaler to reduce bronchial constriction

h. X-ray of lung blood vessels

i. diagnostic tool that uses nuclear medicine, or the use of radioactive material, to evaluate pulmonary function

j. use of spirometry to evaluate lung function

Break the Chain

Analyze these medical terms:

    a)   Separate each term into its word parts; each word part is labeled for you (**p** = prefix, **r** = root, **cf** = combining form, and **s** = suffix).

    b)   For the Bonus Question, write the requested definition in the blank that follows.

1. a) tracheotomy   _____/__/_____
                                    cf   s

    b) *Bonus Question:* What is the definition of the suffix? _____

2. a) thoracentesis   _____/_____
                               r   s

    b) *Bonus Question:* What is the definition of the word root? _____

3. a) pneumonectomy   _____/_____
                               r   s

    b) *Bonus Question:* What is the definition of the word root? _____

4. a) bronchoscopy   _____/__/_____
                                  cf   s

    b) *Bonus Question:* What is the definition of the suffix? _____

5. a) adenoidectomy   _____/_____/_____
                               r   s   s

    b) *Bonus Question:* What is the definition of the first suffix? _____

6. a) bronchodilation   _____/__/_____/__
                               cf   r   s

    b) *Bonus Question:* What is the definition of the suffix? _____

7. a) lobectomy   _____/_____
                               r   s

    b) *Bonus Question:* What is the definition of the word root? _____

8. a) rhinoplasty   _____/__/_____
                                cf   s

    b) *Bonus Question:* What is the definition of the combining form? _____

9. a) septoplasty   _____/__/_____
                                cf   s

    b) *Bonus Question:* What is the definition of the suffix? _____

Abbreviations of the Respiratory System

The abbreviations that are associated with the respiratory system are summarized here. Study these abbreviations, and review them in the exercise that follows.

Abbreviation	Definition
ABGs	arterial blood gases
ARDS	adult (acute) respiratory distress syndrome
AFB	acid-fast bacilli
CF	cystic fibrosis
COPD	chronic obstructive pulmonary disease
CPR	cardiopulmonary resuscitation
CXR	chest X-ray
HMD	hyaline membrane disease

Abbreviation	Definition
LTB	laryngotracheobronchitis
NRDS	neonatal respiratory distress syndrome
PE	pulmonary embolism
PPD	purified protein derivative
RDS	respiratory distress syndrome
SARS	severe acute respiratory syndrome
TB	tuberculosis
URI	upper respiratory infection
VPS or V/Q scan	ventilation-perfusion scanning

PRACTICE: Abbreviations

Fill in the blanks with the abbreviation or the complete medical term.

Abbreviation

1. _____

2. HMD

3. _____

4. ARDS

5. _____

6. CPR

7. _____

8. URI

Medical Term

laryngotracheobronchitis

_____

tuberculosis

_____

chest X-ray

_____

cystic fibrosis

_____

▶▶▶▶▶ Chapter Review

Word Building

Construct medical terms from the following meanings. (Some are built from word parts, some are not.) The first question has been completed as an example.

1. inflammation of the larynx   *laryngitis*_____

2. absence of oxygen   _____oxia

3. inflammation of the bronchi   bronch_____

4. respiratory failure characterized by atelectasis syndrome   respiratory _____

5. physical exam that includes listening to body sounds   _____ (do this one on your own!)

6. deficient oxygen levels in the blood   hyp_____

7. difficulty breathing   _____pnea

8. excessive carbon dioxide levels in the blood   hyper_____

9. dilation of the bronchi   bronchi _____

10. lung inflammation due to dust inhalation   _____coniosis

11. cancer in the cells within the bronchi   bronchogenic _____

12. an inherited disease of excessive mucus production   cystic _____

13. inflammation of the trachea   trache_____

14. the absence of respiratory ventilation   _____sphyxia

15. X-ray image of the bronchi   broncho_____

16. surgical puncture and aspiration of fluid from the pleural cavity   pleuro_____

17. measurement of oxygen levels in the blood   oxi_____

▶▶▶▶▶ Clinical Application Exercises

Medical Report

Read the following medical report, then answer the questions that follow.

University Hospital

5500 University Avenue
Metropolis, TX

Phone: (211) 594-4000
Fax: (211) 594-4001

Medical Consultation: ENT

Date: 2/15/2008

Patient: Geoffrey Piscotti

Patient Complaint: Dyspnea, leading to thoracalgia. General malaise, nasal congestion, and nasal discharge with occasional epistaxis.

History: 6-year-old male with no prior medical history.

Family History: Father, 37 years, 9th-grade teacher in public school system. Mother, 32 years, respiratory therapist in downtown clinic. No surgeries or major medical concerns.

Allergies: None.

Evidences: Initial laryngotracheobronchitis, followed later by general malaise and coughing. TB skin test positive; TB confirmed with blood test. Active form confirmed with chest scan.

Treatment: Inpatient care with oxygen assist and antibiotic cocktail IV drip. Follow with long-term oral AT cocktail. Inform County Health and CDC of incident and potential exposures.

Maria S. Zayas, M.D.

---

1. What complaints support the diagnosis? _____

_____

2. Based on the family history, how do you think the TB infection originated? _____

_____

3. Although the patient is treated with antibiotic therapy, what factor will most likely threaten full

recovery? _____

_____

Medical Report Case Study

The following Case Study provides further discussion regarding the patient in the medical report. Fill in the blanks with the correct terms. Choose your answers from the following list of terms. (Note that some terms may be used more than once.)

acid-fast	chest X-rays	laryngotracheobronchitis
bronchodilating	coryza (or acute rhinitis)	tuberculosis (TB)

Geoffrey Piscotti, a 6-year-old boy with a previous healthy history, was admitted into an emergency clinic when his mother became concerned about his respiratory function. She explained that he had come home from school three weeks ago with a common cold, or (a) _____. He began coughing violently shortly afterward, preventing him from sleeping. Physical exams showed an acute inflammation of the larynx, trachea, and bronchi, indicating the acute condition known as (b) _____, which was bacterial in origin. Following the prescribed use of antibiotic therapy and the use of inhaled (c) _____ agents to reduce bronchial constriction, the patient recovered initially. Several months passed and then the coughing returned and the boy complained of low energy. Following a (d) _____ skin test and a sputum test that included (e) _____-_____ bacilli, positive results indicated an active lung infection known as (f) _____. TB was confirmed with the use of radiographic images of the thorax, or (g) _____ _____. The course of treatment included a cocktail of antibiotics administered over a six-month period.

▶▶▶▶ Key Terms Double-Check

Remember that the chapter's key terms appeared alphabetically throughout this chapter. This exercise helps you to check your knowledge AND review for tests.

1. First, fill in the missing word in the definitions for the chapter's key terms.
2. Then, check your answers using Appendix F.
3. If you got the answer right, put a check mark in the right column.
4. If your answer was incorrect, go back to the frame number provided and review the content.

Use the checklist to study the terms you don't know until you're confident you know them all.

Key Term	Frame	Definition	Know It?
1. acapnia	9.8	the _____ of carbon dioxide	☐
2. acid-fast bacilli smear	9.68	clinical test performed on sputum to identify presence of bacteria that react to acid; used to confirm _____ diagnosis	☐
3. adenoidectomy	9.69	surgical removal of a chronically inflamed _____ (pharyngeal tonsil)	☐
4. anoxia	9.9	the absence of _____	☐
5. antihistamine	9.70	a therapeutic drug that inhibits the effects of _____	☐
6. aphonia	9.10	the absence of _____	☐
7. apnea	9.11	the _____ to breathe or inhale	☐
8. arterial blood gases	9.71	clinical test to identify levels of oxygen and _____ _____ in arterial blood	☐
9. asphyxia	9.31	_____ of respiratory ventilation, or suffocation	☐
10. aspiration	9.72	a procedure that removes fluid, air, or foreign bodies with _____	☐
11. asthma	9.32	condition characterized by widespread _____ of the bronchioles and formation of mucous plugs	☐
12. atelectasis	9.33	condition in which trauma or disease causes the _____ to collapse and prevents air from entering	☐
13. auscultation	9.73	procedure that listens to _____ within the body, often with the aid of a stethoscope	☐
14. bradypnea	9.12	an abnormal _____ of the breathing rhythm	☐
15. bronchiectasis	9.34	abnormal _____ of the bronchi	☐
16. bronchitis	9.35	_____ of the bronchi	☐
17. bronchodilation	9.74	procedure that uses a bronchodilating agent in an _____ to reduce bronchial constriction	☐
18. bronchogenic carcinoma	9.36	aggressive form of _____ in cells of the bronchi	☐
19. bronchography	9.75	the _____ imaging of the bronchi	☐
20. bronchopneumonia	9.37	acute inflammatory disease that involves the bronchioles and alveoli; also called _____ pneumonia	☐
21. bronchoscopy	9.76	evaluation of the bronchi using a flexible fiber-optic tube with a small lens and eyepiece for _____ on a computer monitor	☐

Key Term	Frame	Definition	Know It?
22. bronchospasm	9.13	a narrowing of the airway caused by _____ of smooth muscles in the bronchioles	☐
23. chest CT scan	9.77	diagnostic imaging of the chest by _____ _____ (CT)	☐
24. chest X-ray	9.78	X-ray image of the thoracic cavity used to diagnose TB, tumors, and other lung conditions; also called chest _____	☐
25. Cheyne-Stokes respiration	9.14	a sign characterized by a repeated pattern of distressed _____ with a gradual increase of deep breathing, then shallow breathing, and apnea	☐
26. chronic obstructive pulmonary disease	9.38	general term for several different forms of pulmonary _____, including chronic bronchitis, bronchospasm, cystic fibrosis, and emphysema	☐
27. coccidioidomycosis	9.39	_____ infection of the upper respiratory tract; caused by *Coccidioides immitis* organism	☐
28. coryza	9.40	a(n) _____ of the upper respiratory tract that causes local inflammation and a runny nose; also called rhinitis	☐
29. croup	9.41	viral infectious disease that produces a characteristic barklike, hoarse _____ due to acute obstruction of the larynx	☐
30. cystic fibrosis	9.42	hereditary disease characterized by excess _____ production in the respiratory and digestive tracts, and elsewhere in the body	☐
31. dysphonia	9.15	hoarse _____	☐
32. dyspnea	9.16	difficult _____	☐
33. ears, nose, and throat specialist	9.79	physician who specializes in treatment of upper _____ tract disease; also called an otolaryngologist	☐
34. emphysema	9.43	_____ lung disease characterized by dyspnea, chronic cough, barrel chest, and chronic hypoxemia and hypercapnia	☐
35. endotracheal intubation	9.80	insertion of a noncollapsible breathing tube into the _____ by way of the nose or mouth	☐
36. epiglottitis	9.44	_____ of the epiglottis	☐
37. epistaxis	9.17	_____ bleed	☐
38. expectorant	9.81	a drug that breaks up mucus and promotes the coughing reflex in order to _____ the mucus	☐
39. hemoptysis	9.18	coughing up and spitting out _____	☐
40. hemothorax	9.19	blood pooling within the _____ cavity	☐
41. hypercapnia	9.20	_____ levels of carbon dioxide in the blood	☐
42. hyperpnea	9.21	abnormally deep _____ or an increased rate of breathing	☐
43. hyperventilation	9.21	abnormally _____ breathing	☐
44. hypopnea	9.22	abnormally _____ breathing	☐

Key Term	Frame	Definition	Know It?
45. hypoventilation	9.23	reduced breathing rhythm that fails to meet the body's _____ exchange demands	☐
46. hypoxemia	9.24	abnormally _____ levels of oxygen in the blood	☐
47. incentive spirometry	9.82	a postoperative breathing therapy that uses a portable spirometer to improve lung _____ after an operation	☐
48. laryngectomy	9.83	surgical _____ of the larynx	☐
49. laryngitis	9.45	_____ of the larynx	☐
50. laryngoscopy	9.84	diagnostic procedure that uses a(n) _____ to view the larynx	☐
51. laryngospasm	9.25	closure of the glottis due to muscular _____ of the throat	☐
52. laryngotracheotomy	9.85	surgical _____ into the larynx and trachea	☐
53. legionellosis	9.46	form of _____ caused by the *Legionella pneumophilia* bacterium; also called Legionnaires' disease	☐
54. lobectomy	9.86	surgical removal of a single _____ of a lung	☐
55. lung cancer	9.47	cancer that arises from the soft tissues of the lung; also called _____ of the lung	☐
56. mechanical ventilation	9.87	medical treatment that provides supplemental oxygen to patients in _____ distress with a ventilator	☐
57. nasopharyngitis	9.48	inflammation of the _____ and pharynx	☐
58. nebulizer	9.88	a device that converts a liquid medication into a(n) _____ and delivers it to the lungs through deep inhalation	☐
59. orthopnea	9.26	limited ability to _____ when lying down	☐
60. oximetry	9.89	procedure that measures _____ levels in the blood using an oximeter	☐
61. paroxysm	9.27	sudden, sharp reoccurence of symptoms or a _____	☐
62. pertussis	9.49	acute infectious disease that causes inflammation of the larynx, trachea, and bronchi with spasmodic _____	☐
63. pharyngitis	9.50	inflammation of the _____	☐
64. pleural effusion	9.51	a disease in which _____ leaks into the pleural cavity due to injury or infection of the pleural membranes	☐
65. pleuritis	9.52	_____ of the pleural membranes; also called pleurisy	☐
66. pleurocentesis	9.90	surgical _____ and aspiration of fluid from the pleural cavity	☐
67. pneumoconiosis	9.53	inflammation of the lungs caused by chronic inhalation of fine particles (literally, _____)	☐
68. pneumonectomy	9.91	surgical removal of a(n) _____; also called pneumectomy	☐
69. pneumonia	9.54	inflammation of soft lung tissue caused by bacterial, _____, or fungal pathogens that results in the formation of an exudate within alveoli	☐

Key Term	Frame	Definition	Know It?
70. pneumonitis	9.55	inflammatory condition of the lungs that is independent of a particular _____	☐
71. pneumothorax	9.56	abnormal presence of _____ or gas within the pleural cavity	☐
72. pulmonary angiography	9.92	diagnostic procedure that evaluates the blood _____ in the lungs	☐
73. pulmonary edema	9.57	accumulation of fluid within the interstitial spaces surrounding the alveoli as response to infection or _____	☐
74. pulmonary embolism	9.58	a blockage in the pulmonary circulation due to a mobile blood _____	☐
75. pulmonary function tests	9.93	a series of diagnostic tests that determine the cause of lung disease by evaluating lung _____ through spirometry	☐
76. pulmonary specialist	9.94	physician who specializes in treatment of diseases that affect the lower _____ tract	☐
77. pyothorax	9.59	the presence of _____ in the pleural cavity; also called empyema	☐
78. respiratory distress syndrome	9.60	respiratory disease characterized by atelectasis; one form affects new-borns, another affects _____	☐
79. resuscitation	9.95	artificial respiration used to restore _____	☐
80. rhinitis	9.61	inflammation of the mucous membrane lining the _____ cavity	☐
81. rhinoplasty	9.96	surgical _____ of the nose	☐
82. severe acute respiratory syndrome	9.62	a(n) _____ infection that causes lung inflammation, alveolar damage, and atelectasis	☐
83. sinusitis	9.63	_____ of the mucous membranes of the nasal cavity and paranasal sinuses	☐
84. sputum	9.28	expectorated matter that is coughed out from the _____	☐
85. tachypnea	9.29	_____ breathing	☐
86. TB skin test	9.97	simple skin test used to determine the presence of a _____ infection; also called PPD skin test and Mantoux skin test	☐
87. thoracalgia	9.30	_____ in the chest region	☐
88. thoracentesis	9.98	surgical puncture using a needle and syringe into the thoracic cavity to aspirate pleural _____ for diagnosis or treatment; also called thoracocentesis or pleurocentesis	☐
89. thoracostomy	9.99	surgical _____ into the chest cavity, usually for insertion of a drainage or air tube	☐
90. thoractomy	9.100	surgical _____ into the chest wall	☐
91. tonsillitis	9.64	_____ of one or more tonsils	☐
92. tracheitis	9.65	inflammation of the _____	☐

Key Term	Frame	Definition	Know It?
93. tracheoplasty	9.101	surgical _____ of the trachea	☐
94. tracheostenosis	9.65	_____ of the trachea due to inflammation	☐
95. tracheostomy	9.102	surgical creation of an _____ into the trachea, usually for insertion of a breathing tube	☐
96. tracheotomy	9.103	_____ incision into the trachea	☐
97. tuberculosis	9.66	_____ of the lungs by *Mycobacterium tuberculosis* bacterium	☐
98. upper respiratory infection	9.67	generalized infection of the _____ cavity, pharynx, and larynx	☐
99. ventilation-perfusion scanning	9.104	diagnostic tool that uses _____ medicine, or radioactive material, to evaluate pulmonary function	☐

Multimedia Preview ▶▶▶▶▶

Additional interactive resources and activities for this chapter can be found on the Companion Website. For videos, audio glossary, and review, access the accompanying DVD-ROM in this book.

DVD-ROM Highlights

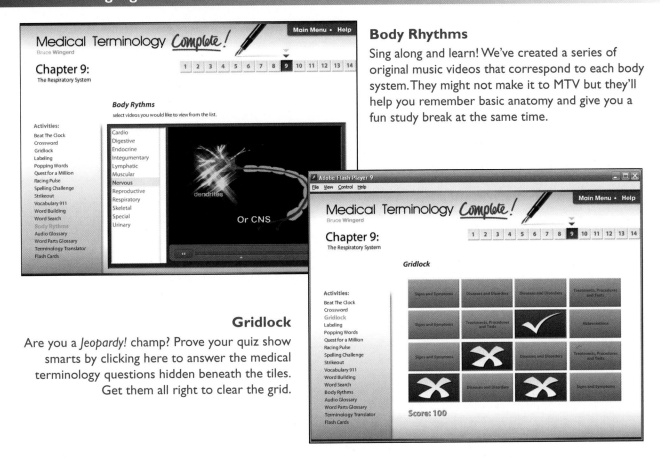

Body Rhythms

Sing along and learn! We've created a series of original music videos that correspond to each body system. They might not make it to MTV but they'll help you remember basic anatomy and give you a fun study break at the same time.

Gridlock

Are you a *Jeopardy!* champ? Prove your quiz show smarts by clicking here to answer the medical terminology questions hidden beneath the tiles. Get them all right to clear the grid.

Website Highlights—www.prenhall.com/wingerd

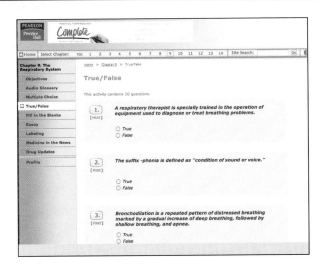

True/False Quiz

Take advantage of the free-access online study guide that accompanies your textbook. You'll find a true/false quiz that provides instant feedback, allowing you to check your score and see what you got right or wrong. By clicking on this URL you'll also access links to download mp3 audio reviews, current news articles, and an audio glossary.

The Digestive System ▶▶▶▶▶

Learning Objectives

After completing this chapter, you will be able to:

- Define and spell the word parts used to create terms for the digestive system.

- Break down and define common medical terms used for symptoms, diseases, disorders, procedures, treatments, and devices associated with the digestive system.

- Build medical terms from the word parts associated with the digestive system.

- Pronounce and spell common medical terms associated with the digestive system.

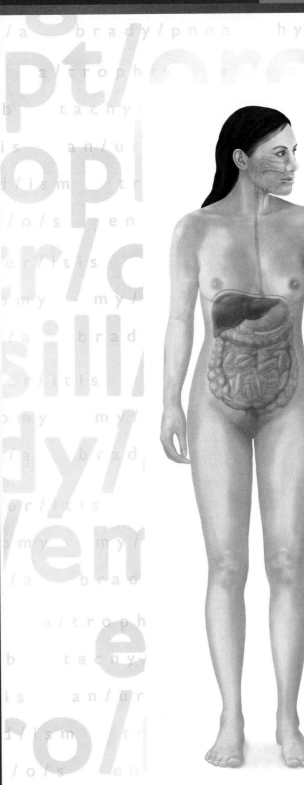

Anatomy and Physiology Terms ▶▶▶▶▶

The following table provides the combining forms that specifically apply to the anatomy and physiology of the digestive system. Note that the combining forms are colored red to help you identify them when you see them again later in the chapter.

Combining Form	Definition	Combining Form	Definition
abdomin/o	abdomen, abdominal cavity	gloss/o	tongue
an/o	anus	hepat/o	liver
append/o or appendic/o	appendix	ile/o	to roll, ileum
bil/i	bile	jejun/o	empty, jejunum
cec/o	blind intestine, cecum	lingu/o	tongue
chol/e	bile, gall	or/o	mouth
choledoch/o	common bile duct	pancreat/o	sweetbread, pancreas
col/o, colon/o	colon	peps/o, pept/o	digestion
cyst/o	bladder	periton/o	stretch over, peritoneum
dent/o	teeth	proct/o	rectum or anus
duoden/o	twelve, duodenum	pylor/o	pylorus
enter/o	small intestine	rect/o	rectum
esophag/o	gullet, esophagus	sial/o	saliva
gastr/o	stomach	sigm/o	the letter S, sigmoid colon
gingiv/o	gums	stomat/o	mouth

digestive

dye JEST iv

GI

10.1 The _____ system converts food into a form the body can use for energy, growth, and repair. It derives its name from its primary function, digestion. The term is from the Latin word *digestus*, which means "to divide, dissolve, or set in order." The digestive system performs all three: When the body digests food, it divides and dissolves it into simpler parts, setting the food parts in order for powering other body functions. Digestion occurs gradually, as food is passed from one organ to the next through the digestive tract, or gastrointestinal (GI) tract. The organs of the _____ tract include the mouth, pharynx, esophagus, stomach, small intestine, and large intestine. Accessory organs contribute to digestion by secreting enzymes and other chemicals into the GI tract. They include the salivary glands, liver, gallbladder, and pancreas.

FUNCTION ▶▶▶
digestion

10.2 You have just learned that _____, which is the break-down of food particles into their small subunits, is the primary function of the digestive system. Chemical digestion is performed by enzymes, and mechanical digestion is achieved by chewing in the mouth and mixing and churning actions produced by muscles in the walls of the stomach. Other important functions of the digestive system include:

- Absorption of nutrients, which occurs across the wall of the small intestine
- Regulation of sugar levels in the blood, which is achieved by endocrine cells of the pancreas and by liver cells
- Conservation of water, which is provided by water absorption across the walls of the small and large intestines

10.3 Use the anatomy terms that appear in the left column to fill in the corresponding blanks in Figures 10.1■ and 10.2■.

1. **pharynx**
2. **esophagus**
3. **stomach**
4. **duodenum (of small intestine)**
5. **tongue**
6. **liver**
7. **cecum**
8. **colon**

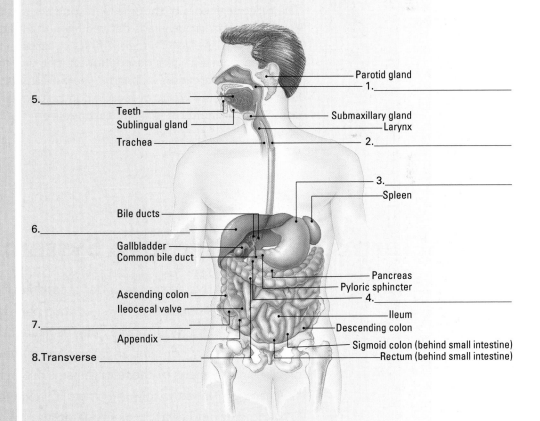

Figure 10.1 ■
Organs of the digestive system.

9. teeth (incisor)
10. palate
11. uvula
12. pharynx
13. tongue

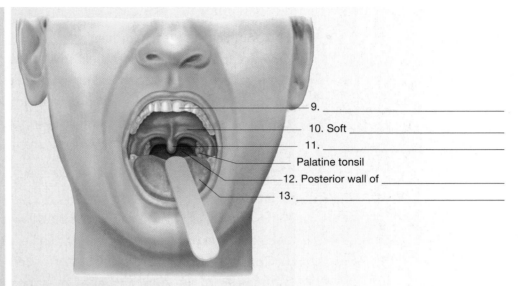

9. _____

10. Soft _____

11. _____

Palatine tonsil

12. Posterior wall of _____

13. _____

Figure 10.2 ■
The oral cavity. Anterior view of the open mouth.

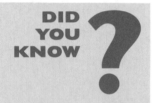

DID YOU KNOW?

Duodenum, Jejunum, and Ileum

The three segments of the small intestine are the duodenum, jejunum, and ileum. The term *duodenum* is derived from the Medieval Latin word, *duodeni*, which means "twelve." This word first appeared in the anatomical texts in 1050 AD, taken from a monk's description of it as the "first part of the small intestine, about 12 fingerbreadths in length." *Ileum* means "to roll" in Greek and is named after its peristaltic waves of muscle contraction that roll through the organ like ocean waves. The term *jejunum* is named from the Latin word *jejunus,* meaning "empty."

Medical Terms of the Digestive System ▶▶▶▶

digestive flora

10.4 The digestive system is under a constant risk of infection because food and other substances that often contain pathogens are introduced into the body through the mouth every day. To make matters even more risky, the GI tract normally contains an enormous number of bacteria. Known as the digestive flora, most of these organisms are beneficial when their populations are contained within the tract. For example, *E. coli* assists in the breakdown of indigestible plant materials and synthesizes vitamin K. But if the _____ _____ is allowed to increase in density or spread to other body areas, severe infections can result.

infections	**10.5** In addition to _____, the GI tract organs are also susceptible to inherited defects and the development of tumors. In each case, the result of the disease may be a reduction of the body's ability to digest food, eliminate wastes, absorb and conserve water, or perform other specific functions. Most digestive disorders affect overall health rather than remain localized, due to the abundance of blood vessels and lymphatics associated with GI tract organs and the functional importance of accessory organs like the liver and pancreas.
disease	**10.6** The clinical treatment of a digestive disorder is performed by a physician with a specialization in treating the body region or organ, the particular disorder, or a set of disorders. For example, a _____ of the mouth or throat is treated by a **head and neck specialist**, stomach or intestinal disease is treated by a **gastroenterologist** (GAS troh EN ter AL oh jist), a disease of the rectum is treated by a **proctologist** (prok TALL oh jist), and a disease of the liver is treated by a **hepatobiliary** (heh PAT oh BIL ee air ee) **specialist**. Cancer is treated by an **oncologist**, often in association with a regional specialist. The area within a hospital that treats digestive disorders is often called **internal medicine**.
digestive **eating**	**10.7** Because most digestive organs are located deep within the body, the diagnosis of _____ disorders can benefit from noninvasive imaging procedures. Consequently, magnetic resonance imaging (MRI), computed axial tomography (CAT) scans, and specialized X-ray techniques are often used. Once diagnosed, most disorders may be treated with therapeutic agents or by surgery. Some disorders, such as _____ disorders, are treated with psychological counseling and a strict diet regimen.
	10.8 In the following sections, you will study the prefixes, combining forms, and suffixes that combine to build the medical terms of the digestive system. Complete the frames and review exercises that follow. You are on your way to mastery of the medical terms related to the digestive system!

Signs and Symptoms of the Digestive System

Following are the word parts that specifically apply to the signs and symptoms of the digestive system that are covered in the following section. Note that the word parts are color-coded to help you identify them: prefixes are blue, combining forms are red, and suffixes are purple.

Prefix	Definition
a-	without or absence of
dia-	through
dys-	bad, abnormal, painful, or difficult
re-	back

Combining Form	Definition
bil/i	bile
flux/o	flow
gastr/o	stomach
halit/o	breath
hemat/o	blood
hepat/o	liver
peps/o, pept/o	digestion
phag/o	eat, swallow
steat/o	fat

Suffix	Definition
-algia	condition of pain
-dynia	pain
-emesis	vomiting
-emia	condition of blood
-ia	condition of
-megaly	abnormally large
-osis	condition of
-rrhea	excessive discharge

KEY TERMS A-Z

aphagia
ah FAY jee ah

10.9 The prefix *a-* means "without or absence of," and the combining form *phag/o* means "eat, swallow." Combining these word parts forms the term _____, which is the inability to swallow. This constructed term contains three word parts, as shown when it is written a/phag/ia. Although the literal meaning is "without eating or swallowing," clinical use of the term has changed its meaning to "inability to swallow."

ascites
ah SIGH teez

10.10 The Greek word for "bag" is *askos*. It is used to create the term **ascites**, which is an accumulation of fluid within the peritoneal cavity that produces an enlarged abdomen. _____ is a sign of liver disease, congestive heart failure, or both.

constipation
kon stih PAY shun

10.11 Infrequent or incomplete bowel movements are characteristic of the condition **constipation**. It is a sign of an intestinal disorder. The term _____ is derived from the Latin word *constipatus*, which means "to press together."

diarrhea
dye ah REE ah

10.12 An opposite condition to constipation is **diarrhea**, in which a frequent discharge of watery fecal material occurs. It is a constructed term, written dia/rrhea. _____ literally means "excessive discharge through" and may be caused by an improper diet, but it is more commonly a sign of infection by virus, bacteria, or protozoa. It is particularly dangerous to infants, who are in danger of severe dehydration. Approximately 2 million children die across the world each year from dehydration resulting from diarrhea.

dyspepsia
diss PEPP see ah

10.13 A common symptom of digestive difficulty that literally translates to "condition of difficult digestion" is _____. This constructed term contains three word parts, as shown in dys/peps/ia. Commonly called indigestion, it is accompanied by stomach or esophageal pain or discomfort.

dysphagia
diss FAY jee ah

10.14 Difficulty in swallowing is called **dysphagia**. It often accompanies a sore throat, although its chronic form can be a sign of oral or pharyngeal cancer. _____ is a constructed term and is written dys/phag/ia.

flatus
FLAY tuss

10.15 The term *flatus* is a Latin word that means "a blowing." It is used to describe the presence of gas, or air, in the GI tract, which is simply called _____. Gas is expelled through the anus as **flatulence** (FLAT yoo lens).

gastrodynia
GAS troh DINN ee ah

10.16 The combining form for stomach is *gastr/o*, and a suffix that means "pain" is *-dynia*. Therefore, the symptom of stomach pain is known as _____. This constructed term includes three word parts and is written gastr/o/dynia. It is also known as **gastralgia** (gast RAL jee ah).

halitosis
hal ih TOH siss

10.17 The word root *halit* means "breath." It is derived from the Latin word for breath, *halitus*. Adding the suffix *-osis* forms the term **halitosis**. Although there is no word part included to give the term a negative meaning, nonetheless _____ means "bad breath." The constructed form is written halit/osis.

hematemesis
hee mah TEM eh siss

10.18 Vomiting blood is a sign of a severe digestive disorder, such as a bleeding peptic ulcer (Frame 10.61) or stomach cancer (Frame 10.42). It is called **hematemesis**, which is a constructed term written hemat/emesis. The literal meaning of _____ is "vomiting blood."

hepatomegaly
HEPP ah toh MEG ah lee

10.19 A sign of liver disease is abnormal enlargement of the liver, called _____. This constructed term is written hepat/o/megaly, which literally means "abnormally large liver."

jaundice
JAWN diss

10.20 A yellowish-orange coloration of the skin, sclera of the eyes, and deeper tissues is a collective sign of liver disease called **jaundice**. The condition of _____ results from the accumulation of bile pigments in the bloodstream that are normally removed by the liver.

DID YOU KNOW ?

Jaundice

The term *jaundice* is derived from the French word for yellow, *jaune,* to describe the yellowing appearance of the skin and sclera. An alternate term for this symptom is *icterus,* which is the Greek word meaning "yellow bird."

nausea
NAW see ah

10.21 A symptom of dizziness that includes an urge to vomit is called **nausea**. When _____ is accompanied by vomiting, it is abbreviated **N&V**. Nausea is derived from the Latin and Greek words for seasickness, *nausia*.

reflux
REE fluks

10.22 A backward flow of material in the GI tract, or regurgitation, is called **reflux**. This constructed term is written re/flux. The literal meaning of _____ is "back flow."

steatorrhea
STEE at oh REE ah

10.23 Abnormal levels of fat in the feces is a sign of digestive malfunction. It is called **steatorrhea**, which is a constructed term written steat/o/rrhea. Because *steat/o* is the combining form for "fat," _____ literally means "excessive discharge of fat."

PRACTICE: Signs and Symptoms of the Digestive System

The Right Match

Match the term on the left with the correct definition on the right.

_____ 1. dysphagia

_____ 2. reflux

_____ 3. flatus

_____ 4. halitosis

_____ 5. ascites

_____ 6. diarrhea

_____ 7. nausea

_____ 8. constipation

_____ 9. jaundice

a. backward flow of material in the GI tract

b. gas trapped in the GI tract

c. difficulty in swallowing

d. infrequent or incomplete bowel movements

e. frequent discharge of watery fecal material

f. bad breath

g. from the French word for "yellow"

h. a symptomatic urge to vomit

i. accumulation of fluid in the peritoneal cavity

Break the Chain

Analyze these medical terms:

  a) Separate each term into its word parts; each word part is labeled for you (**p** = prefix, **r** = root, **cf** = combining form, and **s** = suffix).

  b) For the Bonus Question, write the requested definition in the blank that follows.

The first set has been completed for you as an example.

1. a) aphagia

    a/phag/ia
    p   r   s

    b) *Bonus Question:* What is the definition of the suffix? *condition of* _____

2. a) dyspepsia

    ____/_____/____
     p   r   s

    b) *Bonus Question:* What is the definition of the word root? _____

3. a) gastrodynia

    _____/__/_____
        cf   s

    b) *Bonus Question:* What is the definition of the combining form? _____

4. a) hematemesis

    _____/_____
     r   s

    b) *Bonus Question:* What is the definition of the suffix? _____

5. a) steatorrhea

    _____/__/_____
        cf   s

    b) *Bonus Question:* What is the definition of the combining form? _____

6. a) hepatomegaly

    _____/__/_____
        cf   s

    b) *Bonus Question:* What is the definition of the combining form? _____

Diseases and Disorders of the Digestive System

Following are the word parts that specifically apply to the diseases and disorders of the digestive system that are covered in the following section. Note that the word parts are color-coded to help you identify them: prefixes are blue, combining forms are red, and suffixes are purple.

Prefix	Definition
an-	not
dys-	bad, abnormal, painful, or difficult
mal-	bad

Combining Form	Definition
aden/o	gland
appendic/o	appendix
cheil/o	lip
chol/e	bile, gall
choledoch/o	common bile duct
cirrh/o	orange
col/o	colon
cyst/o	bladder
diverticul/o	diverticulum
duoden/o	twelve, duodenum
enter/o	small intestine
esophag/o	esophagus
gastr/o	stomach
gingiv/o	gums
gloss/o	tongue
hem/o	blood
hepat/o	liver
lip/o	fat
lith/o	stone
orex/o	appetite
pancreat/o	pancreas
parot/o	parotid gland
pept/o	digestion
periton/o	peritoneum
polyp/o	small growth
proct/o	rectum or anus
rect/o	rectum

Suffix	definition
-al	pertaining to
-ectasis	expansion or dilation
-ia	condition of
-ic	pertaining to
-itis	inflammation
-malacia	softening
-megaly	abnormally large
-oid	resembling
-oma	tumor
-osis	condition of
-pathy	disease
-penia	abnormal reduction in number or deficiency
-ptosis	drooping
-sis	state of
-y	process of

KEY TERMS A-Z

anorexia nervosa
AN or EKS ee ah * nerv OH sah

10.24 An emotional eating disorder in which the patient avoids food due to a compulsion to become thin in appearance is known as **anorexia nervosa**. The medical term _____ _____ is a constructed term written an/orex/ia nervosa and literally means "nervous cause of condition of no appetite." It results in extreme weight loss and nutritional deficiencies and can become fatal if left untreated.

appendicitis
ah pen dih SIGH tiss

10.25 Inflammation of the appendix is called _____. It is a constructed term written appendic/itis and is illustrated in Figure 10.3■.

Figure 10.3 ■
Appendicitis. (a) A normal appendix. (b) An inflamed appendix in appendicitis.

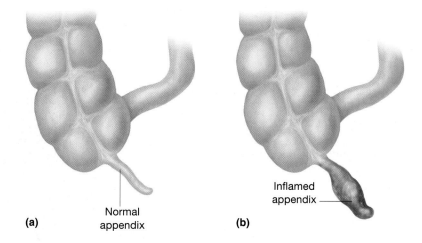

(a) Normal appendix

Inflamed appendix

(b)

bulimia
boo LEEM ee ah

10.26 A common eating disorder involving repeated gorging with food followed by induced vomiting or laxative abuse is known as **bulimia**. Commonly known as "binging and purging," the term _____ is derived from the Greek word for "ravenous hunger," *boulimia*.

cheilitis
kye LYE tiss

10.27 Because the combining form for lip is *cheil/o*, inflammation of the lip is called _____, a constructed term written cheil/itis. Another term using this combining form is **cheilosis** (kye LOH siss). It is a general condition of the lip, which often includes splitting of the lips and corners of the mouth, usually resulting from vitamin B deficiency.

cholecystitis
koh lee siss TYE tiss

10.28 The combining form for gall or bile is *chol/e*, and the form for bladder is *cyst/o*. Thus, the gallbladder is chol/e/cyst/o, which literally means "bladder of gall." Inflammation of the gallbladder is therefore called _____, which can be written chol/e/cyst/itis. It is usually caused by stones lodged within the gallbladder, which are commonly called gallstones.

choledochitis
KOH leh dok EYE tiss

choledoch/o/lith/ia/sis

10.29 The combining form for common bile duct is *choledoch/o*. Thus, inflammation of the common bile duct is called _____. Adding the term *lithiasis* to the word root to describe the presence of stones within the common bile duct forms the term **choledocholithiasis** (KOH leh doh koh lith EYE ah siss). This constructed term is written _____/__/_____/_____/_____.

cholelithiasis
KOH lee lith EYE ah siss

10.30 A generalized condition of stones lodged within the gallbladder or bile ducts is called _____. It is illustrated in Figure 10.4■. This constructed term includes five word parts, as shown when it is written chol/e/lith/ia/sis.

Figure 10.4 ■
Cholelithiasis. Common sites of gallstones in the generalized condition.
(a) Stones in the hepatic duct.
(b) Stones in the gallbladder.
(c) Stones in the common bile duct.

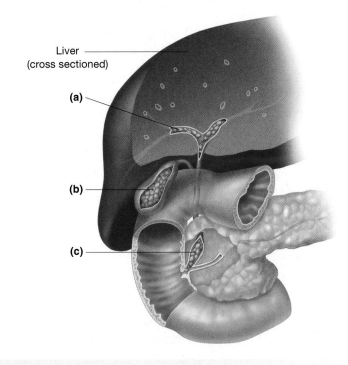

Liver (cross sectioned)

(a)

(b)

(c)

cirrhosis
ser ROH siss

10.31 A chronic, progressive liver disease characterized by the gradual loss of liver cells and their replacement by fat and other forms of connective tissue is known as **cirrhosis**. It is shown in Figure 10.5■. The constructed form of _____ is written cirrh/osis. It literally means "condition of orange," referring to the common symptom of a yellowish-orange coloration of the skin (jaundice, Frame 10.20). Chronic alcoholism is responsible for about 75% of cirrhosis cases. The remainder are usually caused by viral infections, such as hepatitis B and C.

Figure 10.5 ■
Cirrhosis. Cirrhosis is characterized by a chronic deterioration of the liver, replacing healthy cells with connective tissue that causes a mottled appearance. In this photograph, the liver was removed from a deceased patient in an advanced state of cirrhosis.

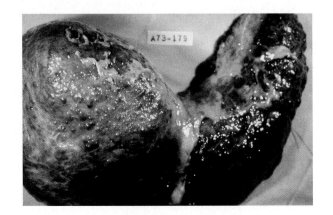

colitis
koh LYE tiss

10.32 Inflammation of the colon is called _____. Colitis often includes excessive peristaltic contractions, mucus production, and cramping pain. If chronic bleeding of the colon wall occurs to form bloody diarrhea, the condition is called **ulcerative colitis** (UHL ser ah tiv * koh LYE tiss). Ulcerative colitis is a form of chronic **inflammatory bowel disease**, or **IBD** (Frame 10.54). *Colitis* is a constructed term, written col/itis.

colorectal cancer
kohl oh REK tal * KAN ser

10.33 Cancer of the colon often includes cancer of the rectum, forming the life-threatening disease known as **colorectal cancer**. *Colorectal* is a constructed term written col/o/rect/al. This form of cancer often arises as a **polyp** (Frame 10.63), which is an abnormal mass of tissue that projects from the wall of the organ into the interior like a mushroom, to become an aggressive, metastatic tumor. The most common sites of _____ _____ are illustrated in Figure 10.6■.

Figure 10.6 ■
Colorectal cancer. The most common sites of tumor development are shown.

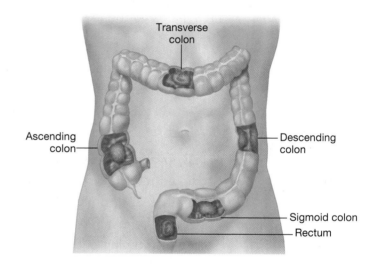

Transverse colon

Ascending colon

Descending colon

Sigmoid colon

Rectum

10.34 A chronic inflammation of any part of the GI tract, most commonly the ileum of the small intestine, that involves ulcerations, scar tissue formation, and thickening adhesions of the organ wall, is called **Crohn's disease**. Also known as **regional ileitis** or **regional enteritis**, it is believed to be an inherited condition. _____ _____ is a form of chronic **inflammatory bowel disease**, or **IBD** (Frame 10.54).

Crohn's disease
KRONZ * dih ZEEZ

DID YOU KNOW ?

Crohn's Disease
Dr. B. B. Crohn first described the disease that bears his name in 1932. At the time, he believed this chronic form of IBD was caused by a pathogen. New evidence suggests that he may have been correct, although the causative organism has not yet been identified.

diverticulosis
DYE ver tik yoo LOH siss

diverticul/itis

10.35 In some individuals, small pouches called **diverticula** form on the wall of the colon. The combining form of this term is *diverticul/o*. The presence of diverticula is often without symptoms or with mild bowel discomfort, and is called _____. This constructed term is written *diverticul/osis*. If the pouches become inflamed, it produces a more painful condition known as **diverticulitis** (DYE ver tik yoo LYE tiss). The constructed form of this term is _____/_____.

duodenal ulcer
doo ODD eh nal * UL ser

10.36 An ulcer, or erosion, in the wall of the duodenum of the small intestine is called a _____ _____. The constructed form of duodenal is written *duoden/al*.

dysentery
DIS en tair ee

10.37 An acute inflammation of the GI tract that is caused by bacteria, protozoa, or chemical irritants is called **dysentery**. This constructed term is written *dys/enter/y* and literally means "difficult intestine." _____ is characterized by severe diarrhea and can become a life-threatening disease by causing dehydration.

enteritis
EHN ter EYE tiss

10.38 The word root for intestine is *enter*. Thus, inflammation of the small or large intestine is called _____, which can be written *enter/itis* to show the word parts.

esophagitis
eh soff ah JYE tiss

esophag/o/malacia

10.39 Inflammation of the esophagus is called **esophagitis**. This constructed term is written *esophag/itis*. It is often caused by acid reflux (Frame 10.22) from the stomach, which burns the esophageal lining to produce the inflammation. Chronic _____ may lead to a morbid softening of the esophageal wall, called **esophagomalacia** (eh soff ah go mah LAY shee ah). This constructed term is written _____/__/_____.

food-borne illness

10.40 Ingestion of food contaminated with harmful bacteria can cause symptoms of diarrhea and vomiting, even in otherwise healthy people, but in the very young, elderly, and immunosuppressed it can become life threatening. Common causes of **food-borne illness**, or food poisoning, include *E. coli*, *Salmonella*, and *Staphylococci*. In addition, the extremely toxic anaerobic bacterium, *Clostridium botulinum*, is a severe form of _____-_____ _____, due to its presence in improperly prepared home-canned foods. The life-threatening disease caused by this organism is called **botulism** (BOTT yoo lizm).

gastrectasis gas TREK tah siss	**10.41** Abnormal stretching, or dilation, of the stomach is called **gastrectasis**. This constructed term uses the suffix *-ectasis* (meaning "expansion or dilation") and is written gastr/ectasis. _____ may be caused by overeating, obstruction of the pyloric opening, or hiatal hernia (Frame 10.53). The related condition of **gastromegaly** (GAS troh MEG ah lee) is an abnormal enlargement of the stomach.
gastric cancer GAS trik * KAN ser	**10.42** Commonly known as stomach cancer, _____ _____ is an aggressive, metastatic cancer arising from cells lining the stomach. Risk of developing gastric cancer increases with chronic infection of the stomach by the bacterium *Helicobacter pylori*.
gastric ulcer GAS trik * UL ser	**10.43** An ulcer, or erosion, in the wall of the stomach is commonly called a _____ _____. It is often caused by an imbalance between the secretion of the protective mucous layer and the secretion of hydrochloric acid in the stomach, which is often the result of infection by the bacterium *Helicobacter pylori* (*H. pylori*).
gastritis gas TRY tiss **gastroenteritis** GAS troh en ter EYE tiss	**10.44** Inflammation of the stomach is called **gastritis**. The constructed form of this term is written gastr/itis. The acute form of _____ is usually caused by an improper diet or an infection, and the chronic form may be caused by a chronic bacterial infection, peptic ulcers (Frame 10.61), or gastric cancer (Frame 10.42). If the small intestine is involved in the inflammation, it is called _____. This constructed term is written gastr/o/enter/itis. If the first segment of the small intestine, the duodenum, is specifically involved, it is called **gastroduodenitis** (GAS troh doo oh den EYE tiss), written gastr/o/duoden/itis. Inflammation of the stomach, small intestine, and colon all at once is called **gastroenterocolitis** (GAS troh EN ter oh koh LYE tiss). The constructed form of this term reveals six word parts and is written gastr/o/enter/o/col/itis.
gastroesophageal GAS troh eh SOFF ah JEE al	**10.45** A recurring backflow, or reflux, of stomach contents into the esophagus is a condition called **gastroesophageal reflux disease,** or **GERD**. It is usually the result of a weakened esophageal sphincter and produces the burning pain of indigestion. The term _____ is constructed of word parts and is written gastr/o/esophag/e/al.

gastromalacia
GAS troh mah LAY shee ah

10.46 The suffix -*malacia* means "softening." The softening of the stomach wall may occur during advanced stages of stomach cancer and other chronic diseases of the stomach. It is called _____. The constructed form of this term is written gastr/o/malacia.

giardiasis
jee ahr DYE ah siss

10.47 Infection by the intestinal protozoa *Giardia intestinalis* or *Giardia lamblia* produces symptoms of diarrhea, cramps, nausea, and vomiting. The disease is usually contracted by drinking contaminated water and is known as _____. This constructed term is written giardia/sis.

gingivitis
jin jih VYE tiss

10.48 Inflammation of the gums, or gingiva, is called _____. It is usually caused by chronic bacterial activity at the junction of the teeth and gums. The constructed form of this term is gingiv/itis.

glossitis
gloss EYE tiss

gloss/itis

10.49 A combining form for tongue, *gloss/o*, is derived from the Greek word *glossa*. Any disease of the tongue is called a **glossopathy** (gloss AH path ee). This constructed term is written gloss/o/pathy. An example of a glossopathy is _____, which is an inflammation of the tongue often caused by exposure to allergens, toxic substances, or extreme heat or cold. The constructed form of glossitis is _____/_____.

hemorrhoids
HEM oh roydz

10.50 A varicose, or swollen, condition of the veins in the anus produces painful swellings that may break open and bleed, known as **hemorrhoids**. This term literally means "resembling leakage of blood." _____ are commonly called *piles*.

hepatitis

10.51 A viral-induced inflammation of the liver is called viral _____. This constructed term is written hepat/itis. There are five known forms of hepatitis, which are categorized with the letters *A* through *E* and described in the Did You Know? box.

DID YOU KNOW ?

Hepatitis Types

There are five main categories of hepatitis, all caused by related forms of a virus. Type A (infectious hepatitis) is transmitted by eating contaminated food. Type B (serum hepatitis) is transmitted via body fluids, such as blood or semen. Type C is mainly transmitted through the blood and often causes permanent liver damage. Type D is similar to type B and may combine with it to severely damage the liver. Type E is similar to type A and is the most common form in countries that have contaminated water supplies.

hepatoma
hepp ah TOH mah

10.52 The suffix that means "tumor" is -*oma*. A tumor arising from cells within the liver is called a _____. The constructed form of this term is hepat/oma. The disease is also called hepatocellular carcinoma, or **HCC**. The malignant form of this cancer accounts for about 85% of the cases and is often associated with alcoholic cirrhosis or hepatitis B.

hiatal hernia
high A tahl * HER nee ah

10.53 Protrusion of the cardiac portion of the stomach through the hiatus of the diaphragm to enter the thoracic cavity is called a _____ _____. It causes the symptom of heartburn that results from the movement of stomach acids into the esophagus and is illustrated in Figure 10.7■. Another type of digestive system hernia, called **inguinal hernia**, is a protrusion of a small intestinal segment through the abdominal wall in the inguinal region. A **direct inguinal hernia** occurs in males and is a protrusion into the scrotal cavity. Also, an **umbilical hernia** occurs when a small intestinal segment enters through a tear in the membrane covering the abdominal wall at the umbilical (navel) region. In each of these cases, the hernia may become strangulated, which restricts blood flow to the protruding organ. A **strangulated hernia** requires medical intervention to avoid loss of the affected organ.

Figure 10.7 ■
Hiatal hernia. (a) The hernia occurs when the stomach protrudes through the diaphragm and into the thoracic cavity, often leading to the movement of stomach fluids into the esophagus that creates esophageal reflux and esophagitis.
(b) A close-up of a hiatal hernia.

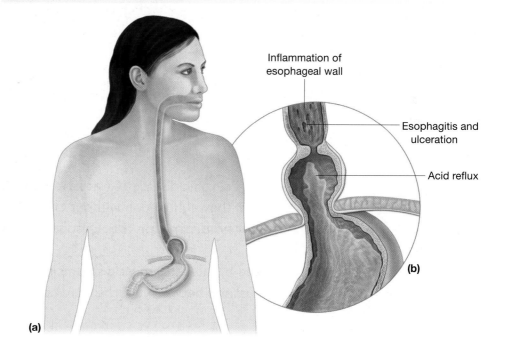

Inflammation of esophageal wall

Esophagitis and ulceration

Acid reflux

(b)

(a)

inflammatory bowel disease

10.54 You have learned from Frames 10.32 and 10.34 that

_____ _____ _____,

or **IBD**, is a general term that includes the conditions ulcerative colitis and Crohn's disease. IBD is a syndrome affecting different patients in different ways. It includes a wide spectrum of conditions and symptoms that range from chronic diarrhea and enteritis to ulcerative colitis and Crohn's disease.

intussusception
IN tuh suh SEP shun

10.55 Although the small intestine is anchored to the abdominal wall by the peritoneal membranes, it is subject to infolding. Infolding of a segment of the small intestine within another segment is a condition called **intussusception** and results in a reduction of intestinal motility. It is illustrated in Figure 10.8■. The term _____ is a combination of Latin words that collectively mean "to take within."

Figure 10.8 ■
Intussusception. The condition is caused by an infolding of the small intestine, which often causes a reduction of intestinal motility.

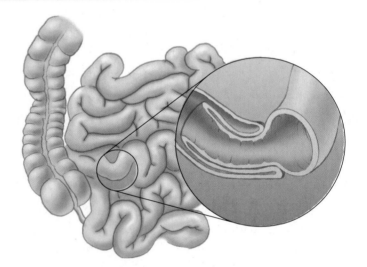

irritable bowel syndrome

10.56 A chronic disease characterized by periodic disturbances of large intestinal (bowel) function without clear physical damage is called **irritable bowel syndrome**, or **IBS**. Episodes of _____ _____ _____ include abdominal pain caused by intestinal muscle spasms and flatus, and are often associated with fluctuations between diarrhea and constipation.

lactose intolerance
LAHK tos * in TOHL er ans

10.57 Most people produce an enzyme in the small intestine that breaks down lactose, the primary sugar in milk and milk products. A lack of this enzyme results in the uncomfortable symptoms of flatus and diarrhea when dairy foods are consumed. This condition is called _____ _____.

malabsorption syndrome
MAL ab sorp shun * SIN drom

10.58 The prefix *mal-* means "bad." A disorder that is characterized by difficulty absorbing one or more nutrients is called **malabsorption syndrome**. It can have severe consequences, depending on the nutrients that cannot be absorbed. An example of _____ _____ is the inability to absorb fat molecules, resulting in a life-threatening disease called **lipopenia** (LYE poh PEE nee ah). This is a constructed term written as lip/o/penia.

pancreatitis
PAN kree ah TYE tiss

10.59 Inflammation of the pancreas is called **pancreatitis**. This constructed term is written pancreat/itis. Possible causes include tumor development and bacterial infection. If pancreatic functions are affected, the complications of acute _____ can become life threatening.

parotitis
pahr oh TYE tiss

10.60 The largest salivary glands are called parotid glands and are located around the angle of the jaw. Inflammation of one or both parotid glands is called _____. If caused by a virus, it is usually referred to as **mumps**. The term *parotitis* is a constructed term, written parot/itis. It may also be referred to as **sialoadenitis** (sigh AL oh add eh NYE tiss). The constructed form of this term, written sial/o/aden/itis, literally means "inflammation of saliva gland."

peptic ulcer

PEPP tik * UL ser

10.61 The term *peptic* is a constructed term, pept/ic, that means "pertaining to digestion." An erosion into the inner wall of an organ along the GI tract is generally called a _____ _____.

Usually, a peptic ulcer occurs in the wall of the stomach as a gastric ulcer (Frame 10.43), or in the wall of the duodenum as a duodenal ulcer (Frame 10.36). A gastric ulcer is shown in Figure 10.9■. The ulcer is formed when the protective mucous layer becomes eroded, exposing the inner lining to the caustic effects of hydrochloric acid. Roughly 80% of peptic ulcers are associated with an infection of *Helicobacter pylori* (*H. pylori*), which triggers an immune response that reduces mucus production.

Figure 10.9 ■

Peptic ulcer.

(a) Peptic ulcer may occur in the stomach (gastric ulcer), as shown here, or in the duodenum (duodenal ulcer). The most common cause is associated with infection by *H. pylori*.

(b) Gastroscopic photograph of a gastric ulcer.

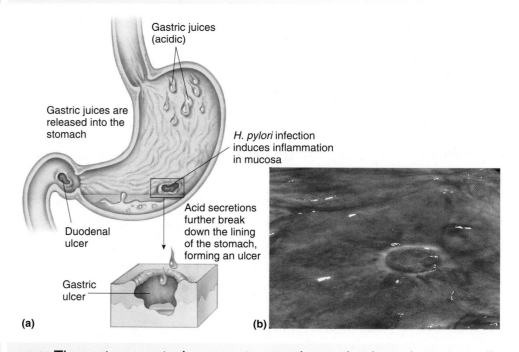

Gastric juices (acidic)

Gastric juices are released into the stomach

H. pylori infection induces inflammation in mucosa

Duodenal ulcer

Acid secretions further break down the lining of the stomach, forming an ulcer

Gastric ulcer

(a)   (b)

peritonitis

pair ih toh NYE tiss

10.62 The peritoneum is the extensive membrane that lines the inner wall of the abdominopelvic cavity and covers most of its organs. Inflammation of this membrane is called _____. This constructed term is written periton/itis. The inflammation is the body's response to an infection of the peritoneum, usually bacterial, that can become life threatening without medical intervention.

polyposis
pall ee POH siss

10.63 Any abnormal mass of tissue that projects inward from the wall of a hollow organ is called a **polyp** (PALL ip). The term means "small growth." It is usually a benign growth that may occur in the nose, throat, or large intestine. The presence of many polyps is called _____ and is illustrated in Figure 10.10■. The constructed form of this term is polyp/osis, which literally means "condition of polyps." Polyposis usually occurs in the colon or rectum of the large intestine, where it increases the risk for colorectal cancer (Frame 10.33).

Figure 10.10 ■
Polyps and polyposis. A polyp is a protruding growth from a mucous membrane lining a hollow organ. In the disease polyposis, multiple polyps develop, usually along the inner wall of the large intestine.

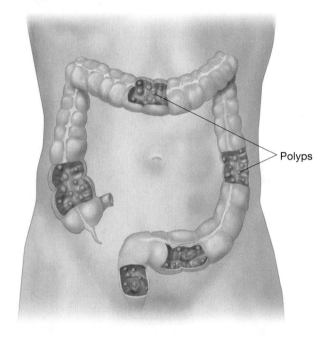

Polyps

proctitis
prok TYE tiss

10.64 A combining form meaning "rectum" or "anus" is proct/o. Inflammation of the anus, and usually the rectum as well, is called _____. This constructed term is written proct/itis.

proctoptosis
PROK top TOH siss

10.65 Recall that the suffix -ptosis means "drooping." A drooping, or prolapse, of the rectum is a condition called _____. The constructed form of this term is proct/o/ptosis.

volvulus

VOLL vyoo lus

10.66 A severe twisting of the intestine that leads to obstruction is called **volvulus**. The term is derived from the Latin word that means "to roll." A _____ that has caused a severe obstruction is illustrated in Figure 10.11 ■.

Figure 10.11 ■
Volvulus. A volvulus results when the small intestine twists, causing an obstruction that can lead to severe complications.

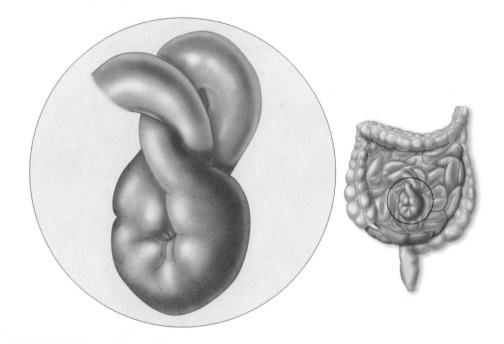

DID YOU KNOW ?

Liver Failure

The leading cause of acute liver failure in the United States is acetaminophen overdose. This drug has been sold over the counter since its discovery as a "safe" analgesic in 1970. Its most popular market name is Tylenol.

PRACTICE: Diseases and Disorders of the Digestive System

The Right Match

Match the term on the left with the correct definition on the right.

_____ 1. gastrectasis

_____ 2. polyp

_____ 3. gingivitis

_____ 4. giardiasis

_____ 5. bulimia

_____ 6. duodenal ulcer

_____ 7. volvulus

_____ 8. intussusception

_____ 9. cirrhosis

_____ 10. Crohn's disease

_____ 11. irritable bowel syndrome

_____ 12. hernia

_____ 13. gastroenterocolitis

_____ 14. cheilitis

_____ 15. choledocholithiasis

_____ 16. colitis

_____ 17. diverticulitis

_____ 18. gastroesophageal reflux disease

a. infolding of a segment of the small intestine within another segment

b. a chronic inflammation of any part of the GI tract, usually of the ileum

c. intestinal infection by the protozoa _Giardia intestinalis_ or _Giardia lamblia_

d. inflammation of abnormal pouches in the colon

e. twisting of the intestine causing an obstruction

f. a protrusion of intestine through connective tissue or a wall of the cavity in which it is normally enclosed

g. characterized by periodic bowel disturbances

h. a chronic liver disease

i. abnormal stretching of the stomach

j. an abnormal mass projecting inward

k. an eating disorder of binging and purging

l. an erosion in the wall of the duodenum of the small intestine

m. inflammation of the colon

n. inflammation of the gums

o. inflammation of the stomach and intestines

p. presence of stones in the common bile duct

q. recurring backflow of stomach contents into the esophagus

r. inflammation of the lips

Linkup

Link the word parts in the list to create the terms that match the definitions. You may use word parts more than once. Remember to add combining vowels when needed—and that some terms do not use any combining vowel. The first one is completed as an example.

Prefix	Combining Form	Suffix
an-	appendic/o	-ia
dys-	chol/e	-itis
	enter/o	-malacia
	esophag/o	-oma
	gastr/o	-osis
	gloss/o	-sis
	hepat/o	-y
	lith/o	
	orex/o	
	pancreat/o	
	polyp/o	
	proct/o	

Definition   Term

1. inflammation of the appendix   *appendicitis*

2. inflammation of the tongue   _____

3. condition of stones lodged within the gallbladder or bile ducts   _____

4. condition of prolapse of the rectum   _____

5. tumor within the liver   _____

6. softening of the stomach wall   _____

7. inflammation of the esophagus   _____

8. inflammation of the stomach and small intestine   _____

9. inflammation of the pancreas   _____

10. acute inflammation of the GI tract caused by bacteria, protozoa,   _____
    or chemical irritants

11. eating disorder in which the patient refuses food due to a compulsion   _____
    to become thin

12. condition of many polyps   _____

Treatments, Procedures, and Devices of the Digestive System

Following are the word parts that specifically apply to the treatments, procedures, and devices of the digestive system that are covered in the following section. Note that the word parts are color-coded to help you identify them: prefixes are blue, combining forms are red, and suffixes are purple.

Prefix	Definition
an-	without or absence of
anti-	against
endo-	within

Combining Form	Definition
abdomin/o	abdomen, abdominal cavity
acid/o	a solution or substance with a pH less than 7
append/o	appendix
cheil/o	lip
cholecyst/o	gallbladder
choledoch/o	common bile duct
col/o	colon
fec/o	feces
gastr/o	stomach
gingiv/o	gums
gloss/o	tongue
ile/o	to roll, ileum
lapar/o	abdomen
lith/o	stone
nas/o	nose
polyp/o	small growth
pylor/o	pylorus
vag/o	vagus nerve

Suffix	Definition
-al, ic	pertaining to
-centesis	surgical puncture
-ectomy	surgical removal
-emetic	pertaining to vomiting
-gram	a record or image
-graphy	measurement or recording process
-plasty	surgical repair
-rrhaphy	suturing
-scopy	to view
-spasmodic	pertaining to a sudden, involuntary contraction
-stomy	surgical creation of an opening
-tomy	incision or to cut

KEY TERMS A-Z

abdominocentesis
ab DOM ih noh sehn TEE siss

10.67 Because the suffix *-centesis* means "surgical puncture," a surgical puncture through the abdominal wall to remove fluid is a procedure called _____. This constructed term is written abdomin/o/centesis. An alternate term for this procedure is **paracentesis** (pair ah sehn TEE siss).

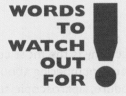

abdomen and *abdomin/o*

The combining form meaning "abdomen" is *abdomin/o*, which is found in terms such as abdominocentesis. Notice that the combining form uses a letter *i* and not an *e*, as in *abdomen*.

antacid
ant ASS id

10.68 An agent that reduces the acidity of the stomach cavity is called an **antacid**. Note that the letter *i* is deleted from the prefix *anti-* to make _____ easier to pronounce. Most mild medications neutralize the acid pH of the stomach, whereas stronger medications inhibit the amount of acid produced and are called proton pump inhibitors. *Antacid* is a constructed term, written as ant/acid.

vagotomy
vay GOTT oh mee

10.94 The vagus nerve is a cranial nerve that innervates much of the GI tract, providing sensory information to the brain relating to digestion and stimulating peristalsis of GI tract organs. The surgical dissection of branches of the vagus nerve may be performed in an effort to reduce gastric juice secretion as a treatment for chronic gastric ulcers (Frame 10.43). This procedure is called _____. The constructed form of this term is vag/o/tomy.

PRACTICE: Treatments, Procedures, and Devices of the Digestive System

The Right Match

Match the term on the left with the correct definition on the right.

_____ 1. colonoscopy

_____ 2. abdominocentesis

_____ 3. antacid

_____ 4. gastric lavage

_____ 5. cholecystography

_____ 6. cheilorrhaphy

_____ 7. ileostomy

_____ 8. stool culture and sensitivity

_____ 9. upper GI series

_____ 10. gavage

a. test that uses a stool sample to grow and identify microorganisms in a culture

b. process of feeding a patient through a tube inserted into the nose that descends into the stomach

c. also known as paracentesis

d. procedure of suturing a lip

e. procedure of producing an X-ray image of the gallbladder

f. endoscopy of the colon

g. cleansing procedure in which the stomach is irrigated with a prescribed solution

h. an agent that neutralizes stomach acid

i. surgical creation of an opening through the abdominal wall and into the ileum of the small intestine

j. a barium substance is ingested to provide X-ray images of the esophagus, stomach, and duodenum

Break the Chain

Analyze these medical terms:

   a)   Separate each term into its word parts; each word part is labeled for you (**p** = prefix, **r** = root, **cf** = combining form, and **s** = suffix).

   b)   For the Bonus Question, write the requested definition in the blank that follows.

1.   a)   antiemetic   _____/_____
                                      p   s

   b)   *Bonus Question:* What is the definition of the suffix? _____

2.   a)   glossorrhaphy   _____/__/____
                                      cf   s

   b)   *Bonus Question:* What is the definition of the combining form? _____

3.   a)   sigmoidoscopy   _____/__/_____
                                      cf   s

   b)   *Bonus Question:* What is the definition of the combining form? _____

4.   a)   hemorrhoidectomy   _____/_____
                                      (noun)   s

   b)   *Bonus Question:* What is the definition of the second suffix? _____

5.   a)   laparotomy   _____/__/_____
                                      cf   s

   b)   *Bonus Question:* What is the definition of the combining form? _____

6.   a)   pyloroplasty   _____/__/_____
                                      cf   s

   b)   *Bonus Question:* What is the definition of the suffix? _____

7.   a)   antidiarrheal   _____/_____/___
                                      p   r   s

   b)   *Bonus Question:* What is the definition of the prefix? _____

8.   a)   gingivectomy   _____/_____
                                      r   s

   b)   *Bonus Question:* What is the definition of the word root? _____

9.   a)   vagotomy   _____/__/_____
                                      cf   s

   b)   *Bonus Question:* What is the definition of the suffix? _____

Abbreviations of the Digestive System

The abbreviations that are associated with the digestive system are summarized here. Study these abbreviations, and review them in the exercise that follows.

Abbreviation	Definition
BE	barium enema
EGD	esophagogastroduodenoscopy
FOBT	fecal occult blood test
GI	gastrointestinal
GERD	gastroesophageal reflux disease

Abbreviation	Definition
IBD	inflammatory bowel disease
IBS	irritable bowel syndrome
LGI	lower GI series
N&V	nausea and vomiting
SCS	stool culture and sensitivity
UGI	upper GI series

PRACTICE: Abbreviations

Fill in the blanks with the abbreviation or the complete medical term.

Abbreviation

1. BE

2. _____

3. UGI

4. _____

5. N&V

6. _____

7. IBS

8. _____

9. SCS

10. _____

11. FOBT

12. _____

Medical Term

_____

inflammatory bowel disease

_____

gastroesophageal reflux disease

_____

upper GI series

_____

lower GI series

_____

gastrointestinal

_____

esophagogastroduodenoscopy

▶▶▶▶ Chapter Review

Word Building

Construct medical terms from the following meanings. (Some are built from word parts, some are not.) The first question has been completed as an example.

1. indigestion   _dys_pepsia

2. enlargement of the liver   _____y

3. difficulty swallowing   _____phag_____

4. inflammation of the lip   _____itis

5. inflammation of the gallbladder   cholecyst_____

6. condition of gallstones   chole_____

7. inflammation of the colon   _____itis

8. cancer of the colon and rectum   _____al cancer

9. inflammation of the small intestine   enter_____

10. softening of the stomach wall   gastro_____

11. condition of diverticula   diverticul_____

12. tumor of the liver   _____oma

13. inflammation of a salivary gland   _____itis

14. surgical removal of hemorrhoids   _____ectomy

15. surgical creation of an opening into the colon   _____ostomy

16. endoscopic evaluation of the rectum   proct_____

17. endoscopic evaluation of the abdominal cavity   _____oscopy

18. surgical repair of the tongue with sutures   gloss_____

19. surgical removal of a polyp   polyp_____

▶▶▶▶ Clinical Application Exercises

Medical Report

Read the following medical report, then answer the questions that follow.

University Hospital

5500 University Avenue
Metropolis, TX

Phone: (211) 594-4000
Fax: (211) 594-4001

Medical Consultation: Internal Medicine

Date: 4/05/2008

Patient: Maria Nguygen

Patient Complaint: Diarrhea, flatus, abdominal cramping, with occasional vomiting for approximately four weeks prior to initial office visit.

History: 10-year-old female, showing normal height but underweight by 15 pounds; otherwise no prior medical concerns.

Family History: Father of Asian descent, 42 years old, with food allergies to milk products; suspect ulcer tested positive for *H. pylori* but declined treatment. Mother of Hispanic descent, 38 years old, with no reported medical concerns.

Allergies: Suspected lactose intolerance.

Evidences: Progressive intestinal pain with diarrhea and cramping. Colonoscopy positive for inflamed diverticula of colon; BE test reveals inflammation of ileum as diagnostic of CD with intussusception of ileum, confirmed with laparoscopy.

Treatment: Admit patient for additional tests in preparation for possible radical colectomy with ileostomy.

Joanne M. Winegard, M.D.

---

1. What is the diagnosis? _____

    _____

2. Which findings support the diagnosis? _____

    _____

3. Can you think of an additional diagnostic exam that might be used before a conclusive treatment plan is begun?

    _____

    _____

Medical Report Case Study

The following Case Study provides further discussion regarding the patient in the medical report. Fill in the blanks with the correct terms. Choose your answers from the following list of terms. (Note that some terms may be used more than once.)

barium enema	diarrhea	intussusception
colectomy	diverticulitis	irritable bowel syndrome
constipation	flatus	lactose intolerance
Crohn's disease	inflammatory bowel	laparoscopy

A 10-year-old female named Maria Nguygen was admitted following a history of four weeks of intermittent watery

stools, or (a) _____, accompanied with trapped gas, or (b) _____, occasional reduced

peristalsis of the large intestine, or (c) _____, abdominal pain, and vomiting. Initial diagnosis by her

personal GP was the lack of the digestive enzyme lactase, known as (d) _____ _____,

although IBS, or (e) _____ _____ _____, was ruled as another pos-

sibility. With time, symptoms of pain and bowel irregularity increased, raising the concern that the child might be suffering

from a chronic inflammation of the ileum, or (f) _____ _____, a type of IBD, or

(g) _____ _____ disease. Once admitted, thorough testing including a lactase enzyme

test, BE (also known as (h) _____ _____), a UGI series, and an endoscopy into the

abdomen, called a (i) _____ ensued. The BE revealed the presence of inflamed diverticula, leading to the

diagnosis of (j) _____. The laparoscopy indicated an infolding of a segment of the small intestine into

another segment, a condition known as (k) _____, which had led to an intestinal obstruction.

Because both the colon and ileum are diseased, the recommended treatment was surgery for the removal of the colon in

the (l) _____ procedure with establishment of ileostomy.

▶▶▶▶ Key Terms Double-Check

Remember that the chapter's key terms appeared alphabetically throughout this chapter. This exercise helps you to check your knowledge AND review for tests.

1. First, fill in the missing word in the definitions for the chapter's key terms.
2. Then, check your answers using Appendix F.
3. If you got the answer right, put a check mark in the right column.
4. If your answer was incorrect, go back to the frame number provided and review the content.

Use the checklist to study the terms you don't know until you're confident you know them all.

Key Term	Frame	Definition	Know It?
1. abdominocentesis	10.67	surgical puncture through the abdominal wall to remove fluid, also known as _____	☐
2. anorexia nervosa	10.24	emotional _____ _____ in which the patient avoids food due to a compulsion to become thin in appearance	☐
3. antacid	10.68	an agent that reduces the _____ of the stomach cavity	☐
4. antiemetic	10.69	a drug that prevents or stops the _____ reflex	☐
5. antispasmodic	10.70	a drug that reduces _____ activity in the GI tract	☐
6. aphagia	10.9	inability to swallow, literally "without _____"	☐
7. appendectomy	10.71	surgical _____ of the appendix	☐
8. appendicitis	10.25	inflammation of the _____	☐
9. ascites	10.10	an accumulation of fluid within the peritoneal cavity that produces an enlarged _____	☐
10. bulimia	10.26	eating disorder involving repeated _____ with food followed by induced vomiting or laxative abuse	☐
11. cathartic	10.72	an agent that stimulates strong _____ of peristalsis of the colon	☐
12. cheilitis	10.27	_____ of the lip	☐
13. cheilorrhaphy	10.73	procedure of _____ a lip	☐
14. cholecystectomy	10.74	surgical _____ of the gallbladder	☐
15. cholecystitis	10.28	inflammation of the gallbladder, usually caused by _____ lodged within it	☐
16. cholecystography	10.75	procedure of producing an X-ray image, or _____, of the gallbladder	☐
17. choledochitis	10.29	presence of stones within the _____ _____ _____ causing inflammation	☐
18. choledocho-lithotomy	10.76	surgery that involves the removal of one or more obstructive _____ from the common bile duct	☐
19. cholelithiasis	10.30	generalized condition of stones lodged within the _____ or bile ducts	☐
20. cirrhosis	10.31	chronic, progressive liver disease characterized by the gradual loss of liver cells and their replacement by fat and other forms of _____ tissue	☐

Key Term	Frame	Definition	Know It?
21. cleft palate	10.77	a congenital defect in which the bones supporting the roof of the mouth, or hard palate, fail to fuse during fetal development, leaving a _____ between the oral cavity and nasal cavity	☐
22. colectomy	10.78	surgical removal of a segment of the _____	☐
23. colitis	10.32	inflammation of the colon; if chronic bleeding of the colon wall produces bloody diarrhea, the condition is called _____ _____	☐
24. colorectal cancer	10.33	cancer of the colon and the rectum often arises as a _____ becomes an aggressive, metastatic tumor	☐
25. colostomy	10.79	surgical creation of an opening in the colon to serve as an artificial _____	☐
26. constipation	10.11	_____ or incomplete bowel movements	☐
27. Crohn's disease	10.34	chronic inflammation of any part of the GI tract that involves ulcerations, scar tissue formation, and thickening adhesions of the organ wall, also known as _____ _____	☐
28. diarrhea	10.12	frequent discharge of _____ fecal material	☐
29. diverticulosis	10.35	presence of small pouches called _____ on the wall of the colon, often without symptoms or with mild bowel discomfort	☐
30. duodenal ulcer	10.36	ulcer, or erosion, in the wall of the _____ of the small intestine	☐
31. dysentery	10.37	acute inflammation of the _____ tract that is caused by bacteria, protozoa, or chemical irritants	☐
32. dyspepsia	10.13	commonly called _____, it is accompanied by stomach or esophageal pain or discomfort	☐
33. dysphagia	10.14	difficulty in _____	☐
34. enteritis	10.38	inflammation of the _____ or large intestine	☐
35. esophagitis	10.39	inflammation of the esophagus often caused by acid _____	☐
36. fecal occult blood test	10.80	clinical lab test performed to detect blood in the feces, abbreviated _____	☐
37. flatus	10.15	presence of _____, or air, in the GI tract	☐
38. food-borne illness	10.40	ingestion of food contaminated with harmful bacteria can cause symptoms of diarrhea and vomiting; *Clostridium botulinum* causes food-borne illness known as _____	☐
39. gastrectasis	10.41	abnormal _____ of the stomach	☐
40. gastrectomy	10.81	surgical removal of part of the stomach or, in extreme cases, the _____ organ	☐
41. gastric cancer	10.42	an aggressive, metastatic cancer arising from cells lining the stomach, commonly known as _____ cancer	☐
42. gastric lavage	10.82	cleansing procedure in which the stomach is _____ with a prescribed solution	☐

Key Term	Frame	Definition	Know It?
43. gastric ulcer	10.43	_____, or erosion, in the wall of the stomach	☐
44. gastritis	10.44	inflammation of the _____	☐
45. gastrodynia	10.16	symptom of stomach pain, also known as _____	☐
46. gastroenteritis	10.44	inflammation of the stomach and _____ intestine	☐
47. gastroesophageal reflux disease	10.45	recurring reflux of stomach contents into the esophagus is a condition that is abbreviated _____	☐
48. gastromalacia	10.46	_____ of the stomach wall	☐
49. gavage	10.83	process of feeding a patient through a tube inserted into the _____ that extends through the esophagus to enter the stomach	☐
50. giardiasis	10.47	_____ by the intestinal protozoa *Giardia intestinalis* or *Giardia lamblia* produces symptoms of diarrhea, cramps, nausea, and vomiting	☐
51. GI endoscopy	10.84	visual examination of the GI tract made possible by the use of an _____	☐
52. GI series	10.85	diagnostic techniques that provide radiographic examination of the GI tract, usually by means of barium swallow, barium _____, or barium meal (upper GI), or barium enema (BE) (lower GI)	☐
53. gingivectomy	10.86	surgical removal of diseased tissue in the _____, or gingiva	☐
54. gingivitis	10.48	inflammation of the gums, or _____	☐
55. glossitis	10.49	inflammation of the _____ often caused by exposure to allergens, toxic substances, or extreme heat or cold	☐
56. glossorrhaphy	10.87	_____ of the tongue	☐
57. halitosis	10.17	condition of bad _____	☐
58. hematemesis	10.18	vomiting _____, a sign of a severe digestive disorder	☐
59. hemorrhoidectomy	10.88	surgical removal of _____	☐
60. hemorrhoids	10.50	varicose, or _____, condition of the veins in the anus that produces painful swellings that may break open and bleed	☐
61. hepatitis	10.51	_____-_____ inflammation of the liver; the five known forms are categorized with the letters *A* through *E*	☐
62. hepatoma	10.52	tumor arising from cells within the liver; also called _____ carcinoma, or HCC	☐
63. hepatomegaly	10.19	abnormal _____ of the liver	☐
64. hiatal hernia	10.53	protrusion of the cardiac portion of the stomach through the _____ of the diaphragm to enter the thoracic cavity	☐
65. ileostomy	10.89	surgical creation of an _____ through the abdominal wall and into the ileum of the small intestine to establish an alternative anus for the passage of feces	☐
66. inflammatory bowel disease	10.54	general term that includes the conditions ulcerative colitis and Crohn's disease, abbreviated _____	☐

Key Term	Frame	Definition	Know It?
67. intussusception	10.55	condition of _____ of a segment of the small intestine within another segment	☐
68. irritable bowel syndrome	10.56	_____ disease characterized by periodic disturbances of large intestinal (bowel) function without clear physical damage, abbreviated IBS	☐
69. jaundice	10.20	yellowish-orange coloration of the skin, sclera of the eyes, and deeper tissues that is a collective sign of _____ disease	☐
70. lactose intolerance	10.57	lack of an _____ in the small intestine that breaks down lactose, the primary sugar in milk and milk products	☐
71. laparotomy	10.90	surgical procedure that involves an _____ through the abdominal wall, often from the base of the sternum to the pubic bone	☐
72. malabsorption syndrome	10.58	disorder that is characterized by difficulty in _____ one or more nutrients	☐
73. nausea	10.21	symptom of dizziness that includes an urge to vomit; when accompanied by vomiting, it is abbreviated _____	☐
74. pancreatitis	10.59	inflammation of the _____	☐
75. parotitis	10.60	inflammation of one or both parotid glands; if caused by a virus, it is usually referred to as _____	☐
76. peptic ulcer	10.61	erosion into the inner wall of an organ along the GI _____	☐
77. peritonitis	10.62	inflammation of the extensive _____ that lines the inner wall of the abdominopelvic cavity and covers most of its organs	☐
78. polypectomy	10.91	surgical removal of _____	☐
79. polyposis	10.63	condition of polyps, usually occurring in the colon or rectum of the large intestine, where it increases the risk for colorectal _____	☐
80. proctitis	10.64	inflammation of the _____, and usually the rectum as well	☐
81. proctoptosis	10.65	_____ of the rectum	☐
82. pyloroplasty	10.92	surgical repair of the pylorus region of the stomach, which may include repair of the pyloric _____	☐
83. reflux	10.22	backward flow of material in the GI tract, or _____	☐
84. steatorrhea	10.23	abnormal levels of fat in the _____, literally "discharge of fat"	☐
85. stool culture and sensitivity	10.93	test that includes obtaining stool (fecal) samples, using the samples to grow microorganisms in culture, and identifying the microorganisms, abbreviated _____	☐
86. vagotomy	10.94	surgical dissection of branches of the _____ nerve	☐
87. volvulus	10.66	severe _____ of the intestine that leads to obstruction	☐

Multimedia Preview ▶▶▶▶▶

Additional interactive resources and activities for this chapter can be found on the Companion Website. For videos, audio glossary, and review, access the accompanying DVD-ROM in this book.

DVD-ROM Highlights

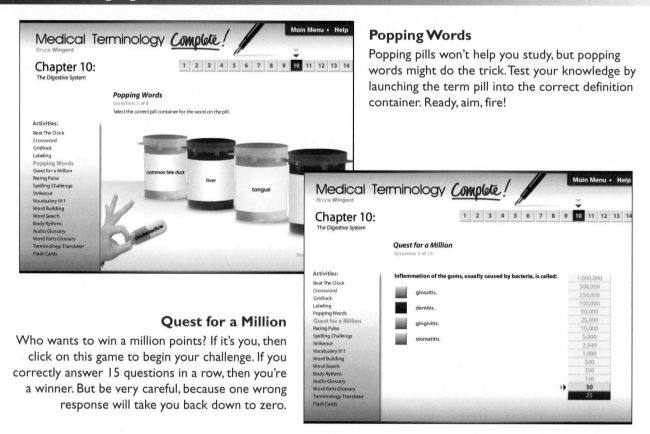

Popping Words

Popping pills won't help you study, but popping words might do the trick. Test your knowledge by launching the term pill into the correct definition container. Ready, aim, fire!

Quest for a Million

Who wants to win a million points? If it's you, then click on this game to begin your challenge. If you correctly answer 15 questions in a row, then you're a winner. But be very careful, because one wrong response will take you back down to zero.

Website Highlights—www.prenhall.com/wingerd

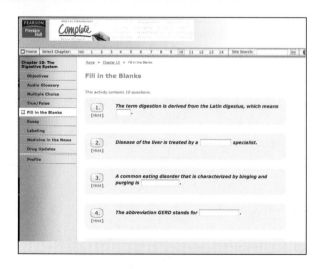

Fill-in-the-Blanks Exercise

Take advantage of the free-access online study guide that accompanies your textbook. You'll find a fill in the blanks quiz that provides instant feedback, allowing you to check your score and see what you got right or wrong. By clicking on this URL you'll also access links to download mp3 audio reviews, current news articles, and an audio glossary.

The Urinary System ▶▶▶▶▶

Learning Objectives

After completing this chapter, you will be able to:

- Define and spell the word parts used to create terms for the urinary system.

- Break down and define common medical terms used for symptoms, diseases, disorders, procedures, treatments, and devices associated with the urinary system.

- Build medical terms from the word parts associated with the urinary system.

- Pronounce and spell common medical terms associated with the urinary system.

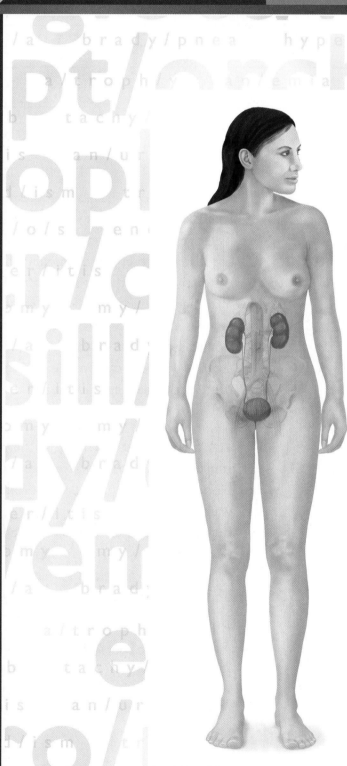

Anatomy and Physiology Terms ▶▶▶▶▶

The following table provides the combining forms that specifically apply to the anatomy and physiology of the urinary system. Note that the combining forms are colored red to help you identify them when you see them again later in the chapter.

Combining Form	Definition	Combining Form	Definition
albumin/o	protein	pyel/o	renal pelvis
blast/o	developing cell	ren/o	kidney
glomerul/o	little ball, glomerulus	ureter/o	ureter
gluc/o, glyc/o, glycos/o	sweet, sugar	urethr/o	urethra
meat/o	opening, passage	ur/o, urin/o	urine
nephr/o	kidney		

urinary
YOU rih nair ee

11.1 The _____ system functions as the sanitation engineer of the body, maintaining the purity and health of the body's fluids by removing unwanted waste materials and recycling other materials. The kidneys are its most important organs. They filter gallons of fluids from the bloodstream every day, removing metabolic wastes, toxins, excess ions, and water that leave the body as urine, while returning needed materials back into the blood. Because waste removal is essential for your survival, the kidneys are vital organs; a loss of both kidneys requires medical intervention to sustain life. Other organs of the urinary system transport urine or store it before it can be released to the exterior. They are the paired ureters, the urinary bladder, and the urethra.

FUNCTION ▶▶▶

urine

11.2 You have just learned that the primary function of the kidneys is the removal of metabolic wastes, toxins, excess ions, and water from the bloodstream. This function is performed by the formation of urine as a watery waste. _____ is formed by three processes occurring in the kidneys: filtration of the blood to produce a filtrate, reabsorption of excess water in the filtrate to return it to the bloodstream, and secretion of excess ions as waste into the filtrate. In addition to forming urine, the kidneys also perform other vital functions:

- Regulation of blood pressure
- Regulation of pH within body fluids
- Regulation of water and salt concentrations
- Regulation of red blood cell production

11.3 Use the anatomy terms that appear in the left column to fill in the corresponding blanks in Figures 11.1■ through 11.3■.

1. **kidney**
2. **artery**
3. **ureter**
4. **bladder**
5. **urethra**

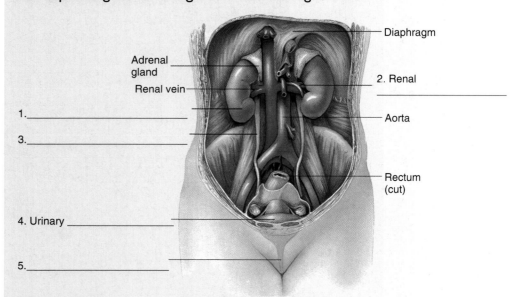

Adrenal gland

Renal vein

Diaphragm

2. Renal _____

Aorta

Rectum (cut)

1. _____

3. _____

4. Urinary _____

5. _____

Figure 11.1 ■

Organs of the urinary system. This illustration is an anterior view of a female with the abdominal wall and digestive organs removed.

6. **renal**
7. **pelvis**
8. **ureter**

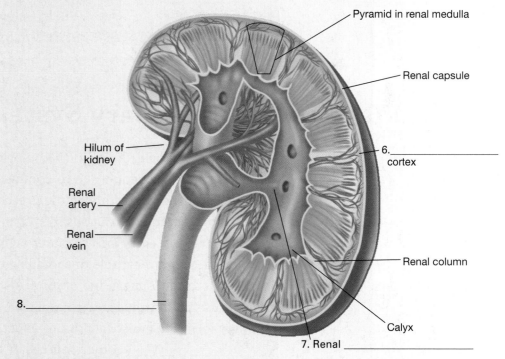

Pyramid in renal medulla

Renal capsule

Hilum of kidney

Renal artery

Renal vein

6. _____ cortex

Renal column

8. _____

Calyx

7. Renal _____

Figure 11.2 ■

The kidney. Illustration of a sectioned kidney, which reveals its internal features.

9. **distal**
10. **duct**
11. **glomerulus**

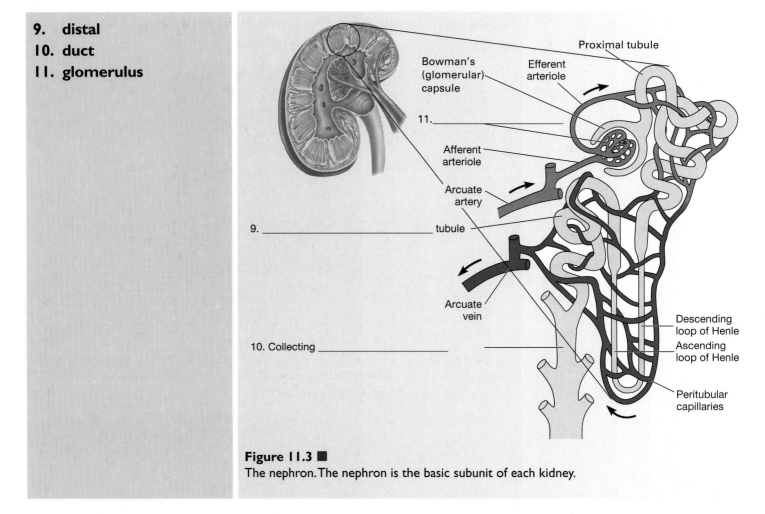

Bowman's (glomerular) capsule

Proximal tubule

Efferent arteriole

11. _____

Afferent arteriole

Arcuate artery

9. _____ tubule

Arcuate vein

Descending loop of Henle

Ascending loop of Henle

Peritubular capillaries

10. Collecting _____

Figure 11.3 ■
The nephron. The nephron is the basic subunit of each kidney.

Medical Terms for the Urinary System ▶▶▶▶▶

infections

11.4 For most people, the major pathological challenge to the health of the urinary system is infection, due to communication to the exterior by way of the urinary meatus. Although the urethra, urinary bladder, and ureters are each protected by a mucous membrane, bacteria and viruses are sometimes able to gain entry into the internal organs through the meatus. Once established, they are capable of spreading through the urinary tract, bringing disease to the kidneys and beyond. Also, the close location of the urinary meatus to the anus in females enables some bacterial populations that normally form the intestinal flora to infect the urinary tract. In addition to _____, other sources of disease may afflict the urinary system, including tumors, stones, inherited disorders, and cardiovascular disease.

urine

11.5 Because _____ originates from the bloodstream and the urinary system releases urine on a regular basis, urine testing provides a convenient means for testing general health. Many diseases can be diagnosed from a urine sample that contains abnormal contents, such as blood cells, bacteria, albumin (a protein normally found in blood), glucose, and high levels of creatinine (a protein product of metabolism).

nephrology
neh FROL oh jee

11.6 The clinical treatment of urinary disease is a medical discipline known as **urology** (yoo RAHL oh jee). In most hospitals and clinics, the unit specializing in the treatment of urinary diseases is simply called urology. A physician specializing in this field of medicine is called a **urologist**. The field that specializes in the treatment of kidney disease is _____. A physician specializing in this field is a **nephrologist.**

11.7 In the following sections, you will study the prefixes, combining forms, and suffixes that combine to build the medical terms of the urinary system. Complete the frames and review exercises that follow. You are on your way to mastery of the medical terms related to the urinary system!

Signs and Symptoms of the Urinary System

Following are the word parts that specifically apply to the signs and symptoms of the urinary system that are covered in the following section. Note that the word parts are color-coded to help you identify them: prefixes are blue, combining forms are red, and suffixes are purple.

Prefix	Definition
an-	without or absence of
dia-	through
dys-	bad, abnormal, painful, or difficult
poly-	excessive, over, or many

Combining Form	Definition
albumin/o	albumin (a protein)
azot/o	urea or nitrogen
bacteri/o	bacteria
glycos/o	sweet or sugar
hem/o, hemat/o	blood
ket/o, keton/o	ketone
noct/o	night
olig/o	few in number
prote/o	protein
py/o	pus

Suffix	Definition
-emia	condition of blood
-urea	urine
-uresis	urination
-uria	pertaining to urine or urination

albuminuria
AL byoo men YOO ree ah

11.8 A **urinalysis** (Frame 11.82) is a clinical procedure that examines the composition of urine using a variety of tests, including microscopy. Diseases of the urinary system and other parts of the body may be diagnosed with this valuable clinical tool. For example, albumin is a protein normally present in the bloodstream. If it appears in the urine, it is a physical sign of abnormal renal filtration. The condition is called _____. This constructed term contains two word parts and is written albumin/uria.

anuresis
an yoo REE siss

anuria
an YOO ree ah

11.9 The inability to pass urine is a sign of a blockage of the urinary tract or kidney failure. It is called _____, which is a constructed term written as an/uresis. It literally means "without urination." Alternatively, the suffix -uria may be substituted to form the term _____ and is written an/uria. It means "without urine." Clinically, anuria is the production of less than 100 mL of urine per day.

azotemia
az oh TEE mee ah

11.10 The sign of abnormally high levels of urea and other nitrogen-containing compounds in the blood is called **azotemia**. _____ is a constructed term and is written azot/emia.

bacteriuria
bak ter ee YOO ree ah
bacter/i/uria

11.11 The abnormal presence of bacteria in the urine is a sign of a urinary tract infection and is called _____. This constructed term includes three word parts, which are revealed when the term is written as _____/__/_____.

diuresis
DYE yoo REE siss

11.12 The excessive discharge of urine is a sign of the endocrine disorders known as diabetes insipidus and diabetes mellitus. This is known as **diuresis**, which literally means "urination through." (Note that, in this term, the *a* in the prefix *dia-* is not used.) The constructed form of _____ is written di/uresis. It may also be called **polyuria** (Frame 11.19).

dysuria
diss YOO ree ah

11.13 Recall that the prefix *dys-* means "bad, abnormal, painful, or difficult." When *dys-* is combined with the suffix for "urination," the resulting term refers to difficulty or pain experienced during urination. It is a symptom of a urinary tract disease often caused by a bacterial infection. The symptom is called _____. It is a constructed term written dys/uria.

glycosuria
glye kohs YOO ree ah

11.14 The combining form *glycos/o* means "sweet or sugar." The abnormal presence of glucose (sugar) in the urine is a sign of an endocrine disease, such as diabetes mellitus, or a kidney disorder, or perhaps both. The sign is called _____, which is a constructed term written *glycos/uria*.

hematuria
HEE mah TOO ree ah

11.15 The abnormal presence of blood in the urine is a sign of urinary disease. It is called _____, which means "pertaining to bloody urination." The constructed form of this term is written *hemat/uria*.

ketonuria
kee tohn YOO ree ah

11.16 The abnormal presence of ketone bodies in the urine is called **ketonuria**. The constructed form of _____ uses the combining form for ketone bodies (*keton/o*) and is written *keton/uria*. It is a common sign of a metabolic disorder, a high-protein/low-carbohydrate diet, starvation, or diabetes mellitus.

WORDS TO WATCH OUT FOR !

Terms with No Combining Vowels

Most of the terms related to the signs and symptoms of the urinary system contain no combining vowel. For example, terms such as *ketonuria* and *anuresis* only contain a word root and suffix. This is because the suffixes in this section (*-emia, -urea, -uresis, -uria*) all begin with a vowel, so no combining vowel is needed to make the terms easier to pronounce.

nocturia
nok TOO ree ah

11.17 The need to urinate frequently at night is a possible symptom of diabetes mellitus or benign prostate hyperplasia (BPH). It is called **nocturia**. As a constructed term, _____ includes two word parts and is written *noct/uria*.

oliguria
all ig YOO ree ah

11.18 Reduced urination becomes a clinical problem when the volume of urine declines to less than 500 mL within a 24-hour period. It is known as **oliguria** and is a possible sign of a kidney disorder. _____ may also be a sign of congestive heart failure, dehydration, or a blockage in the urinary tract. This constructed term is written *olig/uria*.

polyuria
pall ee YOO ree ah

11.19 Chronic excessive urination is a common sign of an endocrine disease, usually diabetes insipidus or diabetes mellitus. The sign is called _____, which is a constructed term written *poly/uria*. It is also known as **diuresis** (Frame 11.12).

proteinuria proh tee NYOO ree ah	**11.20** In Frame 11.8 you learned that albuminuria is the presence of the protein albumin in the urine. The presence of any protein in the urine is called _____. This constructed term is written protein/uria.
pyuria pye YOO ree ah	**11.21** Pus is a mixture of white blood cells, bacteria, and cell debris that forms during an infection. Its appearance in the urine indicates a urinary tract infection. The presence of pus in urine is called _____, which is a constructed term written py/uria. The combining form that means "pus" is py/o.

PRACTICE: Signs and Symptoms of the Urinary System

The Right Match

Match the term on the left with the correct definition on the right.

_____ 1. albuminuria	a. urination at night
_____ 2. bacteriuria	b. presence of blood in the urine
_____ 3. diuresis	c. presence of bacteria in the urine
_____ 4. glycosuria	d. chronic excessive urination
_____ 5. hematuria	e. ketone bodies in the urine
_____ 6. ketonuria	f. presence of sugar in the urine
_____ 7. nocturia	g. presence of albumin in the urine
_____ 8. oliguria	h. reduced urination
_____ 9. polyuria	i. literally "urination through"

Break the Chain

Analyze these medical terms:

    a) Separate each term into its word parts; each word part is labeled for you (**p** = prefix, **r** = root, **cf** = combining form, and **s** = suffix).

    b) For the Bonus Question, write the requested definition in the blank that follows.

The first set has been completed as an example.

1. a) proteinuria

                     protein/uria
                           r   s

    b) *Bonus Question:* What is the definition of the suffix? *pertaining to urine or urination*

2. a) azotemia

                       ____/_____
                        r   s

    b) *Bonus Question:* What is the definition of the word root? _____

3. a) dysuria

                       _____/_____
                       p   s

    b) *Bonus Question:* What is the definition of the suffix? _____

4. a) anuresis

                       _____/_____
                       p   s

    b) *Bonus Question:* What is the definition of the prefix? _____

5. a) pyuria

                       _____/_____
                       r   s

    b) *Bonus Question:* What is the definition of the word root? _____

Diseases and Disorders of the Urinary System

Review some of the word parts that specifically apply to the diseases and disorders of the urinary system that are covered in the following section. Note that the word parts are color-coded to help you identify them: prefixes are blue, combining forms are red, and suffixes are purple.

Prefix	Definition
an-	without or absence of
dia-	through
dys-	bad, abnormal, painful, or difficult
en-	within, upon, on, or over
epi-	upon, over, above, or on top
hypo-	deficient, abnormally low, or below
poly-	excessive, over, or many

Combining Form	Definition
albumin/o	albumin (a protein)
azot/o	urea or nitrogen
bacter/o	bacteria
blast/o	germ or bud
cyst/o	bladder
glomerul/o	ball or glomerulus
hemat/o	blood
hydr/o	water
ket/o, keton/o	ketone
lith/o	stone
nephr/o	kidney
olig/o	few in number
prote/o	protein
py/o	pus
pyel/o	renal pelvis
ren/o	kidney
spadias/o	rip or tear
sten/o	narrow
ur/o	urine
ureter/o	ureter
urethr/o	urethra

Suffix	Definition
-al	pertaining to
-cele	hernia, swelling, or protrusion
-emia	condition of blood
-ia	condition of
-iasis	condition of
-ic	pertaining to
-itis	inflammation
-megaly	abnormally large
-oma	tumor
-osis	condition of
-pathy	disease
-ptosis	drooping
-sis	state of
-urea	urine
-uria	pertaining to urine or urination

KEY TERMS A-Z

cystitis
siss TYE tiss

11.22 The combining form for bladder is cyst/o. An inflammation of the urinary bladder is called _____. This constructed term is written cyst/itis. It is usually caused by a bacterial infection that travels up the urethra. An infection of the urinary bladder and the urethra is called **urethrocystitis** (yoo REE throh siss TYE tiss), which is written urethr/o/cyst/itis.

cystocele
SISS toh seel

11.23 A herniation of the urinary bladder is called a **cystocele**. In females, the protrusion pushes into the adjacent vagina. The term _____ is a constructed term with three word parts, written cyst/o/cele.

cystolith
SISS toh lith

11.24 A _____ is a stone, or calculus, in the urinary bladder. If it is too large to pass through the urethra, medical intervention is required to eliminate it. This constructed term is written cyst/o/lith.

enuresis
ehn yoo REE siss

11.25 An involuntary release of urine, which usually occurs due to a lack of bladder control among children or the elderly, is known as **enuresis**. When this occurs during sleep, it is known as **nocturnal** _____, or bedwetting. This constructed term is written en/uresis.

epispadias
EP ih SPAY dee ass

11.26 A congenital defect resulting in the abnormal positioning of the urinary meatus is known as **epispadias**. In males, the meatus opens on the dorsal (upper) surface of the penis, and in females the meatus opens dorsal to the clitoris. _____ is a constructed term written epi/spadias, which literally means "a rip or tear upon."

glomerulonephritis
gloh MAIR yoo loh neh FRYE tiss

11.27 Recall that a glomerulus is a ball of specialized capillaries within a kidney nephron. Any disease of the glomeruli is called a **glomerulonephropathy** (gloh MAIR yoo loh neh FROH path ee), which is a constructed term written glomerul/o/nephr/o/pathy. An example is inflammation of the glomeruli, which is known as _____. It is usually caused by a bacterial infection. The constructed term is written glomerul/o/nephr/itis.

hydronephrosis
HIGH droh neh FROH siss

11.28 The production of urine by the kidneys is a physiological process that is continual throughout your lifetime. If the exit of urine out of the kidneys becomes blocked by an obstruction in a ureter, the urine will back up to cause distension of the renal pelvis. This condition is known as **hydronephrosis** and is illustrated in Figure 11.4■. The term _____ contains five word parts and is written hydr/o/nephr/o/sis. Recall that *hydr/o* means "water," which refers to the fluid (urine) blockage that occurs in this condition.

Figure 11.4 ■
Hydronephrosis. External (left) and internal (right) views of a kidney with hydronephrosis. Note the distension (swelling) of the renal pelvis. In this illustration, the distension was caused by the constriction of the ureter, causing urine to back up in the renal pelvis.

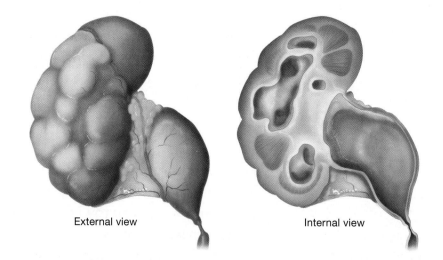

External view   Internal view

hypospadias
HIGH poh SPAY dee ass

11.29 You learned in Frame 11.26 that epispadias is a congenital defect in which the urinary meatus has shifted dorsally. In **hypospadias**, the change in location of the urinary meatus is ventral. In males, it opens on the underside of the penis, and in females the meatus is within the vagina. _____ is a constructed term written hypo/spadias, which literally means "a rip or tear below."

incontinence
in KON tih nens

11.30 The inability to control urination is called **urinary** _____. In **stress incontinence**, an involuntary discharge of urine occurs during a cough, sneeze, or strained movement.

nephritis
neh FRYE tiss

11.31 One word root for kidney is *nephr*, and is found in many terms describing a kidney disease or procedure. For example, inflammation of a kidney is known as **nephritis**. Its usual cause is a bacterial infection, and if left untreated it can lead to the more serious condition of glomerulonephritis (Frame 11.27). _____ is a constructed term written nephr/itis.

11.32 A **nephroblastoma** is a tumor originating from kidney tissue that includes developing embryonic cells (Figure 11.5■). It is also called **Wilms' tumor** after the 19th-century German physician who published the first description of the disease. _____ is a constructed term written nephr/o/blast/oma.

nephroblastoma
NEFF roh blass TOH mah

Figure 11.5 ■
Nephroblastoma. A sectioned kidney reveals the presence of a very large tumor, which arose from fetal cells during development. A newborn with nephroblastoma is illustrated to show the location and relative size of the tumor.

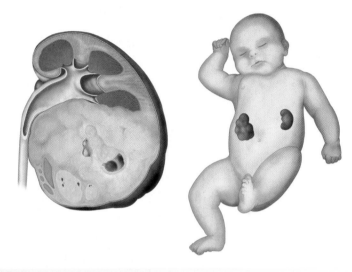

11.33 The presence of one or more stones, or calculi, within a kidney is called **nephrolithiasis**. This constructed term is written nephr/o/lith/iasis. An alternate term for _____ is **renal calculi** (REE nal * KAL kyoo lye) and is further described in Figure 11.6■.

nephrolithiasis
NEFF roh lith EYE ah siss

Figure 11.6 ■
Nephrolithiasis. Stones, or calculi, may form in several areas within the urinary tract. When they form in the kidney, they usually arise within the renal pelvis to form the condition nephrolithiasis. Kidney stones may dislocate to form obstructions in the ureter, urinary bladder, or urethra, usually at their junctions.

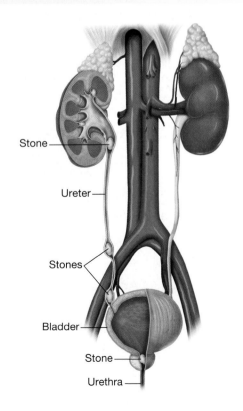

Stone
Ureter
Stones
Bladder
Stone
Urethra

nephroma neff ROH mah	**11.34** A general term for a tumor arising from kidney tissue is _____. This constructed term is written nephr/oma.
nephromegaly neff roh MEG ah lee	**11.35** The suffix -*megaly* means "abnormally large." An abnormal enlargement of one or both kidneys is called _____. The three word parts of this term can be shown as nephr/o/megaly.
nephroptosis neff ropp TOH siss	**11.36** The condition of a downward displacement ("drooping") of a kidney is known as **nephroptosis**. The constructed form of this term is nephr/o/ptosis. It occurs when the kidney is no longer held in its proper position against the posterior abdominal wall. _____ is commonly called **floating kidney**.
polycystic PALL ee SISS tik	**11.37** A kidney condition characterized by the presence of numerous cysts (fluid-filled capsules) occupying much of the kidney tissue is called **polycystic kidney disease**. The cysts replace normal tissue, resulting in a loss of kidney function (Figure 11.7■). The term _____ is a constructed term composed of three word parts, poly/cyst/ic, and literally means "pertaining to many bladders."

Figure 11.7 ■
Polycystic kidney disease. A polycystic kidney on the left is compared to a normal kidney on the right.

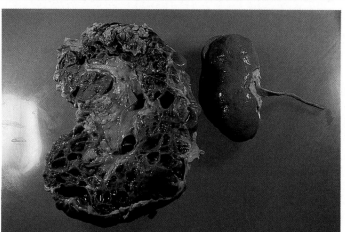

pyelitis PYE eh LYE tiss	**11.38** The combining form for renal pelvis is *pyel/o*. Inflammation of the renal pelvis is called _____. It is usually caused by a bacterial infection. The constructed form of this term is pyel/itis.
pyelonephritis PYE eh loh neh FRYE tiss	**11.39** An inflammatory condition of the renal pelvis and nephrons is called **pyelonephritis**. The constructed form of _____ is written pyel/o/nephr/itis.

strictures
STRIK cherz

11.40 A condition of abnormal narrowing is known as a **stricture**. Examples of urinary _____ include **ureteral stricture**, in which the ureter is narrowed; **urethral stricture**, in which the urethra is narrowed; and a **ureterovesical stricture**, in which the junction of the ureter and bladder is narrowed. Because the medical term **stenosis** also refers to an abnormal narrowing, it may be used as an alternative term to *stricture* in each of these terms. An example term is **ureterostenosis** (yoo REE ter oh steh NOH siss), which is a ureteral stricture, or narrowing. The constructed form of this term is ureter/o/sten/osis.

uremia
yoo REE mee ah

11.41 In the condition **uremia**, an excess of urea and other nitrogenous wastes are present in the blood. The constructed form of this term is ur/emia. _____ is caused by failure of the kidneys to remove urea and is associated with renal insufficiency or renal failure.

ureteritis
yoo REE ter EYE tiss

11.42 The ureters are the paired narrow tubes that transport urine from the kidneys to the urinary bladder. Inflammation of a ureter is called _____ and is often the result of a bacterial infection. This constructed term is written ureter/itis.

ureterocele
yoo REE ter oh seel

11.43 A herniated ureter is called a **ureterocele**. The constructed form of _____ is ureter/o/cele.

ureterolithiasis
yoo REE ter oh lith EYE ah siss

11.44 The presence of one or more stones, or calculi, within a ureter is called **ureterolithiasis**. The constructed form of _____ includes a combining form *and* a word root, and is written ureter/o/lith/iasis.

urinary retention
YOO rih nair ee * ree TEN shun

11.45 The abnormal accumulation of urine within the urinary bladder is called **urinary retention**. The condition of _____ _____ results from an inability to void, or urinate.

urinary suppression
YOO rih nair ee * suh PREH shun

11.46 An acute stoppage of urine formation by the kidneys is known as **urinary suppression**. The condition of _____ _____ is a consequence of **acute renal failure**, in which kidney function ceases.

urinary tract infection
YOO rih nair ee * trakt * in FEK shun

11.47 Commonly called by its abbreviation of **UTI**, a _____ _____ _____ is an infection of urinary organs, usually the urethra and urinary bladder. The symptoms are illustrated in Figure 11.8■ and include fever, dysuria (Frame 11.13), and lumbar or abdominal pain. It is more common in females and is usually caused by staphylococci or *E. coli* bacteria.

Figure 11.8 ■
Urinary tract infection. A UTI is characterized by fever, lumbar or abdominal pain, and pain or burning during urination. A diagnosis may be confirmed in a urine exam that reveals the presence of bacteria (bacteriuria) and white blood cells (pyuria).

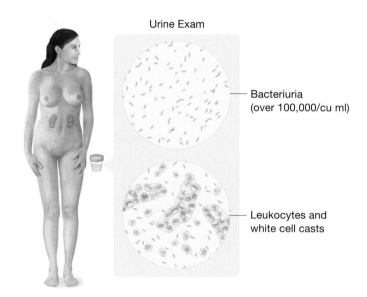

Urine Exam

Bacteriuria (over 100,000/cu ml)

Leukocytes and white cell casts

PRACTICE: Diseases and Disorders of the Urinary System

The Right Match

Match the term on the left with the correct definition on the right.

_____ 1. cystocele

_____ 2. cystolith

_____ 3. nephritis

_____ 4. nephromegaly

_____ 5. uremia

_____ 6. hypospadias

_____ 7. polycystic kidney disease

_____ 8. renal calculi

_____ 9. urinary incontinence

_____ 10. urinary retention

_____ 11. urinary suppression

_____ 12. stricture

_____ 13. acute renal failure

a. condition of excess urea in the blood

b. protrusion of the urinary bladder

c. stone(s) in the urinary bladder

d. urinary meatus opens on the penis underside

e. inflammation of a kidney

f. enlargement of a kidney

g. a condition of stones in the kidneys

h. an acute stoppage of urine formation

i. involuntary discharge of urine

j. a condition of many cysts within a kidney

k. abnormal accumulation of urine in the bladder

l. a condition in which kidney function ceases

m. condition of abnormal narrowing

Linkup

Link the word parts in the list to create the terms that match the definitions. You may use word parts more than once. Remember to add combining vowels when needed—and that some terms do not use any combining vowel. The first one is completed as an example.

Combining Form	Suffix
cyst/o	-ia
glomerul/o	-itis
hydr/o	-oma
lith/o	-sis
nephr/o	
pyel/o	

Definition   Term

1. **inflammation of the urinary bladder**   *cystitis*

2. inflammation of the glomeruli   _____

3. inflammation of the renal pelvis and the nephrons   _____

4. presence of one or more stones within a kidney   _____

5. condition of blockage of urine (water) in the kidney   _____

6. tumor that arises from kidney tissue   _____

7. inflammation of the renal pelvis   _____

Treatments, Procedures, and Devices of the Urinary System

Review some of the word parts that specifically apply to the treatments, procedures, and devices of the urinary system that are covered in the following section. Note that the word parts are color-coded to help you identify them: prefixes are blue, combining forms are red, and suffixes are purple.

Prefix	Definition
a-	without or absence of
dia-	through

Combining Form	Definition
cyst/o	bladder
hemat/o, hem/o	blood
lith/o	stone
meat/o	opening
nephr/o	kidney
peritone/o	peritoneum
pyel/o	renal pelvis
ren/o	kidney
son/o	sound
tom/o	to cut
ureter/o	ureter
urethr/o	urethra
ur/o, urin/o	urine
vesic/o	bladder

Suffix	Definition
-al	pertaining to
-ectomy	surgical excision or removal
-gram	a record or image
-graphy	recording process
-is	pertaining to
-lysis	loosen or dissolve
-meter	measuring instrument
-pexy	surgical fixation
-plasty	surgical repair
-rrhaphy	suturing
-scopy	process of viewing
-stomy	surgical creation of an opening
-tomy	incision or to cut
-tripsy	surgical crushing

KEY TERMS A-Z

blood urea nitrogen
blud * YOO ree ah

11.48 A clinical lab test that measures urea concentration in a sample of blood as an indicator of kidney function is **blood urea nitrogen.** Abbreviated **BUN**, elevated values of _____ _____ _____ indicate kidney disease.

creatinine
kree ATT ih neen

11.49 The protein **creatinine** is a normal component of urine and is a by-product of muscle metabolism. It may be measured in a urine sample. Elevated levels of _____ indicate a problem during kidney filtration, suggesting kidney disease.

cystectomy
siss TEK toh mee

11.50 Because the combining form cyst/o means "urinary bladder" and the suffix -ectomy means "surgical removal," the surgical removal of the urinary bladder is called _____. This constructed term is written cyst/ectomy.

cystogram
SISS toh gram

cystourethrogram
SISS toh you REE throh gram

11.51 An X-ray procedure producing an image of the urinary bladder with injection of a contrast medium or dye is called **cystography** (siss TOG rah fee). This constructed term is written cyst/o/graphy. The X-ray image is called a _____. If the procedure includes the ureters, it is called a **cystoureterography** (SISS toh yoo REE ter OG rah fee), and the image obtained is a **cystoureterogram** (SISS toh yoo REE ter oh gram). The constructed form of the term *cystoureterography* is cyst/o/ureter/o/graphy. If the procedure includes the urethra, it is a **cystourethrography** (SISS toh yoo reeth ROG rah fee), and the image is a **cystourethrogram**. The constructed form of the term *cystourethrogram* is written cyst/o/urethr/o/gram. In a **voiding** _____ (**VCUG**), X-rays are taken before, during, and after urination to observe bladder function.

WORDS TO WATCH OUT FOR !

-graphy or -gram?
Remember that the suffix *-graphy* means "a recording process," whereas the suffix *-gram* means "a record or image." In each of these procedures, switching the suffix from *-graphy* to *-gram* creates the term that refers to the *record* that is a result of the *recording process*.

cystolithotomy
siss toh lith OTT oh mee
cyst/o/lith/o/tomy

11.52 A procedure in which an incision is made through the urinary bladder wall to remove a stone is called _____. The constructed form of this term includes five word parts and is written _____/__/_____/__/_____.

cystoplasty
SISS toh plass tee

11.53 Surgical repair of the urinary bladder is a procedure called _____. The constructed form of this term is cyst/o/plasty, which reveals three word parts.

cystorrhaphy
sist OR ah fee

11.54 Suturing the urinary bladder wall is a procedure called _____. The constructed form of the term is cyst/o/rrhaphy, which literally means "suturing bladder."

cystoscopy
siss TOSS koh pee

11.55 A procedure using a modified endoscope to view the interior of the urinary bladder is known as _____. The instrument is inserted through the urinary meatus and urethra to enter the bladder cavity (Figure 11.9■). The constructed form of this term is cyst/o/scopy. The cystoscope may also be used as a surgical instrument.

Figure 11.9 ■
Cystoscopy. In this procedure, a specialized endoscope with a rigid tube, known as a cystoscope, is used to view the internal environment of the urinary bladder. As shown, the cystoscope may be outfitted to include surgical devices to remove tumors or stones.

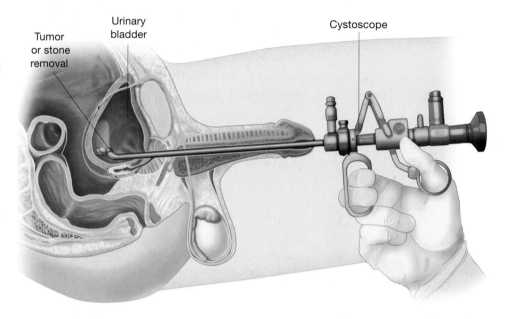

Urinary bladder

Tumor or stone removal

Cystoscope

cystostomy
siss TOSS toh mee

11.56 Recall that the suffix -stomy means "surgical creation of an opening." The surgical creation of an artificial opening into the urinary bladder is a procedure called _____. It is performed to provide an alternate exit pathway for urine if the normal passageway through the urethra is blocked or the urethra is surgically removed (Figure 11.10■). Cystostomy is a constructed term written cyst/o/stomy.

Figure 11.10 ■
Cystostomy. An artificial opening is made through the urinary bladder wall during this procedure. As the illustration suggests, it is often performed to enable a patient to bypass obstructions for voiding.

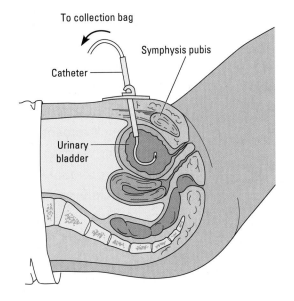

To collection bag

Catheter

Symphysis pubis

Urinary bladder

---

cystotomy

siss TOTT oh mee

11.57 The suffix *-tomy* means "incision" or "to cut." Therefore, the term _____ is an incision through the urinary bladder wall. It is also called **vesicotomy** (VESS ih KOTT oh mee), because both *cyst* and *vesic* are word roots meaning "bladder."

---

fulguration

full guh RAY shun

11.58 A surgical procedure that destroys living tissue with an electric current is called **fulguration**. _____ is commonly used to remove tumors and polyps from the interior wall of the urinary bladder.

DID YOU KNOW ?

Fulguration

Fulguration is derived from the Latin word *fulguratio*, which means "flash of lightning."

hemodialysis
HEE moh dye AL ih siss

11.59 The general term dia/lysis means "dissolving through" and refers to the movement of substances across a permeable membrane during the process of filtration. Also, *hem/o* is the combining form that means "blood." Combining these word parts forms the term _____, which is a procedure that pushes a patient's blood through permeable membranes within an instrument (Figure 11.11■). It is performed to artificially remove nitrogenous wastes and excess ions that accumulate during normal body metabolism, temporarily replacing the function of kidney filtration for patients with kidney disease or kidney failure. Hemodialysis is a constructed term, written hem/o/dia/lysis.

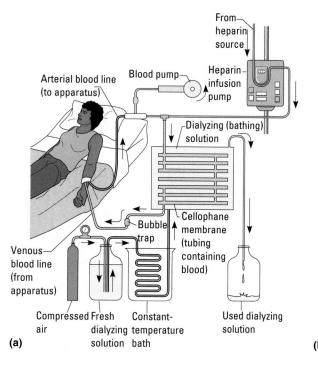

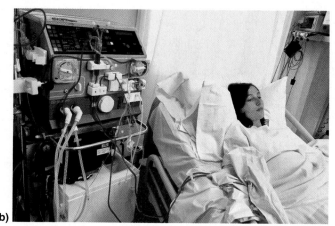

Figure 11.11 ■

Hemodialysis. (a) The process of hemodialysis replaces the kidney function of blood filtration by forcing blood from the patient through cellophane membranes, as shown in this schematic.
(b) A patient undergoing hemodialysis.
Source: Southern Illinois University/Photo Researchers, Inc.

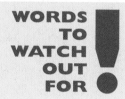

WORDS TO WATCH OUT FOR

A Misplaced Prefix?

Most prefixes appear in the very beginning of a term, but in the term *hemodialysis*, note that the prefix (*dia-*) appears as the second word part (just after the combining form *hem/o*).

11.60 The suffix *-tripsy* means "surgical crushing." A surgical technique that applies concentrated sound waves to pulverize or dissolve stones into smaller pieces that may then pass with urine through the urethra is called _____. This constructed term is written lith/o/tripsy. In the procedure **extracorporeal shock wave lithotripsy (ESWL)**, ultrasonic energy from a source outside of the body is used on stones that are too large to pass through the urethra. It is a noninvasive technique and therefore avoids the risks of surgery. Both procedures are shown in Figure 11.12■.

lithotripsy
LITH oh trip see

Figure 11.12 ■
Lithotripsy. The direction of a sound pulse crushes the stones into smaller fragments that can be passed with urine. It includes invasive and noninvasive procedures. (a) During the invasive procedure, the ultrasound device is surgically inserted near the stone.
(b) When applied through the skin, the noninvasive procedure is called extracorporeal shock wave lithotripsy, or ESWL.
Source: Visuals Unlimited.

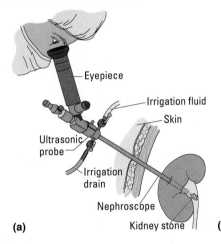
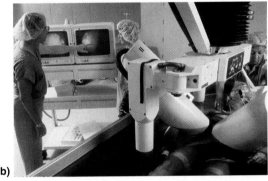

- Eyepiece
- Irrigation fluid
- Skin
- Ultrasonic probe
- Irrigation drain
- Nephroscope
- Kidney stone

(a)   (b)

nephrectomy
neh FREK toh mee

11.61 Recall that one of the combining forms for kidney is *nephr/o*. A surgical procedure that removes a kidney is called _____. This constructed term is written nephr/ectomy.

nephrogram
NEFF roh gram

11.62 An X-ray technique producing an image of a kidney after injection of a contrast medium or dye is called **nephrography** (neh FROG rah fee). It is a constructed term written nephr/o/graphy. The X-ray image of the kidney obtained in this procedure is called a _____.

nephrology
neff ROL oh jee

11.63 The medical field that studies and treats disorders associated with the kidneys is called _____. This constructed term is written nephr/o/logy. A physician specializing in this field is a **nephrologist** (neff ROL oh jist).

nephrolysis
neh FRALL ih siss

11.64 The suffix *-lysis* means "loosen or dissolve." Combining it with the combining form for kidney, *nephr/o*, forms the constructed term _____. It is a surgical procedure during which abnormal adhesions are removed from a kidney, loosening the organ. This constructed term is written nephr/o/lysis.

nephropexy
NEFF roh pek see

11.65 The suffix that means "surgical fixation" is -*pexy*. Surgical fixation of a kidney is sometimes necessary if the kidney is abnormally loose within the abdominal cavity, such as in the condition nephroptosis or floating kidney (Frame 11.36). The procedure is called _____, and the constructed form of this term is written nephr/o/pexy.

nephroscopy
neh FROSS koh pee

11.66 Remember that the suffix -*scopy* means "process of viewing." Therefore, visual examination of kidney nephrons may be performed in the procedure known as _____, during which a modified fiber-optic endoscope called a **nephroscope** (NEFF roh skope) is used.

nephrosonography
neff roh son OG rah fee

11.67 An ultrasound procedure that provides an image of a kidney for diagnostic analysis is known as **nephrosonography**. _____ is a constructed term that contains five word parts and is written nephr/o/son/o/graphy.

nephrostomy
neff ROSS toh mee

nephr/o/stomy

11.68 A procedure that surgically creates an opening through the body wall and into a kidney is called a _____. It is usually established to allow a catheter to be inserted from the exterior to a renal pelvis for urine drainage and is also called a **pyelostomy** (PYE ell OSS toh mee). The constructed form of nephrostomy is written _____/__/_____, and pyelostomy is pyel/o/stomy.

nephrotomogram
NEH froh toh moh gram

11.69 A diagnostic procedure that images the kidney with sectional X-rays to observe internal details of kidney structure is known as **nephrotomography** (NEH froh toh MOG rah fee). The suffix that means "record" or "image" is -*gram*, so the image obtained from this procedure is a _____. Nephrotomography is a constructed term that is written nephr/o/tom/o/graphy, which literally means "recording process of cut kidney."

peritoneal dialysis
pair ih TOH nee al * dye AL ih siss

11.70 You learned about hemodialysis in Frame 11.59. A similar procedure is **peritoneal dialysis**, which also processes fluids and electrolytes by artificial filtration as a cleansing treatment to compensate for kidney failure. Thus, _____ _____ removes toxins and other wastes as a replacement for kidney function. In contrast to hemodialysis, peritoneal dialysis processes fluids from the peritoneal cavity rather than directly from the bloodstream. The constructed form of this term is written periton/e/al dia/lysis.

pyelogram
PYE ell oh gram

11.71 An X-ray image of the renal pelvis (a **pyelogram**) is a useful diagnostic tool that is often used to examine kidney-related disorders. In obtaining an image called a **retrograde** _____, the procedure involves injection of contrast medium into the ureter using a cystoscope. As the X-ray is taken, it moves in a direction opposite from the norm (retrograde means "opposite of normal"). It is abbreviated **RP**, and an example is shown in Figure 11.13■. In an **intravenous pyelogram**, iodine is used as the contrast medium and is injected into the bloodstream. It is abbreviated **IVP**.

Figure 11.13 ■
Retrograde pyelogram. A contrast medium is injected into the ureter using a cystoscope, and the X-ray moves in a direction opposite from the norm, producing the image that is shown. It serves to highlight the internal features of the renal pelvis and ureters.
Source: Photo Researchers, Inc.

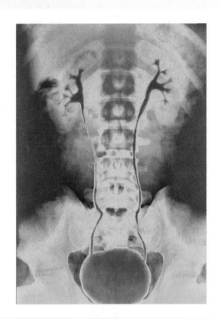

pyelolithotomy
pye ell oh lith OTT oh mee

11.72 A kidney stone may sometimes form within the renal pelvis. A surgery performed to remove the stone from the renal pelvis involves an incision into the kidney and is called a **pyelolithotomy**. The constructed form of the term _____ is written pyel/o/lith/o/tomy, which literally means "incision of stone in renal pelvis."

pyeloplasty
PYE ell oh PLASS tee

11.73 The suffix that means "surgical repair" is -*plasty*. Surgical repair of the renal pelvis is a procedure called _____. This constructed term is written pyel/o/plasty.

renal transplant

11.74 The replacement of a dysfunctioning kidney with a donor kidney is a surgery called _____ _____ (Figure 11.14■). The donated kidney is often provided by a close relative with a similar genetic makeup. Alternatively, a donor kidney can be implanted with the use of cytological drugs that suppress the immune response, reducing the chance of rejection.

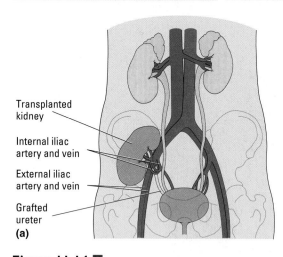

Transplanted kidney

Internal iliac artery and vein

External iliac artery and vein

Grafted ureter
(a)

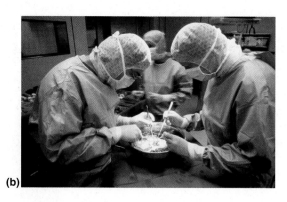

(b)

Figure 11.14 ■
Renal transplant. (a) A transplanted kidney is placed within the pelvic cavity below the location of the kidney requiring replacement. (b) Two nephrologists examine a donated kidney prior to its insertion into the recipient during a renal transplant.
Source: Peter Arnold, Inc.

renography
ree NOG rah fee

11.75 An examination that uses nuclear medicine by IV (intravenous) injection of radioactive material into the patient's kidneys is called **renography**. The radioactive materials highlight internal details of the kidney during the _____. This constructed term is written ren/o/graphy. The recording is called a **renogram** (REE noh gram).

specific gravity

11.76 The measurement of the density of substances in a liquid compared to water is called **specific gravity (SG)**. The _____ _____ of a urine sample is often measured with an instrument called a **urinometer** (Frame 11.85). The specific gravity of a urine sample helps to reveal the efficiency of renal filtration and the reabsorption of water.

ureterectomy
yoo REE ter EK toh mee

11.77 The suffix that means "surgical removal" is *-ectomy*. The surgical removal of a ureter is called _____. The constructed form of this term is written ureter/ectomy.

ureterostomy
yoo REE ter OSS toh mee

ureterotomy
yoo ree ter OTT oh mee

11.78 The surgical creation of an external opening from the ureter to the body surface is called _____. It is performed to provide an alternate exit route for urine that bypasses the urethra. The procedure includes an incision into the wall of the ureter, called _____. Both terms are constructed of word parts: *ureterostomy* is written ureter/o/stomy, and *ureterotomy* is written ureter/o/tomy.

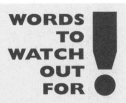

WORDS TO WATCH OUT FOR !

-stomy or -tomy?

The suffix *-stomy* means "surgical creation of an opening," whereas *-tomy* means "incision or to cut." The two suffixes represent two different surgical techniques. In general, an incision is a cut through tissue, whereas the surgical creation of an opening establishes an artificial window into the body, usually for the drainage of fluids or waste. Can you see how the small addition of an *s* makes a big difference in meaning?

urethropexy
yoo REE throh pek see

11.79 Surgical fixation of the urethra is a procedure called **urethropexy**. A _____ is often performed to correct stress incontinence (see Frame 11.30). It is a constructed term written urethr/o/pexy.

urethroplasty
yoo REE throh plass tee

11.80 Surgical repair of the urethra is a procedure called _____. This constructed term is written urethr/o/plasty.

urethrostomy
yoo REE THROSS toh mee

urethrotomy
yoo ree THROTT oh mee

11.81 The surgical creation of an opening through the urethra is called _____. It is performed to provide an alternate exit route for urine. The procedure includes an incision into the wall of the urethra, called _____. Both terms are constructed of word parts: *urethrostomy* is written urethr/o/stomy, and *urethrotomy* is written urethr/o/tomy.

urinalysis
YOO rin AL ih siss

11.82 A combination of clinical lab tests that are performed on a urine specimen is called **urinalysis**. The term _____ is a constructed term written urin/a/lysis, which literally means "dissolve urine." Abbreviated **UA**, it provides information on the quality and composition of urine, including specific gravity, creatinine levels, glucose levels, protein levels, and the presence of red blood cells, white blood cells, and pus for diagnostic purposes.

urinary catheterization
YOO rih nair ee *
KATH eh ter ih ZAY shun

11.83 A **catheter** is a flexible tube that is inserted into an opening of the body to transport fluids in or out. A **urinary catheter** is usually inserted through the urethra to enter the urinary bladder and is often used to drain urine from a patient who is immobile. The process of inserting the urinary catheter is called _____ _____. It is illustrated in Figure 11.15■.

Figure 11.15 ■
Urinary catheterization. The procedure involves the insertion of a flexible tube, or catheter, through the urethra and into the urinary bladder. Voiding occurs through the catheter and is collected in a plastic bag adjacent to the patient.
(a) Catheterization of a female patient.
(b) Catheterization of a male patient.

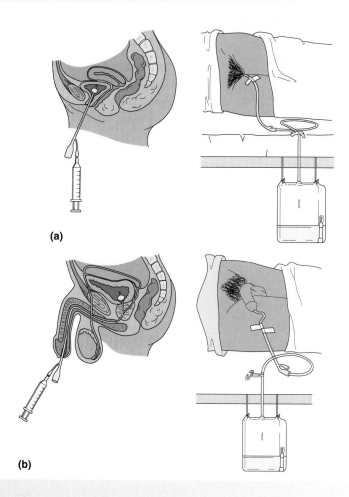

(a)

(b)

DID YOU KNOW ?

Catheter

The term *catheter* is from the Greek word, *katheter,* which means "to send down," so named because it is a flexible tube that lets urine down from the urinary bladder.

urinary endoscopy
YOO rih nair ee * ehn DOSS koh pee

11.84 The procedural use of an endoscope to observe internal structures of the urinary system is generally known as _____ _____. A specialized endoscope is associated with each urinary organ, including a **meatoscope** (mee AT oh skope) for inserting into the urinary meatus, a **nephroscope** (NEFF roh skope) for viewing a kidney, a **urethroscope** (yoo REE throh skope) for viewing the urethra, and a **cystoscope** (SISS toh skope) for observing the interior of the urinary bladder.

urinometer
yoo rih NOM eh ter

11.85 An instrument that measures the specific gravity (density of substances in water) in a sample of urine is known as a **urinometer**. This constructed term is composed of three word parts and is written urin/o/meter. A _____ is illustrated in Figure 11.16■.

Figure 11.16 ■
Urinometer. Specific gravity is a measure of the density of a liquid. In this procedure, a urine sample and urinometer are placed within a tube, and the liquid level is compared to the scale on the urinometer. The procedure provides information on the concentration of solids within a urine sample.

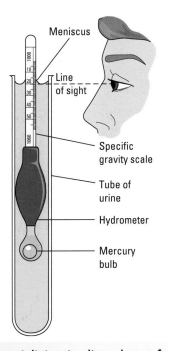

Meniscus

Line of sight

Specific gravity scale

Tube of urine

Hydrometer

Mercury bulb

urologist
yoo RAHL oh jist

11.86 The medical field specializing in disorders of the urinary system is called **urology** (yoo RAHL oh jee). A physician who treats patients in this discipline is called a _____.

vesicourethral
vess ih koh yoo REE thral

11.87 A surgery that is performed to stabilize the position of the urinary bladder is called **vesicourethral suspension**. The term _____ contains four word parts and is written vesic/o/urethr/al. It is performed to treat stress incontinence (Frame 11.30).

PRACTICE: Treatments, Procedures, and Devices of the Urinary System

The Right Match

Match the term on the left with the correct definition on the right.

_____ 1. cystorrhaphy

_____ 2. extracorporeal shockwave lithotripsy

_____ 3. nephrectomy

_____ 4. nephrostomy

_____ 5. vesicourethral suspension

_____ 6. fulguration

_____ 7. renal transplant

_____ 8. blood urea nitrogen

_____ 9. peritoneal dialysis

_____ 10. creatinine

_____ 11. specific gravity

_____ 12. urinary catheter

a. removal of a kidney

b. creates a new opening through the renal pelvis to the outside

c. stabilizes the position of the urinary bladder

d. suture of the urinary bladder

e. technique that uses ultrasonic energy to crush stones

f. test for protein levels in a urine sample

g. test for water concentration in urine

h. electric current that kills unwanted tissue

i. test for urea in the blood

j. insertion of a tube to drain urine

k. surgical procedure replacing a diseased kidney

l. blood filtration using the peritoneal cavity

Break the Chain

Analyze these medical terms:

a) Separate each term into its word parts; each word part is labeled for you (**p** = prefix, **r** = root, **cf** = combining form, and **s** = suffix).

b) For the Bonus Question, write the requested definition in the blank that follows.

1. a) cystography   _____/__/_____
                              cf   s

    b) *Bonus Question:* What is the definition of the suffix? _____

2. a) cystolithotomy   _____/__/_____/__/_____
                              cf   cf   s

    b) *Bonus Question:* What is the definition of the suffix? _____

3. a) lithotripsy   _____/__/_____
                              cf   s

    b) *Bonus Question:* What is the definition of the combining form? _____

4. a) hemodialysis   _____/__/___/_____
                              cf   p   s

    b) *Bonus Question:* What is the definition of the prefix? _____

5. a) cystorrhaphy   _____/__/_____
                              cf   s

    b) *Bonus Question:* Does this term contain a prefix? _____

6. a) nephrolysis   _____/__/_____
                                     cf   s

     b) *Bonus Question*: What is the definition of the suffix? _____

7. a) nephrogram   _____/__/_____
                                   cf   s

     b) *Bonus Question*: What is the meaning of the suffix? _____

8. a) nephrotomography   _____/__/_____/__/_____
                                     cf   cf   s

     b) *Bonus Question*: What is the definition of the *first* combining form? _____

9. a) ureterostomy   _____/__/_____
                                     cf   s

     b) *Bonus Question*: What is the definition of the suffix? _____

Abbreviations of the Urinary System

The abbreviations that are associated with the urinary system are summarized here. Study these abbreviations, and review them in the exercise that follows.

Abbreviation	Definition	Abbreviation	Definition
BUN	blood urea nitrogen	SG	specific gravity
cath	catheter, catheterization	UA	urinalysis
HD	hemodialysis	UTI	urinary tract infection
IVP	intravenous pyelogram	VCUG	voiding cystourethrogram
RP	retrograde pyelogram		

PRACTICE: Abbreviations

Fill in the blanks with the abbreviation or the complete medical term.

Abbreviation   Medical Term

1.   UA   _____

2.   _____   retrograde pyelogram

3.   cath   _____

4.   _____   voiding cystourethrogram

5.   IVP   _____

6.   _____   urinary tract infection

7.   HD   _____

▶▶▶▶▶ Chapter Review

Word Building _____

Construct medical terms from the following meanings. (Some are built from word parts, some are not.) The first question has been completed as an example.

1. inability to pass urine   _an_uresis

2. absence of urine   an_____

3. presence of bacteria in the urine   bacteri_____

4. presence of a stone in the bladder   _____lith

5. inflammation of a kidney   nephr_____

6. presence of blood in the urine   _____uria

7. protrusion of a ureter   uretero_____

8. involuntary release of urine   _____uresis

9. presence of stones in the kidney   nephro_____

10. fixation of an abnormally mobile kidney   nephro_____

11. surgical creation of an opening into the renal pelvis   _____stomy

12. surgical repair of the urethra   urethro_____

13. incision into the ureter wall   uretero_____

14. X-ray image of the urinary bladder   cysto_____

15. X-ray technique imaging a kidney   nephro_____

16. X-ray image of the renal pelvis with iodine   intravenous _____gram

17. an endoscope modified to view a kidney   _____scope

18. lab test measuring urea in the blood   blood urea _____ (BUN)

19. instrument measuring water concentration in urine   urino_____

20. urine test that includes multiple parameters   urin_____

Clinical Application Exercises

Medical Report

Read the following medical report, then answer the questions that follow.

University Hospital

5500 University Avenue
Metropolis, TX

Phone: (211) 594-4000
Fax: (211) 594-4001

Medical Consultation: Internal Medicine

Date: 6/25/2008

Patient: Sylvia Hernandez-Brown

Patient Complaint: Pain in the lower lumbar region (right and left sides), malaise, hematuria, shortness of breath, generalized body aches with mild fever, loss of appetite.

History: 60-year-old Hispanic female, 40 pounds overweight with Type II diabetes without drug assist, history of periodic UTIs.

Family History: Father deceased at 72 years old with COPD and CHF. Mother alive at 77 years with Type II diabetes under care; lost one kidney at age 70 due to polycystic disease.

Allergies: None

Evidences: Elevated urea, albuminuria, hematuria; severe lumbar pain reported by patient. Renal failure of left kidney apparent with increasing insufficiency of right kidney due to PD evident by nephrotomography and confirmed by nephroscopy.

Treatment: Immediate dialysis, to repeat daily until surgery. Admit patient for radical nephrectomy. Schedule dialysis treatments postoperative and include patient to renal transplant database.

Joshua Ryan, M.D.

---

1. What patient complaints point to the kidneys as the source of the disease? _____

_____

2. Does the patient history and family history provide any clues to the diagnosis? _____

_____

3. Why does the urologist order dialysis for the patient prior to surgery? _____

_____

Medical Report Case Study

The following Case Study provides further discussion regarding the patient in the medical report. Fill in the blanks with the correct terms. Choose your answers from the following list of terms. (Note that some terms may be used more than once.)

albuminuria	nephroscopy	renal transplant
hematuria	nephrotomography	urinalysis
hemodialysis	polycystic kidney disease	
nephromegaly	pyelonephritis	

A 60-year-old female, Sylvia Hernandez-Brown, was admitted to urology by her general practitioner following a physical

exam that included blood tests revealing abnormally high levels of urea in the blood. A generalized test of urine

composition, or (a) _____, revealed elevated levels of albumin, a symptom known as

(b) _____, and the presence of red blood cells in the urine, or (c) _____. Following

diagnostic exams that included an X-ray technique imaging the kidney by sections called (d) _____; and

an endoscopic evaluation of the kidney known as (e) _____, the attending physician concluded a

diagnosis of enlargement of both kidneys, or (f) _____, caused by multiple polyps, or

(g) _____ _____ _____, which had resulted in inflammation of

the renal pelvis and nephrons, or (h) _____ and renal failure. Artificial filtration of the blood, or

(i) _____, was ordered, due to a growing insufficiency to reduce blood metabolites (metabolic wastes).

Surgical removal of both diseased kidneys was scheduled immediately, and the patient was placed on a waiting list for a

replacement kidney as a (j) _____ _____.

▶▶▶▶▶ Key Terms Double-Check

Remember that the chapter's key terms appeared alphabetically throughout this chapter. This exercise helps you to check your knowledge AND review for tests.

1. First, fill in the missing word in the definitions for the chapter's key terms.
2. Then, check your answers using Appendix F.
3. If you got the answer right, put a check mark in the right column.
4. If your answer was incorrect, go back to the frame number provided and review the content.

Use the checklist to study the terms you don't know until you're confident you know them all.

	Key Term	Frame	Definition	Know It?
1.	albuminuria	11.8	the condition of albumin in the _____	☐
2.	anuresis	11.9	the _____ to pass urine	☐
3.	anuria	11.9	the production of less than 100 mL of urine per _____	☐
4.	azotemia	11.10	abnormally high levels of urea and other nitrogen-containing compounds in the _____	☐
5.	bacteriuria	11.11	abnormal presence of _____ in the urine	☐
6.	blood urea nitrogen	11.48	a lab test that measures urea concentration in blood as an indicator of _____ function	☐
7.	creatinine	11.49	a(n) _____ that is a normal component of urine and is measured in urine samples	☐
8.	cystectomy	11.50	surgical _____ of the urinary bladder	☐
9.	cystitis	11.22	inflammation of the urinary _____	☐
10.	cystocele	11.23	_____ of the urinary bladder	☐
11.	cystogram	11.51	the X-ray image of the urinary bladder that results from a procedure called _____ that involves the injection of a contrast medium or dye	☐
12.	cystolith	11.24	a(n) _____ in the urinary bladder	☐
13.	cystolithotomy	11.52	the removal of a stone through a(n) _____ in the urinary bladder wall	☐
14.	cystoplasty	11.53	surgical _____ of the urinary bladder	☐
15.	cystorrhaphy	11.54	_____ of the urinary bladder wall	☐
16.	cystoscopy	11.55	a diagnostic procedure that uses a modified endoscope to view the interior of the urinary _____	☐
17.	cystostomy	11.56	the surgical creation of an artificial _____ into the urinary bladder	☐
18.	cystotomy	11.57	a(n) _____ through the urinary bladder wall	☐
19.	cystourethrogram	11.51	the _____ formed during a cystourethrography	☐
20.	diuresis	11.12	excessive discharge of _____	☐
21.	dysuria	11.13	difficulty or _____ during urination	☐
22.	enuresis	11.25	the _____ release of urine	☐
23.	epispadias	11.26	a(n) _____ defect that results in the abnormal positioning of the urinary meatus	☐

Key Term	Frame	Definition	Know It?
24. fulguration	11.58	a surgical procedure that destroys living tissue with _____ current	☐
25. glomerulonephritis	11.27	_____ of the glomeruli	☐
26. glycosuria	11.14	the abnormal presence of _____ (sugar) in the urine	☐
27. hematuria	11.15	the abnormal presence of _____ in the urine	☐
28. hemodialysis	11.59	a procedure that pushes a patient's blood through permeable membranes within an instrument to artificially _____ nitrogenous wastes and excess ions	☐
29. hydronephrosis	11.28	distension of the renal pelvis due to a(n) _____ of urine	☐
30. hypospadias	11.29	a congenital defect in which the urinary meatus is shifted _____	☐
31. incontinence	11.30	the inability to control _____	☐
32. ketonuria	11.16	the _____ presence of ketone bodies in the urine	☐
33. lithotripsy	11.60	a surgical technique that applies concentrated sound waves to pulverize or _____ kidney stones	☐
34. nephrectomy	11.61	the surgical _____ of a kidney	☐
35. nephritis	11.31	inflammation of a(n) _____	☐
36. nephroblastoma	11.32	a(n) _____ that originates from kidney tissue and includes embryonic cells	☐
37. nephrogram	11.62	the X-ray _____ of the kidney from a nephrography	☐
38. nephrolithiasis	11.33	the presence of one or more _____ (or calculi) within a kidney	☐
39. nephrology	11.63	the _____ field that studies and treats disorders associated with the kidneys	☐
40. nephrolysis	11.64	surgical procedure in which abnormal adhesions are removed from a kidney, which _____ the organ	☐
41. nephroma	11.34	a general term for a tumor that arises from _____ tissue	☐
42. nephromegaly	11.35	abnormal _____ of one or both kidneys	☐
43. nephropexy	11.65	surgical _____ of a kidney	☐
44. nephroptosis	11.36	a(n) _____ displacement of a kidney	☐
45. nephroscopy	11.66	visual examination of kidney nephrons using a(n) _____	☐
46. nephrosonography	11.67	an _____ procedure that provides an image of a kidney for diagnostic analysis	☐
47. nephrostomy	11.68	the surgical creation of an opening through the body wall and into a(n) _____	☐
48. nephrotomogram	11.69	the X-ray image obtained from a diagnostic procedure that images the kidney to observe internal details of kidney _____	☐
49. nocturia	11.17	the need to urinate frequently at _____	☐
50. oliguria	11.18	_____ urination	☐
51. peritoneal dialysis	11.70	the use of artificial filtration to _____ fluids from the peritoneal cavity	☐

Key Term	Frame	Definition	Know It?
52. polycystic kidney disease	11.37	a condition in which _____ cysts occupy much of the kidney tissue	☐
53. polyuria	11.19	chronic _____ urination	☐
54. proteinuria	11.20	the presence of any protein in the _____	☐
55. pyelitis	11.38	inflammation of the _____ pelvis	☐
56. pyelogram	11.71	a procedure that injects a contrast medium into the ureter using a(n) _____ to examine kidney-related disorders	☐
57. pyelolithotomy	11.72	surgical _____ of a stone from the renal pelvis	☐
58. pyelonephritis	11.39	inflammation of the renal pelvis and _____	☐
59. pyeloplasty	11.73	surgical _____ of the renal pelvis	☐
60. pyuria	11.21	the presence of _____ in the urine	☐
61. renal transplant	11.74	the replacement of a dysfunctioning kidney with a _____ kidney	☐
62. renography	11.75	an examination that uses nuclear medicine by IV injection of radioactive material into the _____	☐
63. specific gravity	11.76	the measurement of the _____ of substances in a liquid compared to water	☐
64. stricture	11.40	condition of _____ narrowing	☐
65. uremia	11.41	excess urea and other nitrogenous wastes in the _____	☐
66. ureterectomy	11.77	the _____ _____ of a ureter	☐
67. ureteritis	11.42	inflammation of a(n) _____	☐
68. ureterocele	11.43	_____ ureter	☐
69. ureterolithiasis	11.44	one or more _____ (or calculi) within a ureter	☐
70. ureterostomy	11.78	the surgical creation of a(n) _____ through a ureter	☐
71. urethropexy	11.79	surgical _____ of the urethra	☐
72. urethroplasty	11.80	_____ _____ of the urethra	☐
73. urethrostomy	11.81	surgical creation of an opening through the _____	☐
74. urethrotomy	11.81	a(n) _____ into the wall of the urethra	☐
75. urinalysis	11.82	a collection of clinical lab tests that are performed on a(n) _____ specimen	☐
76. urinary catheterization	11.83	the process of inserting a urinary catheter into the urethra to drain urine from an immobile patient's _____	☐
77. urinary endoscopy	11.84	the use of an endoscope to _____ internal structures of the urinary system	☐
78. urinary retention	11.45	abnormal _____ of urine within the urinary bladder	☐
79. urinary suppression	11.46	an acute stoppage of urine formation by the _____	☐
80. urinary tract infection	11.47	an infection of urinary organs, usually the _____ and urinary bladder	☐
81. urinometer	11.85	a(n) _____ that measures the specific gravity of urine	☐
82. urologist	11.86	a physician who treats patients in the discipline of _____	☐
83. vesicourethral suspension	11.87	a surgery that _____ the position of the urinary bladder	☐

Multimedia Preview ▶▶▶▶▶

Additional interactive resources and activities for this chapter can be found on the Companion Website. For videos, audio glossary, and review, access the accompanying DVD-ROM in this book.

DVD-ROM Highlights

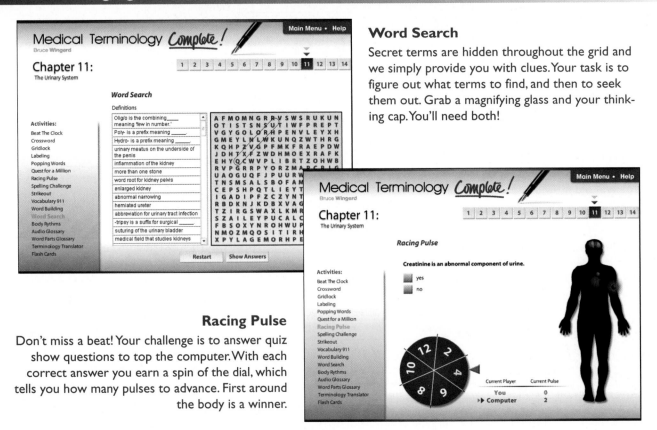

Word Search

Secret terms are hidden throughout the grid and we simply provide you with clues. Your task is to figure out what terms to find, and then to seek them out. Grab a magnifying glass and your thinking cap. You'll need both!

Racing Pulse

Don't miss a beat! Your challenge is to answer quiz show questions to top the computer. With each correct answer you earn a spin of the dial, which tells you how many pulses to advance. First around the body is a winner.

Website Highlights—www.prenhall.com/wingerd

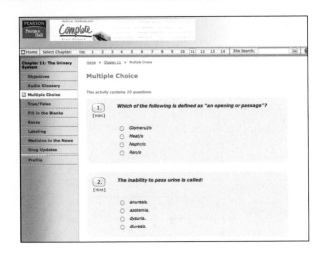

Multiple Choice Quiz

Take advantage of the free-access online study guide that accompanies your textbook. You'll find a multiple-choice quiz that provides instant feedback and allows you to check your score to see what you got right or wrong. By clicking on this URL you'll also access links to download mp3 audio reviews, current news articles, and an audio glossary.

Reproductive System and Obstetrics ▶▶▶▶

Learning Objectives

After completing this chapter, you will be able to:

- Define and spell the word parts used to create terms for the reproductive system and obstetrics.

- Break down and define common medical terms used for symptoms, diseases, disorders, procedures, treatments, and devices associated with the reproductive system and obstetrics.

- Build medical terms from the word parts associated with the reproductive system and obstetrics.

- Pronounce and spell common medical terms associated with the reproductive system and obstetrics.

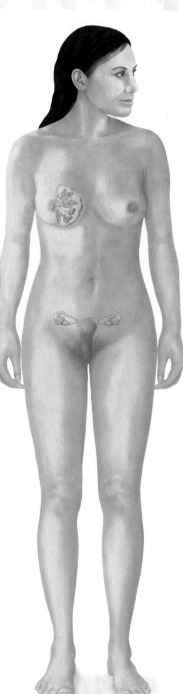

Anatomy and Physiology Terms ▶▶▶▶▶

The following table provides the combining forms that specifically apply to the anatomy and physiology of the reproductive system and obstetrics. Note that the combining forms are colored red to help you identify them when you see them again later in the chapter.

Combining Form	Definition
amni/o, amnion/o	amnion, amniotic fluid
andr/o	male
balan/o	glans penis
cervic/o	neck, cervix
chori/o	membrane, chorion
cyes/o, cyesi/o	pregnancy
embry/o	embryo
epididym/o	epididymis
episi/o	vulva
fet/o	fetus
gravid/o, gravidar/o	pregnancy
mamm/o, mast/o	breast

Combining Form	Definition
men/o, menstru/o	month, menstruation
orch/o, orchid/o	testis
pen/o	penis
prostat/o	prostate gland
semin/o	seed, sperm
sperm/o, spermat/o	seed, sperm
test/o, testicul/o	testis or testicle
urethr/o	urethra
vas/o	vessel or duct

reproductive

obstetrics
ob STET riks

12.1 The reproductive systems are separated in this chapter to reflect the differences between the male and female. In both sexes, the _____ system performs the role of producing sex cells, or gametes (GAH meets), in preparation for fertilization and the development of new offspring. The male gametes are called spermatozoa, or sperm cells, and are produced by the male gonads, the testes. Other male organs include the scrotum that houses the testes, the penis, the tubes that convey sperm (vas deferens and urethra), and the glands that contribute to semen (seminal vesicles, prostate gland, and bulbourethral glands). The male sex hormone, testosterone, is also produced by the testes. The female gametes are called ova and are produced by the female gonads, the ovaries. Other female organs include the fallopian tubes, uterus, vagina, and vulva. The female hormones, estrogen and progesterone, are produced by cells within the ovaries.

Once a new life has been conceived, the developing embryo enters into the segment of life called **prenatal** (pree NAY tal) **development**, which includes the changes in body form that occur through the mother's pregnancy until birth. The clinical field of **obstetrics** is focused on this period of life. _____ is often referred to by its abbreviation, **OB**. It supports the mother during childbirth and during the first month or so following childbirth.

FUNCTION ▶▶▶

gamete
GAMM eet

1. **vas**
2. **prostate**
3. **testis**
4. **epididymis**

12.2 The general function of the reproductive system is the creation of offspring, which occurs when the male gamete (sperm) unites successfully with a female _____ (ovum). The resulting fertilized egg is the origin of a new human life.

12.3 Use the anatomy terms that appear in the left column to fill in the corresponding blanks in Figures 12.1■ through 12.3■.

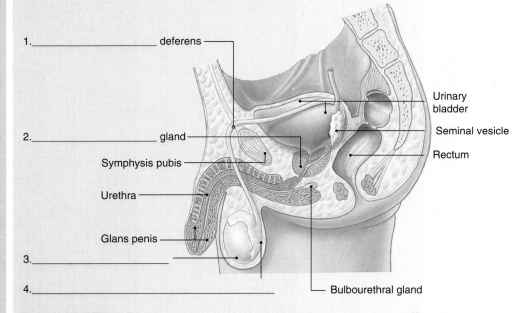

1._____ deferens ____

2._____ gland ____

Symphysis pubis ____

Urethra ____

Glans penis ____

3._____

4._____

Urinary bladder

Seminal vesicle

Rectum

Bulbourethral gland

Figure 12.1 ■
The male reproductive system.

5. vagina
6. majora
7. ovary

8. cervix
9. vagina

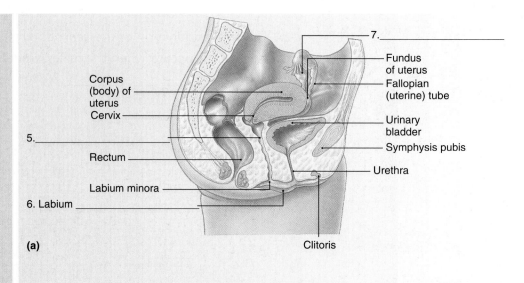

Corpus (body) of uterus
Cervix
5._____
Rectum
Labium minora
6. Labium _____
7._____
Fundus of uterus
Fallopian (uterine) tube
Urinary bladder
Symphysis pubis
Urethra
Clitoris

(a)

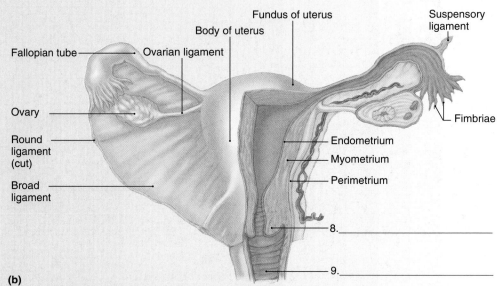

Fallopian tube
Ovary
Round ligament (cut)
Broad ligament
Ovarian ligament
Body of uterus
Fundus of uterus
Suspensory ligament
Fimbriae
Endometrium
Myometrium
Perimetrium
8._____
9._____

(b)

Figure 12.2 ■
The female reproductive system. (a) Sagittal section through the pelvis. (b) Top view of pelvic organs.

10. placenta
11. uterus

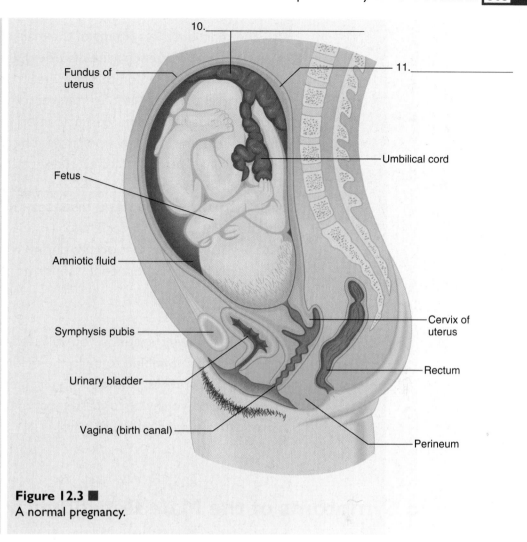

10._____

11._____

Fundus of uterus

Umbilical cord

Fetus

Amniotic fluid

Cervix of uterus

Symphysis pubis

Rectum

Urinary bladder

Vagina (birth canal)

Perineum

Figure 12.3 ■
A normal pregnancy.

Medical Terms for the Reproductive System and Obstetrics ▶▶▶▶

reproductive

12.4 The medical field of **reproductive medicine** manages the health care of both the male and female _____ systems. Because the male urethra is responsible for transporting both urine and semen, diseases of the male reproductive system are usually treated within the field of **urology** (yoo RAHL oh jee) by a _____. Diseases of the female reproductive system are generally treated by a physician called a **gynecologist** (gye neh KAHL oh jist), who specializes within the field of _____. In both sexes, reproductive diseases are often diagnosed initially during a physical examination. The diseases that require confirmation or an internal evaluation may be further analyzed using the noninvasive procedures of MRI, CAT scan, or ultrasound imaging.

urologist
yoo RAHL oh jist

gynecology
GYE neh KALL oh jee

transmitted

12.5 The reproductive systems of the male and female are subject to infections, tumors, injury, endocrine disorders, and inherited diseases. For many people, the most common threat to health is the exposure to pathogens during sexual contact. Although the reproductive tract is lined with a protective mucous membrane, certain bacteria, viruses, fungi, and protozoa are able to gain entry into the bloodstream directly or by way of breaks in the mucosal lining. Once established, these pathogens may spread throughout the body. Most **sexually** _____ **infections (STIs)**, also called **sexually transmitted diseases (STDs)** or venereal diseases, infect the body in this manner. Thus, STIs are infections acquired during intimate physical contact that occurs during sexual intercourse or other sexual activities. The most common forms of STIs are described in this chapter.

12.6 In the following sections, you will study the prefixes, combining forms, and suffixes that combine to build the medical terms of the reproductive system and obstetrics. Complete the frames and review exercises that follow. You are on your way to mastery of the medical terms related to the reproductive system and obstetrics!

Signs and Symptoms of the Male Reproductive System

Following are the word parts that specifically apply to the signs and symptoms of the male reproductive system that are covered in the following section. Note that the word parts are color-coded to help you identify them: prefixes are blue, combining forms are red, and suffixes are purple.

Prefix	Definition
a-	without or absence of
oligo-	little

Combining Form	Definition
balan/o	glans penis
orch/o, orchid/o, test/o	testis
prostat/o	prostate gland
sperm/o	sperm, living seed
urethr/o	urethra
zo/o	animal, living

Suffix	Definition
-ia	condition of
-itis	inflammation
-rrhea	excessive discharge
-algia	condition of pain

KEY TERMS A-Z

aspermia
ah SPER mee ah

12.7 As you know, the prefix *a-* means "without or absence of." Therefore, the inability to produce or ejaculate sperm is a sign of male infertility known as _____. The constructed form of this term is a/sperm/ia, which literally means "condition of without seed."

azoospermia AY zoh oh SPER mee ah a/zo/o/sperm/ia	**12.8** The absence of living sperm in semen is called **azoospermia** and is another sign of infertility. The term _____ literally means "condition of without living seed." This constructed term has five word parts and is written as __/____/__/_____/____.
balanorrhea BAL ah noh REE ah	**12.9** The combining form for the distal end of the penis, known as the glans penis, is balan/o. Recall that the suffix -*rrhea* means "excessive discharge." Therefore, a condition of excessive discharge from the glans is called _____, which is a symptom of the sexually transmitted infection called gonorrhea (Frame 12.135). Balanorrhea is a constructed term that can be written balan/o/rrhea.
chancres SHANG kerz	**12.10** The sexually transmitted infection syphilis (Frame 12.138) may be diagnosed by the presence of small ulcers on the skin of the penis, which are called **chancres**. The term _____ is a French word meaning "cancer."
oligospermia all ih goh SPER mee ah	**12.11** An abnormally low sperm count is the most common sign of male infertility. Combining the prefix that means "little," *oligo-*, with the word parts meaning "pertaining to sperm," the term that results is the condition _____. It is a constructed term that can be represented as oligo/sperm/ia.
papilloma pap ih LOH mah	**12.12 Papillomas** are wartlike lesions on the skin and mucous membranes. A _____ is a sign of infection by the sexually transmitted human papillomaviruses (Frame 12.137), and they are commonly called genital warts.
prostatitis pross tah TYE tiss	**12.13** Inflammation of the prostate gland is called _____. It is usually a sign of either BPH (Frame 12.20) or prostate cancer (Frame 12.28). This constructed term is written prostat/itis.
prostatorrhea PROSS tah toh REE ah	**12.14** An abnormal, excessive discharge from the prostate gland is known as _____. This is a constructed term that is written prostat/o/rrhea.

testalgia test AHL jee ah	**12.15** The suffix that means "condition of pain" is -*algia*. The condition of testicular pain is known as _____, which is written test/algia. It is also known as **orchialgia** (OR kee ALL jee ah) and **orchidalgia** (OR kid ALL jee ah) because *test/o*, *orch/o*, and *orchid/o* are each combining forms of testis.
urethritis yoo ree THRYE tiss	**12.16** Inflammation of the urethra is called _____. It is a symptom of an irritation of the urethra, usually resulting from a sexually transmitted infection. This constructed term is written urethr/itis.

PRACTICE: Signs and Symptoms of the Male Reproductive System

The Right Match

Match the term on the left with the correct definition on the right.

_____ 1. chancres

_____ 2. balanorrhea

_____ 3. prostatitis

_____ 4. papillomas

_____ 5. azoospermia

a. excessive discharge from the glans penis

b. inflammation of the prostate gland

c. absence of living sperm in semen

d. small ulcers on the skin of the penis, sign of syphilis

e. wartlike lesions

Break the Chain

Analyze these medical terms:

a) Separate each term into its word parts; each word part is labeled for you (**p** = prefix, **r** = root, **cf** = combining form, and **s** = suffix).

b) For the Bonus Question, write the requested definition in the blank that follows.

The first set has been completed as an example.

1. a) prostatorrhea

   prostat / o / rrhea
         cf   s

   b) *Bonus Question:* What is the definition of the suffix? *excessive discharge*

2. a) oligospermia

   _____ / _____ / __
     p   r   s

   b) *Bonus Question:* What is the definition of the prefix? _____

3. a) testalgia

   _____ / _____
     r   s

   b) *Bonus Question:* What is the definition of the word root? _____

4. a) urethritis _____/_____
                    r   s

    b) *Bonus Question*: What is the definition of the suffix? _____

5. a) aspermia ____/_____/____
                   p   r   s

    b) *Bonus Question*: What is the definition of the prefix? _____

Diseases and Disorders of the Male Reproductive System

Following are the word parts that specifically apply to the diseases and disorders of the male reproductive system that are covered in the following section. Note that the word parts are color-coded to help you identify them: prefixes are blue, combining forms are red, and suffixes are purple.

Prefix	Definition	Combining Form	Definition	Suffix	Definition
an-	without or absence of	andr/o	male	-cele	hernia, swelling, or protrusion
crypt-	hidden	balan/o	glans penis		
hyper-	excessive, abnormally high, or above	epididym/o	epididymis	-ism	condition
		hydr/o	water	-itis	inflammation
		orch/o, orchid/o	testis	-pathy	disease
		prostat/o	prostate gland		
		varic/o	dilated vein		

KEY TERMS A-Z

andropathy
an DROPP ah thee

12.17 A combining form that means "male" and the suffix meaning "disease" may be combined to form a general term for a disease afflicting only males, _____. This constructed term includes three word parts, which can be represented as andr/o/pathy.

anorchism
an OR kizm

an/orch/ism

12.18 The word root that means "testis" is *orch* or *orchid*. When the prefix meaning "without or absence of" is added along with the suffix *-ism*, the constructed term _____ is created. It means "condition of without testis" and refers to the absence of one or both testes. The constructed form of the term is written ____/_____/____. The term *anorchidism* may also be used with the same meaning.

balanitis
bal ah NYE tiss

12.19 Inflammation of the glans penis is a disorder called _____. It is a constructed term with two word parts, written balan/itis.

prostate cancer
PROSS tayt * KANN ser

12.28 The prostate gland is subject to an aggressive form of cancer, commonly known as _____ _____. Also called **prostatic carcinoma** (pro STAT ik * kar sih NOH mah), it increases the size of the prostate before it spreads into the pelvic region and beyond and can often be felt as a hard nodule on the prostate during a digital rectal exam (Frame 12.35). It is illustrated in Figure 12.6■.

Figure 12.6 ■
Prostate cancer. In this example, a large mass has grown into the urinary bladder. Prostate cancer is highly metastatic, sending tumor cells to the pelvic area and beyond, where they may form secondary tumor sites.

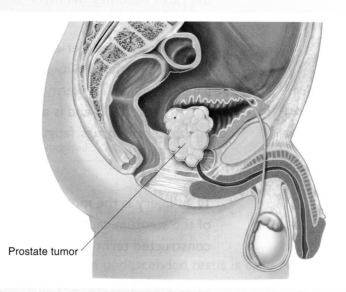

Prostate tumor

testicular carcinoma
tess TIK yoo ler * kar sih NOH mah

12.29 A cancer originating from the testis is known as _____ _____. Its occurrence and mortality rate is highest among the 20- to 29-year-old age group. The most common form is called **seminoma** (sem ih NOH mah), which arises from sperm-forming cells and metastasizes to nearby lymph nodes. It is the most common cancer in American young men, with about 8,000 expected diagnoses in 2007 and roughly 1,000 deaths.

testicular torsion

tess TIK yoo ler * TOR shun

12.30 A **testicular torsion** occurs when the spermatic cord becomes twisted, causing a reduced blood flow to the testis (Figure 12.7■). If _____ _____ is not corrected within a few hours by surgery, the affected testicular tissue can die.

Figure 12.7 ■
Testicular torsion.

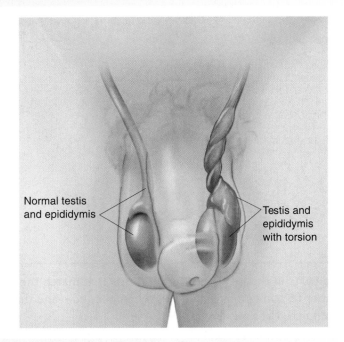

Normal testis and epididymis

Testis and epididymis with torsion

varic/o/cele
varicocele

VAIR ih koh seel

12.31 Herniation of the veins within the spermatic cord is a condition known as **varicocele**. It is a constructed term that uses the combining form for dilated vein, _varic/o_, and can be written _____/__/_____. A _____ is caused by failure of the valves within the veins, allowing blood to pool and dilate the veins.

PRACTICE: Diseases and Disorders of the Male Reproductive System

The Right Match

Match the term on the left with the correct definition on the right.

_____ 1. benign prostatic hyperplasia

_____ 2. erectile dysfunction

_____ 3. Peyronie's disease

_____ 4. priapism

_____ 5. phimosis

_____ 6. testicular torsion

   a. the inability to achieve an erection sufficient to perform sexual intercourse

   b. an abnormally persistent erection of the penis

   c. reduced blood flow to the testis due to a twisted spermatic cord

   d. enlargement of the prostate gland that constricts the urethra

   e. a hardness of the erectile tissue within the penis

   f. a congenital narrowing of the prepuce

Linkup

Link the word parts in the list to create the terms that match the definitions. You may use word parts more than once. Remember to add combining vowels when needed—and that some terms do not use any combining vowel. The first one is completed as an example.

Prefix	Combining Form	Suffix
(none)	andr/o	-pathy
	balan/o	-itis
	epididym/o	-cele
	hydr/o	
	varic/o	

Definition   Term

1. a disease that afflicts only males   *andropathy*

2. inflammation of the glans penis   _____

3. inflammation of the epididymis   _____

4. fluid accumulation in the scrotum   _____

5. herniation of the veins within the spermatic cord   _____

Treatments, Procedures, and Devices of the Male Reproductive System

Following are the word parts that specifically apply to the treatments, procedures, and devices of the male reproductive system that are covered in the following section. Note that the word parts are color-coded to help you identify them: prefixes are blue, combining forms are red, and suffixes are purple.

Prefix	Definition
anti-	against or opposite of
poly-	excessive, over, or many
trans-	through, across, or beyond

Combining Form	Definition
balan/o	glans penis
cyst/o	bladder
hydr/o	water
orch/i, orchid/o	testis
prostat/o	prostate gland
urethr/o	urethra
ur/o	urine
vas/o	vessel
vesicul/o	small bag

Suffix	Definition
-al	pertaining to
-cele	hernia, swelling, or protrusion
-ectomy	surgical removal
-pexy	surgical fixation
-plasty	surgical repair
-stomy	surgical creation of an opening
-tomy	incision or to cut

KEY TERMS A-Z

anti-impotence therapy
an tye IM poh tens * THAIR ah pee

12.32 A collection of therapies that address erectile dysfunction (Frame 12.23) is called **anti-impotence therapy**. _____ _____ includes drugs such as sildenafil (Viagra) or implantation of a penile implant (Frame 12.40).

balanoplasty
BAL ah noh plass tee

12.33 The suffix that means "surgical repair" is -plasty. The surgical repair of the glans penis is therefore called _____. The constructed form of this term is balan/o/plasty.

circumcision
ser kum SIH zhun

12.34 A common, routine procedure in many parts of the world is the removal of the prepuce. Known as **circumcision** after the circular cut that is made around the base of the glans penis, it is usually performed within hours after birth. Alternate procedures of _____ are illustrated in Figure 12.8■.

Figure 12.8 ■
Circumcision. Alternate procedures may be used with the common goal of removing the prepuce from the penis.
(a) Use of the Yellen clamp, in which a cone is inserted over the glans and clamped in place, followed by the excision of the prepuce.
(b) Use of the PlastiBell, which is inserted over the glans and the prepuce cut away. The plastic rim remains in place for three to four days until healing occurs, then falls away.

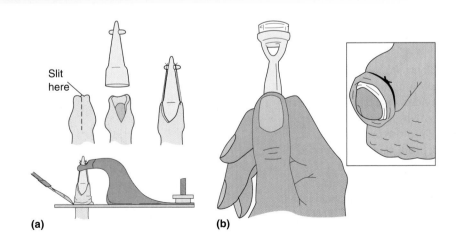

Slit here

(a)　　　(b)

digital rectal examination DIH jih tal * REK tal * eks AM ih NAY shun	**12.35** A **digital rectal examination** is a physical exam that involves the insertion of a finger into the rectum to feel the size and shape of the prostate gland through the wall of the rectum. A _____ _____ _____ is used to screen the patient for BPH (Frame 12.20) and prostate cancer (Frame 12.28), and is abbreviated **DRE**.
hydrocelectomy HIGH droh see LEK toh mee	**12.36** Recall that the suffix -*ectomy* means "surgical removal." The surgical removal of a hydrocele (Frame 12.24) is a procedure called _____. The constructed form of this term is written hydr/o/cel/ectomy.
orchidectomy OR kid EK toh mee	**12.37** The surgical removal of a testis is called _____, or **orchiectomy**. A bilateral orchidectomy is commonly called **castration** (kass TRAY shun).
orchidopexy or KID oh pek see	**12.38** Surgical fixation of a testis is sometimes required to draw an undescended testis into the scrotum. The procedure is called _____, or **orchiopexy**, because the suffix -*pexy* means "surgical fixation." The constructed form of orchidopexy reveals three word parts and is written orchid/o/pexy.
orchidoplasty OR kid oh PLASS tee orchid/o/**tomy**	**12.39** A general term for a surgical repair of a testis is _____, or **orchioplasty**. An incision into the testis is a form of orchidoplasty and is called **orchidotomy** (OR kid OTT oh mee). The constructed form of orchidotomy is written _____/__/_____. Similar to other terms of the testis, an alternate term for orchidotomy is **orchiotomy** (OR kee OTT oh mee).
penile implants PEE nile * IM plants	**12.40** A **penile implant** is the surgical insertion of a prosthesis, or artificial device, to correct erectile dysfunction. Optional _____ _____ include semirigid rods and inflatable balloonlike cylinders (Figure 12.9■).

Figure 12.9 ■

Penile implants. (a) Semirigid rods may be surgically implanted into the penis, which provides a partial erection that is persistent. (b) Inflatable cylinders implanted into the penis may be self-contained, producing an erection when the pump is activated by physical contact. (c) Inflatable cylinders may alternatively include a pump that requires a more directed hand pumping action to activate.

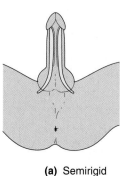

(a) Semirigid

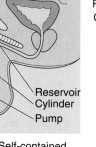

(b) Self-contained

Reservoir
Cylinders

Reservoir
Cylinder
Pump

Pump

(c) Inflatable

prostatectomy
pross tah TEK toh mee

12.41 The surgical removal of the prostate gland is a procedure called _____. This constructed term is written prostat/ectomy. It is a treatment for BPH (Frame 12.20) and prostate cancer (Frame 12.28). During a suprapubic prostatectomy, the prostate gland is removed through an abdominal incision made above the pubic bone and a second incision through the urinary bladder wall. The second incision is called a **prostatocystotomy** (pross TAH toh siss TOTT oh mee).

prostate-specific antigen
PROSS tayt * speh SIH fik *
AN tih jenn

12.42 A **prostate-specific antigen** is a clinical test that measures levels of the protein, prostate-specific antigen, in the blood. _____- _____ _____ is commonly called **PSA**. Elevated levels suggest a presence of prostate cancer and indicate a need for additional tests before a diagnosis can be made.

transurethral resection of the prostate gland
trans you REE thrall

12.43 **Transurethral resection of the prostate gland** is a procedure that treats BPH (Frame 12.20) through the noninvasive removal of prostate tissue. It involves the scraping of the urethral section of prostate tissue using a specialized endoscope, called a retroscope. The retroscope is inserted through the urethra to the prostate wall, where it scrapes the capsule (outer covering) of the prostate while as much inner tissue is left intact as possible. _____ _____ _____ _____ _____ is abbreviated **TURP**. *Transurethral* is a constructed term that can be written as trans/urethr/al.

urology
yoo RAHL oh jee

12.44 The department within a hospital or clinic that treats urinary tract problems (in both sexes) is called **urology**. The constructed form of _____ is written ur/o/logy. A specialist in this field is a **urologist** (yoo RAHL oh jist).

vasectomy

vas EK toh mee

12.45 A male can elect to become **sterile**, or unable to produce and ejaculate sperm, by undergoing a **vasectomy**. This constructed term literally means "surgical removal of vessel," where the "vessel" is the vas deferens. It is a simple, quick procedure in which the vas deferens is severed to block the flow of sperm during ejaculation (Figure 12.10■). A _____ does not affect a man's ability to ejaculate (the fluid is a spermless semen) or his experience of sexual pleasure. Vasectomy is a constructed term with two word parts, written vas/ectomy.

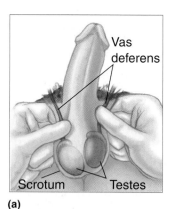
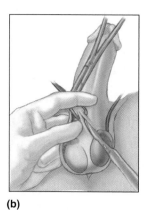
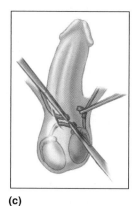
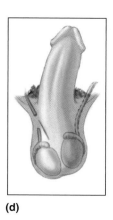

(a) (b) (c) (d)

Figure 12.10 ■
Vasectomy. (a) Vas deferens is located within the spermatic cord on both sides.
(b) A small incision is made through the scrotum, and an instrument is inserted that gently separates the vas deferens from other tissues of the spermatic cord. Once separated, the vas deferens is pulled out gently.
(c) The vas deferens is cut and the exposed ends cauterized to close them.
(d) The vas deferens is returned to the spermatic cord, tucked back into the scrotum, and a single suture closes the incision. The vas deferens on the other side is then cut in a duplicate procedure.

vasovasostomy

VAS oh vah SOSS toh mee

12.46 A surgery to reverse a vasectomy is known as a **vasovasostomy**. This constructed term uses the combining form for "vessel" twice and contains five total word parts, as shown in vas/o/vas/o/stomy. A _____ involves the creation of artificial openings and reconnection of the severed ends of the vas deferens to restore fertility.

vesiculectomy

veh SIK yoo LEK toh mee

12.47 A procedure to remove the seminal vesicles is called a _____. The constructed form of this term is vesicul/ectomy.

PRACTICE: Treatments, Procedures, and Devices of the Male Reproductive System

The Right Match

Match the term on the left with the correct definition on the right.

_____ 1. anti-impotence therapy

_____ 2. circumcision

_____ 3. penile implant

_____ 4. prostate-specific antigen

_____ 5. urology

a. the removal of the prepuce

b. blood protein that is measured in the PSA test

c. a collection of therapies that address erectile dysfunction

d. department that treats urinary tract problems

e. surgical insertion of a prosthesis to correct erectile dysfunction

Break the Chain

Analyze these medical terms:

a) Separate each term into its word parts; each word part is labeled for you (**p** = prefix, **r** = root, **cf** = combining form, and **s** = suffix).

b) For the Bonus Question, write the requested definition in the blank that follows.

1. a) vasectomy   _____/_____
                                r   s

    b) *Bonus Question*: Which vessel does the word root refer to in this procedural term? _____

2. a) hydrocelectomy   _____/___/___/_____
                                cf   s   s

    b) *Bonus Question*: What is the definition of the first suffix? _____

3. a) orchidopexy   _____/___/_____
                                cf   s

    b) *Bonus Question*: What is the definition of the combining form? _____

4. a) prostatectomy   _____/____
                                r   s

    b) *Bonus Question*: What is the definition of the suffix? _____

5. a) vasovasostomy   _____/__/_____/__/_____
                                cf   cf   s

    b) *Bonus Question*: What is the definition of the suffix? _____

fibrocystic breast disease figh broh SISS tik	**12.68** In the condition **fibrocystic breast disease**, one or more benign, fibrous cysts develop within the breast (see Figure 12.11). _____ _____ _____ is an inherited condition that has no known association with breast cancer. The term *fibrocystic* is a constructed term written fibr/o/cyst/ic.
fistulas FISS tyoo lahs	**12.69** A **fistula** is an abnormal passage from one organ or cavity to another. Two major types of vaginal _____ may occur. A **rectovaginal** (rek toh VAJ ih nal) **fistula** occurs between the vagina and rectum, and a **vesicovaginal** (vess ih koh VAJ ih nal) **fistula** is located between the urinary bladder and the vagina.
hysteratresia hiss ter ah TREE zee ah	**12.70** The suffix *-atresia* means "closure or absence of a normal body opening." Adding this suffix to the word root for uterus forms the term _____, which means a closure of the uterus. The closure results in an abnormal obstruction within the uterine canal that may interfere with childbirth. The constructed form of this term is written hyster/atresia.
leiomyoma lye oh my OH mah	**12.71** The muscular wall of the uterus is the origin of benign tumors known as **leiomyomas**. Also known as **fibroid tumors** because of their tough, fibrous structure, their presence can produce abnormal pain during menstruation (Figure 12.13■). _____ is a constructed term written as lei/o/my/oma, which literally means "tumor of smooth muscle."

Figure 12.13 ■
Fibroid tumors, or leiomyomas. Fibroids develop from the uterus to form a variety of hard, round benign structures.

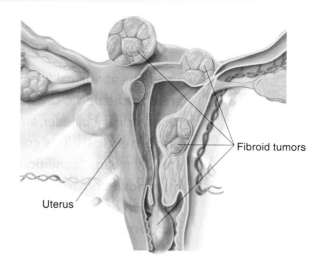

Fibroid tumors

Uterus

mastitis mass TYE tiss	**12.72** Inflammation of the breast is a condition known as _____. It is often caused by bacterial infection of the lactiferous ducts within breast tissue. The constructed form of this term is written mast/itis.
mastoptosis mass top TOH siss	**12.73** The suffix -ptosis means "drooping." A breast that is abnormally pendulous or drooping is the condition known as _____. The constructed form of this term is mast/o/ptosis.
oophoropathy oh OFF or OPP ah thee **oophoritis** oh OFF or EYE tiss	**12.74** The combining form that means "ovary" is oophor/o. Any disease of an ovary is known as _____. An example of an oophoropathy is inflammation of an ovary, which is called _____. This constructed term is written oophor/itis. Inflammation of an ovary and fallopian tube is called **oophorosalpingitis** (oh OFF or oh sal pinj EYE tiss). This term is also constructed of word parts, written as oophor/o/salping/itis.
ovarian cancer oh VAIR ee an * KANN ser	**12.75** The most common form of reproductive cancer in women is **ovarian cancer**. Older women and women who have not given birth are at higher risk, and there is some evidence for a genetic link. The incidences of _____ _____ in 2007 were about 22,000 new diagnoses and roughly 15,000 deaths.
ovarian cyst oh VAIR ee an * sist	**12.76** A cyst is a fluid-filled sac that forms within the body from mutated cells. An _____ _____ is a cyst on an ovary that is usually benign and asymptomatic, although in some cases it may cause pelvic pain and dysmenorrhea (Frame 12.49). The term **polycystic ovary syndrome** is quite different. It is a hormonal disturbance characterized by lack of ovulation (called anovulation), amenorrhea (Frame 12.48), and infertility. Numerous ovarian cysts may develop, sometimes increasing the size of the ovary dramatically. If cyst development spreads into the fallopian tube, the condition is called **parovarian cyst** (par oh VAIR ee an * sist).
pelvic inflammatory disease	**12.77** An inflammation involving some or all of the female organs within the pelvic cavity is called **pelvic inflammatory disease**, abbreviated **PID**. It is usually caused by bacterial infection that spreads from organ to organ. Complications of _____ _____ _____ include obstruction of the fallopian tubes and infertility.

premenstrual syndrome
pre MEN stroo al * SIN drohm

12.78 Premenstrual syndrome is a collection of symptoms, including nervous tension, irritability, breast pain (mastalgia), edema, and headache, which usually occur during the ten days preceding menstruation. _____ _____ is abbreviated **PMS**.

prolapsed uterus

12.79 The uterus is suspended in the pelvic cavity by ligaments. If these ligaments weaken, often due to a congenital deformity or trauma, the uterus may become displaced to droop downward into the vagina. The condition is called **prolapsed uterus**, and in some cases may even fall completely within the vagina (Figure 12.14■). Another term for _____ _____ is **hysteroptosis** (HISS ter op TOH siss), which is a constructed term written hyster/o/ptosis.

Figure 12.14 ■
Prolapsed uterus. (a) A prolapse is the abnormal drop of the uterus into the vagina, representing the most common type of uterine displacement. It is usually caused by weakened uterine ligaments.
(b) A severely prolapsed uterus may extend through the vaginal orifice, as shown.

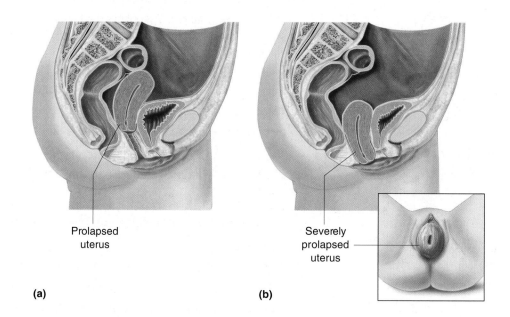

Prolapsed uterus

(a)

Severely prolapsed uterus

(b)

salpingitis
sal pin JYE tiss

12.80 Inflammation of a fallopian tube is called _____. The constructed form of this term is salping/itis. It is usually caused by bacterial infection, and is often associated with PID (Frame 12.77).

salpingocele
sal PING goh seel

12.81 A protrusion, or herniation, of a fallopian tube wall is known as _____. The constructed form is salping/o/cele.

toxic shock syndrome	**12.82 Toxic shock syndrome**, or **TSS**, is a severe bacterial infection characterized by a sudden high fever, skin rash, mental confusion, acute renal failure, and abnormal liver function. _____ _____ _____ is caused by a type of *Staphylococcus* and is most common in menstruating women using non-cotton tampons.
vaginitis vaj ih NYE tiss	**12.83** Inflammation of the vagina is known as _____. Because *colp/o* is an alternate combining form for vagina, it is also called **colpitis** (kol PYE tiss). In a common form known as **atrophic vaginitis** (ay TROH fik * vaj ih NYE tiss), the usual symptoms of redness and swelling are accompanied by thinning of the vaginal wall and loss of moisture, usually due to a depletion of estrogen.
vulvitis vul VYE tiss **vulv/o/vagin/itis**	**12.84** Inflammation of the external genitals, or vulva, is called _____. When the vagina is also inflamed, the condition is known as **vulvovaginitis** (VUL voh vaj ih NYE tiss). The constructed form of this term is written _____/__/_____/____.

PRACTICE: Diseases and Disorders of the Female Reproductive System

The Right Match

Match the term on the left with the correct definition on the right.

_____ 1. breast cancer

_____ 2. carcinoma in situ

_____ 3. cervical cancer

_____ 4. fibrocystic breast disease

_____ 5. fistula

_____ 6. ovarian cancer

_____ 7. ovarian cyst

_____ 8. pelvic inflammatory disease

_____ 9. premenstrual syndrome

_____ 10. prolapsed uterus

_____ 11. toxic shock syndrome

a. a malignant tumor of the cervix

b. the most common form is infiltrating ductal carcinoma

c. a form of cervical cancer

d. the most common form of reproductive cancer in women

e. a condition in which one or more benign, fibrous cysts develop within the breast

f. an abnormal passage from one hollow organ to another

g. inflammation that involves some or all of the female organs within the pelvic cavity

h. a severe bacterial infection caused by a type of *Staphylococcus*

i. a fluid-filled sac on an ovary

j. collection of symptoms that occur during the ten days preceding menstruation

k. displacement of the uterus into the vagina

Break the Chain

Analyze these medical terms:

 a) Separate each term into its word parts; each word part is labeled for you (**p** = prefix, **r** = root, **cf** = combining form, and **s** = suffix).

 b) For the Bonus Question, write the requested words or definition in the blank that follows.

1. a) vulvitis

   _____/_____

     r   s

   b) *Bonus Question:* What is the definition of the word root? _____

2. a) salpingocele

   _____/__/_____

        cf   s

   b) *Bonus Question:* What anatomical part does the combining form refer to? _____

3. a) amastia

   ___/_____/___

    p   r   s

   b) *Bonus Question:* What is the definition of the word root? _____

4. a) endometriosis

   _____/_____/__/_____

      p   cf   s

   b) *Bonus Question:* What is the definition of the prefix? _____

5. a) leiomyoma

   _____/_____/_____/_____

     cf   r   s

   b) *Bonus Question:* What is the definition of the combining form? _____

Treatments, Procedures, and Devices of the Female Reproductive System

Following are the word parts that specifically apply to the treatments, procedures, and devices of the female reproductive system that are covered in the following section. Note that the word parts are color-coded to help you identify them: prefixes are blue, combining forms are red, and suffixes are purple.

Prefix	Definition	Combining Form	Definition	Suffix	Definition
endo-	within	cerv/o	cervix	-al, -ic	pertaining to
trans-	through, across, or beyond	colp/o	vagina	-ectomy	surgical removal
		episi/o	vulva	-gram	a record or image
		gynec/o, gyn/o	woman	-graphy	recording process
		lapar/o	abdomen	-logist	one who studies
		mamm/o, mast/o	breast	-logy	study of
		metr/o, hyster/o	uterus	-pexy	surgical fixation
		oophor/o	ovary	-plasty	surgical repair
		path/o	disease	-rrhaphy	suturing
		salping/o	trumpet tube, fallopian tube	-scopy	viewing
		son/o	sound	-stomy	surgical creation of an opening
		vagin/o	vagina	-tomy	incision or to cut
		vulv/o	vulva		

biopsy
BYE op see

12.85 A minor surgical procedure that involves the surgical extraction of tissue for microscopic analysis is called a _____. Abbreviated **Bx**, the sample may be removed from the cervix, endometrium, or breast. Any one of several procedures may be used, including excision, aspiration, or needle biopsy (Figure 12.15■).

Figure 12.15 ■
Biopsy. The various forms of gynecological biopsy are shown.

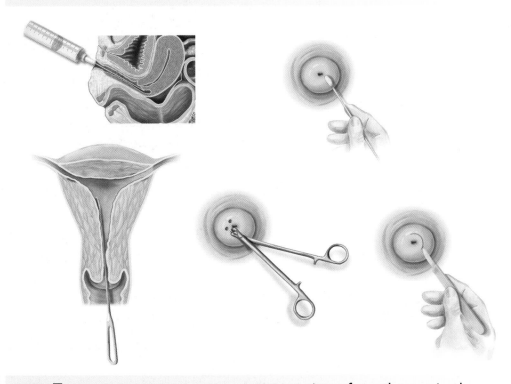

cervicectomy
SER vih SEK toh mee

12.86 To remove precancerous or cancerous tissue from the cervix, the anterior part of the cervix can be removed in a **cervical conization** (SER vih kal * koh nih ZAY shun). In this procedure, a cone-shaped section of the cervix is removed. If the cancer is developed, the cervix may be removed in a _____. The constructed form of this term is written cerv/ic/ectomy.

colpectomy
kol PEK toh mee

12.87 Recall that a word root for vagina is *colp*. Removal of the vagina is a surgery called a _____, or alternatively called **vaginectomy** (VAJ ih NEK toh mee).

colpoplasty
KOL poh plass tee

colporrhaphy
kol POR ah fee

colp/o/scopy

12.88 Surgical repair of the vagina is a procedure called _____. This constructed term may be written as colp/o/plasty. A colpoplasty often includes suturing the wall of the vagina in a procedure called _____. Also a constructed term, it is written colp/o/rrhaphy. Both procedures often follow an endoscopic evaluation of the vagina, called a **colposcopy**. This constructed term is written _____/_/_____.

dilation and curettage
dye LAY shun * and * koo reh TAZH

12.89 A common procedure that is used for both diagnostic and treatment purposes is called **dilation and curettage**, abbreviated **D&C**. During a _____ _____ _____, the cervix is dilated to permit the insertion of a spoon-shaped instrument called a **curette**, which is used to scrape the lining of the endometrium. It is often performed to control bleeding, obtain a tissue sample for biopsy, or remove polyps.

endometrial ablation
ehn doh MEE tree al * ahb LAY shun

12.90 If the endometrium requires more treatment than can be provided by a D&C, an **endometrial ablation** may be applied. In an _____ _____, lasers, electricity, or heat may be used to destroy the endometrium. The procedure is effective in treating dysmenorrhea (Frame 12.49).

gynecology
GYE neh KOL oh jee

gynopathology
GYE no path ALL oh jee

12.91 Two combining forms that mean "woman" are _gynec/o_ and _gyn/o_. The branch of medicine focusing on women is known as _____, abbreviated **GYN**. The constructed form of this term is _gynec/o/logy_. Frequently, a physician known as an obstetrician-gynecologist combines these two areas of expertise; this is abbreviated **OB/GYN**. Also, the study of diseases that afflict women is known as _____. As a constructed term, it is written _gyn/o/path/o/logy_. A physician specializing in this field of medicine is called a **gynopathologist** (GYE no path ALL oh jist).

hormone replacement therapy

12.92 As a common therapy for hormonal management, **hormone replacement therapy**, abbreviated **HRT**, can be very effective in correcting disrupted menstrual and ovarian cycles. In _____ _____ _____, the hormones estrogen and progesterone are frequently prescribed in pill form. It is also the most effective means of **female contraception** for the prevention of unwanted pregnancy.

hysterectomy
HISS teh REK toh mee

12.93 The surgical removal of the uterus is commonly called
_____. The surgery may involve surrounding structures, as
shown in Figure 12.16■.

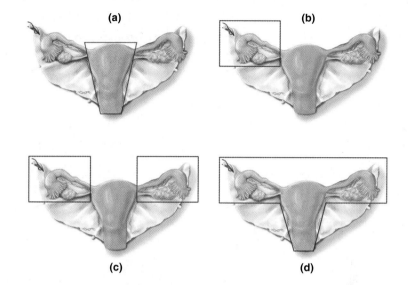

Figure 12.16 ■
Alternative forms of surgeries
involving the uterus, ovaries, and
fallopian tubes. The solid lines indicate
excision. (a) Hysterectomy. (b) Right
salpingo-oophorectomy.
(c) Bilateral salpingo-oophorectomy.
(d) Bilateral hysterosalpingo-
oophorectomy, or panhysterectomy.

hysteropexy
HISS ter oh PEK see

12.94 The surgical procedure that may be used to correct a prolapsed
uterus (Frame 12.79) by strengthening its connections to the abdominal
wall to correct its position is called _____. This constructed term is written hyster/o/pexy and means "surgical fixation of the
uterus."

WORDS TO WATCH OUT FOR ❗

***-pexy* or *-plasty*?**

The meanings of these two suffixes both relate to surgery—but they are very different forms of surgery. Remember that *-pexy* means "surgical *fixation*," and *-plasty*
means "surgical *repair*." One way to remember the meaning of *-pexy* is that it uses
an *x*, as does the word *fixation* in its definition. Similarly, a way to remember the
meaning of *-plasty* is that it uses a *p*, as does the word *repair* in its definition.

hysteroscopy
HISS ter OSS koh pee

laparoscopy
lap ahr OSS koh pee

12.95 A noninvasive diagnostic technique that uses a modified endoscope, called a **hysteroscope** (HISS ter oh skope), to evaluate the uterine cavity is called _____. The constructed form is hyster/o/scopy. In order to evaluate the external appearance of the uterus and other organs of the pelvic cavity, a **laparoscope** (LAP ahr oh skope) is inserted through a small incision through the lower abdominal wall during a _____. The procedure is shown in Figure 12.17■. This is also a constructed term, written as lapar/o/scopy (the word root *lapar* means "abdomen").

Figure 12.17 ■
Laparoscopy. (a) A lighted endoscope specialized for insertion into the abdomen, called a laparoscope, is used to view reproductive organs. The laparoscope may also be outfitted with surgical devices for excision of structures.
(b) Laparoscopic surgery, as seen from the monitor attached to the laparoscope.
Source: Southern Illinois University/Photo Researchers, Inc.

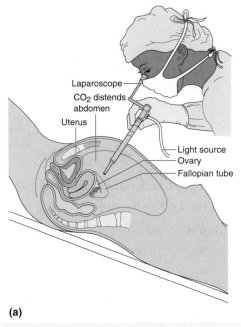

Laparoscope
CO_2 distends abdomen
Uterus
Light source
Ovary
Fallopian tube

(a)

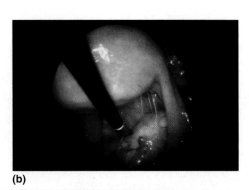

(b)

mammography
mam OG rah fee

12.96 An X-ray procedure that produces an X-ray image of a breast, called a **mammogram**, is called _____. The procedure and a mammogram are shown in Figure 12.18■. The procedure is an early screening for breast cancer. The term mammography is a constructed word, written as mamm/o/graphy.

Figure 12.18 ■
Mammography. (a) A healthcare professional assists the patient to ensure the breast is placed ideally for the X-ray.
(b) A mammogram. A tumor is visible in this mammogram as the darkened oval structure near the center.

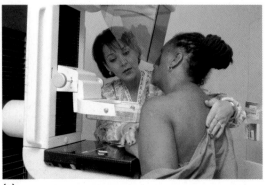

(a)

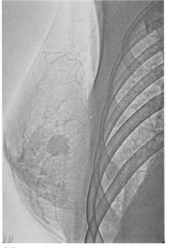

(b)

WORDS TO WATCH OUT FOR !

-graph, -graphy, or -gram?

Remember that the suffix *-y* means "process of." Thus, because the suffix *-graph* means "instrument for recording," the suffix *-graphy* means "recording process" and a "process of a recording instrument." In a slightly different twist, the suffix *-gram* means "a record or image." In each of these suffixes, switching the ending creates the term used for recording information.

mammoplasty
MAM moh PLASS tee

12.97 The surgical repair of one or both breasts is called a _____. It involves either the enlargement or reduction of breast size or, in some cases, removal of a tumor. Mammoplasty is also an important reconstructive procedure for women who have had a mastectomy (Frame 12.98).

mastectomy
mass TEK toh mee

12.98 In addition to the combining form *mamm/o*, the combining form *mast/o* also means "breast." Thus, a procedure involving the removal of breast tissue is a _____. In a **simple mastectomy**, one entire breast is removed while leaving underlying muscles and lymph nodes intact. In a **radical mastectomy** (or Halsted mastectomy), the entire affected breast is removed along with muscles and lymph nodes of the chest. In a **modified radical mastectomy,** the affected breast and lymph nodes are removed but the muscles are left intact. Finally, a **lumpectomy** is the removal of the cancerous lesions only, which conserves the breast.

oophorectomy
oh OFF oh REK toh mee

12.99 Surgical removal of an ovary is performed in an _____. This constructed term is written oophor/ectomy.

Pap smear

12.100 A common diagnostic procedure that screens for precancerous cervical dysplasia and cervical cancer is known as the **Papanicolaou smear** (pap an IK oh law * smeer), commonly called a _____ _____. It involves the gentle scraping of cells from the cervix and vagina followed by their microscopic examination.

DID YOU KNOW ?

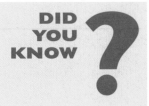

Papanicolaou Smear

Named after Dr. George Papanicolaou, an anatomist and cytologist, the Pap smear is a screening test for ovarian cancer that has made early detection possible. The American Cancer Society recommends annual tests at ages 20 and 21, followed by tests at two-year or three-year intervals throughout later years.

salpingectomy
SAL pin JEK toh mee

salping/o-oophor/ectomy

12.101 The surgical removal of a fallopian tube is performed in the procedure called a _____. This constructed term is written salping/ectomy. If an ovary is also removed, the procedure is called a **salpingo-oophorectomy** (sal ping goh oh OFF oh REK toh mee). Also a constructed term, it includes four word parts and is written _____/__-_____/_____.

WORDS TO WATCH OUT FOR

The Os in Salpingo-oophorectomy

When two combining forms are joined together to form a term, the first combining form keeps its combining vowel, even if the second begins with a vowel. Thus, in the term *salpingo-oophorectomy*, the combining form *salping/o* retains its combining vowel. In this long term, the hyphen is included to distinguish between the two adjacent combining forms and to make pronunciation easier. This makes for a lot of o's, so be careful when you spell this term.

salpingopexy
sal PING oh PEK see

salping/o/stomy

12.102 Surgical fixation of a fallopian tube may become necessary if the ligaments that support the tube within the pelvic cavity weaken. The procedure is called _____. This constructed term is written salping/o/pexy. Often, a salpingopexy is accompanied by a procedure to open a blocked fallopian tube or to drain fluid from an inflamed tube. This procedure is called a **salpingostomy** (SAL ping GOSS toh mee), which can be written as _____/__/_____.

sonohysterography
son oh HIST er OG rah fee

12.103 A noninvasive diagnostic procedure that uses ultrasound waves to visualize the uterus within the pelvic cavity is called **sonohysterography**. The constructed term _____ contains five word parts, represented as son/o/hyster/o/graphy. In the diagnostic procedure known as **transvaginal sonography** (trans VAJ ih nal * son OG rah fee), an ultrasound probe is inserted through the vagina to record images of the uterine cavity and fallopian tubes. The constructed form of these terms is trans/vagin/al son/o/graphy. In addition to its use for observing tumors or cysts, it is used to monitor pregnancy.

tubal ligation
TOO bal * lye GAY shun

12.104 The most common form of female sterilization as a contraceptive measure is called **tubal ligation**, during which the fallopian tubes are severed and closed to prevent the migration of sperm upward into the tubes (Figure 12.19■). The term _____ _____ includes the word that means "to tie up," *ligate*.

Figure 12.19 ■
Tubal ligation. To minimize the size of the incisions necessary, laparoscopic surgery may be used to enter the abdominal cavity through a small incision, cut the fallopian tubes, and ligate (tie off).

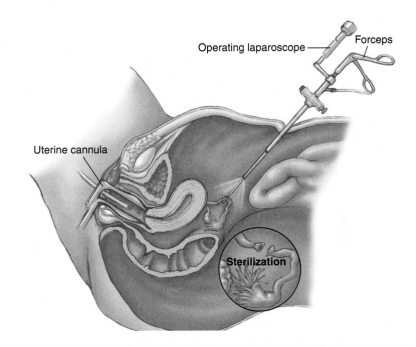

Operating laparoscope — Forceps

Uterine cannula

Sterilization

vaginal speculum
VAJ ih nal * SPEK yoo lum

12.105 A **vaginal speculum** is an instrument used during a gynecological exam. A _____ _____ is used to open the vaginal orifice wide enough to permit visual examination of the vagina and cervix.

vulvectomy
vuhl VEK toh mee

12.106 The surgical removal of the vulva is called a _____. The constructed form of this term is written vulv/ectomy.

PRACTICE: Treatments, Procedures, and Devices of the Female Reproductive System

The Right Match

Match the term on the left with the correct definition on the right.

_____ 1. biopsy

_____ 2. dilation and curettage

_____ 3. cervical conization

_____ 4. Papanicolaou smear

_____ 5. hormone replacement therapy

_____ 6. transvaginal sonography

_____ 7. endometrial ablation

_____ 8. tubal ligation

_____ 9. vaginal speculum

a. removal of the cervix

b. severs and closes the fallopian tubes to prevent migration of sperm

c. common therapy for hormone imbalances

d. destroys the endometrium with a laser

e. a procedure in which the cervix is dilated, and a curette is inserted to scrape the endometrium

f. instrument that opens the vaginal orifice to permit visual examination

g. records images of the uterine cavity and fallopian tubes

h. microscopic examination of cells scraped from the cervix and vagina

i. surgical extraction of tissue for microscopic analysis

Linkup

Link the word parts in the list to create the terms that match the definitions. You may use word parts more than once. Remember to add combining vowels when needed—and that some terms do not use any combining vowel.

Prefix	Combining Form	Suffix
(none)	colp/o	-ectomy
	gynec/o	-gram
	hyster/o	-logy
	mamm/o	-pexy
	oophor/o	-plasty
	salping/o	-rrhaphy
	vulv/o	

Definition

1. surgical removal of the vulva

2. surgical repair of the vagina

3. branch of medicine that focuses on women

4. surgical removal of the uterus

5. suturing the wall of the vagina

6. surgical fixation of the uterus

7. X-ray image of a breast

8. surgical removal of an ovary

9. surgical removal of a fallopian tube

Term

_____

_____

_____

_____

_____

_____

_____

_____

_____

Signs and Symptoms of Obstetrics

Following are the word parts that specifically apply to the signs and symptoms of obstetrics that are covered in the following section. Note that the word parts are color-coded to help you identify them: prefixes are blue, combining forms are red, and suffixes are purple.

Prefix	Definition	Combining Form	Definition	Suffix	Definition
dys-	bad, abnormal, painful, or difficult	amni/o	amnion	-emesis	vomiting
hyper-	excessive, abnormally high, or above	gravid/o, cyes/o	pregnancy	-cyesis	pregnancy
		lact/o	milk	-ia	condition of
		hydr/o	water	-rrhea	excessive discharge
poly-	excessive, over, or many	pseud/o	false	-s	plural
		toc/o	birth		

KEY TERMS A-Z

amniorrhea
AM nee oh REE ah

12.107 Recall that the suffix -rrhea means "excessive discharge." The abnormal discharge of amniotic fluid is a sign of a ruptured amniotic sac. The sign is called _____. This constructed term is written amni/o/rrhea.

dystocia
diss TOH see ah

12.108 The combining form for birth or labor is toc/o. When the prefix dys- and the suffix -ia are added, the new term is _____ and means "condition of difficult labor." The constructed form is written dys/toc/ia.

hyperemesis gravidarum
HIGH per EM eh siss *
grav ih DAR um

12.109 The symptom of severe nausea and emesis (vomiting) during pregnancy is called **hyperemesis gravidarum**. The term literally means "excessive vomiting when pregnant." _____ _____ can cause severe dehydration in the mother and fetus if left untreated.

lactorrhea
LAK toh REE ah

12.110 A normal, spontaneous discharge of milk is known as _____. This constructed term contains three word parts, shown as lact/o/rrhea.

polyhydramnios
PALL ee high DRAM nee ohs

12.111 An excessive production of amniotic fluid during fetal development is called **polyhydramnios**. If left untreated, _____ can cause unwanted pressure on the fetus that can disturb development. The term is a constructed term, written as poly/hydr/amni/o/s.

pseudocyesis
SOO doh sigh EE siss

12.112 A sensation of being pregnant when a true pregnancy does not exist is called **pseudocyesis**, which literally means "false pregnancy." The constructed form of _____ is written pseud/o/cyesis.

PRACTICE: Signs and Symptoms of Obstetrics

Break the Chain

Analyze these medical terms:

 a) Separate each term into its word parts; each word part is labeled for you (**p** = prefix, **r** = root, **cf** = combining form, and **s** = suffix).

 b) For the Bonus Question, write the requested definition in the blank that follows.

1. a) dystocia _____/_____/____
   p   r   s

   b) *Bonus Question:* What is the definition of the suffix? _____

2. a) hyperemesis _____/_____
   p   s

   b) *Bonus Question:* What is the definition of the prefix? _____

3. a) pseudocyesis _____/_____/___
   cf   s

   b) *Bonus Question:* What is the definition of the combining form? _____

4. a) polyhydramnios _____/_____/_____/__/__
   p   r   cf   s

   b) *Bonus Question:* What is the definition of the combining form? _____

Diseases and Disorders of Obstetrics

Following are the word parts that specifically apply to the diseases and disorders of obstetrics that are covered in the following section. Note that the word parts are color-coded to help you identify them: prefixes are blue, combining forms are red, and suffixes are purple.

Combining Form	Definition
amni/o, amnion/o	amnion
blast/o	germ, bud
chori/o	chorion
erythr/o	red
fet/o	fetus
plasm/o	form
tox/o	poison

Suffix	Definition
-al	pertaining to
-itis	inflammation
-osis	condition of
-rrhexis	rupture
-sis	state of

abruptio placentae
ah BRUP shee oh * plah SEN tee

12.113 The premature separation of the placenta from the uterine wall is called **abruptio placentae**. This Latin word means "abrupt (loss) of placenta." _____ _____ results in either a miscarriage, stillbirth, or premature birth and is illustrated in Figure 12.20■.

Figure 12.20 ■
Abruptio placentae. The placenta becomes prematurely detached from the uterine wall.

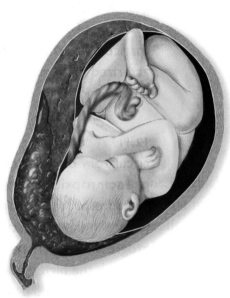

amnionitis
AM nee oh NYE tiss

12.114 Inflammation of the amnion is a condition known as _____. It is a constructed term written amnion/itis. If the chorion is also inflamed, the condition is called **chorioamnionitis** (KOR ee oh AM nee o NYE tiss), which is written as chori/o/amnion/itis. In some cases, either condition leads to a rupture of the amnion, called **amniorrhexis**. This term is also constructed of word parts and is written

amni/o/rrhexis

_____/__/_____.

breech presentation

12.115 An abnormal childbirth in which the buttocks, feet, or knees appear through the birth canal first is commonly called a **breech presentation**. A _____ _____ is relatively common and places the child at risk due to an increased risk of complications during birth.

fetal alcohol syndrome

12.120 A neonatal condition caused by excessive alcohol consumption by the mother during pregnancy is known as **fetal alcohol syndrome**, or **FAS**. The _____ _____

_____ often causes brain dysfunction and growth abnormalities that usually afflict the child throughout life.

hyaline membrane disease

12.121 A lung disorder of neonates, particularly premature infants, in which certain cells of the lungs fail to mature at birth causing lung collapse, is commonly referred to as **hyaline membrane disease** or **HMD**.

_____ _____ _____

contributes to **respiratory distress syndrome of the newborn**, or **RDS**, which is often managed by placing monitors around the baby with alarms that warn when breathing has stopped.

placenta previa

plah SEN tah * PREH vee ah

12.122 A condition in which the placenta is abnormally attached to the uterine wall in the lower portion of the uterus is called **placenta previa**. An example of _____ _____ is illustrated in Figure 12.23■.

Figure 12.23 ■
Placenta previa. The condition is caused by the development of the placenta over the cervical canal, creating an occlusion.

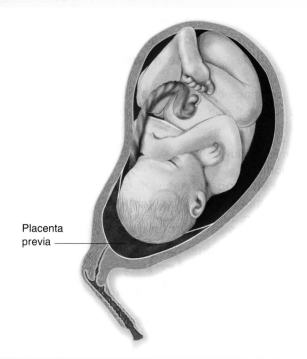

Placenta previa

toxoplasmosis

TAHK soh plaz MOH siss

12.123 Caused by the protozoan *Toxoplasma gondii*, the disease _____ may be contracted by exposure to animal feces, most commonly from household cats. This constructed term is written tox/o/plasm/osis, and means "condition of toxic form." It is a danger to pregnant women because the protozoa are capable of crossing the placental barrier to infect the fetus and cause birth defects.

PRACTICE: Diseases and Disorders of Obstetrics

The Right Match

Match the term on the left with the correct definition on the right.

_____ 1. congenital anomaly

_____ 2. breech presentation

_____ 3. eclampsia

_____ 4. abruptio placentae

_____ 5. ectopic pregnancy

_____ 6. fetal alcohol syndrome

_____ 7. hyaline membrane disease

_____ 8. placenta previa

a. severely high blood pressure in the pregnant woman

b. brain dysfunction and growth abnormalities caused by excessive alcohol consumption by the mother during pregnancy

c. abnormality present at birth

d. placenta is abnormally located

e. lung disorder of neonates

f. abnormal birth position in which the buttocks, feet, or knees appear through the birth canal first

g. pregnancy that occurs outside the uterus

h. premature separation of the placenta from the uterine wall

Treatments, Procedures, and Devices of Obstetrics

Following are the word parts that specifically apply to the treatments, procedures, and devices of obstetrics that are covered in the following section. Note that the word parts are color-coded to help you identify them: prefixes are blue, combining forms are red, and suffixes are purple.

Combining Form	Definition
abort/o	miscarry
amni/o	amnion
episi/o	vulva
fet/o	fetus
obstetr/o	midwife

Suffix	Definition
-centesis	surgical puncture
-ic	pertaining to
-ician	one who practices
-metry	measurement or process of measuring
-tomy	incision or to cut

KEY TERMS A-Z

abortion
ah BOR shun

12.124 A term derived from the Latin word, *aborto*, which means "miscarry," is abortion. It is the termination of pregnancy by expulsion of the embryo or fetus from the uterus. A natural expulsion is called a **miscarriage** or **spontaneous abortion (SAB)**. An _____ induced by surgery or drugs is called a **therapeutic abortion (TAB)**. A drug that induces TAB is called an **abortifacient** (ah BOR tih FAY shent).

amniocentesis
AM nee oh sehn TEE siss

12.125 A procedure that involves penetration of the amnion with a syringe and aspiration of a small amount of amniotic fluid for analysis is known as **amniocentesis**. This constructed term is written amni/o/centesis. _____ literally means "surgical puncture of amnion." It is shown in Figure 12.24■.

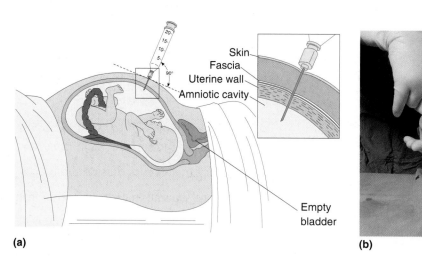

Skin
Fascia
Uterine wall
Amniotic cavity

Empty
bladder

(a)   (b)

Figure 12.24 ■
Amniocentesis. (a) In this examination procedure, amniotic fluid is aspirated with a syringe that is inserted through the abdominal wall, uterine wall, and amnion.
(b) Photograph of the procedure. Amniotic fluid is a slightly yellowish color, which can be seen within the syringe.

cesarean section
seh ZAIR ee an * SEK shun

12.126 An alternative to the nonsurgical birth of a child through the birth canal, birthing can be accomplished surgically by making an incision through the abdomen and uterus. This procedure is called _____ _____; it is abbreviated **C-section**.

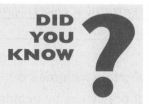

Cesarean section

The term *cesarean section* was first used to describe this surgical alternative to vaginal birth during Roman times, because it was thought that Julius Caesar was born in this way. However, his family name, Caesar, had its origin from such a birth, which literally means *to cut*, centuries before the birth of Julius.

contraception
kon trah SEP shun

12.127 The term **contraception** literally means "against conception," or prevention of birth. It is the use of devices and drugs to prevent fertilization, implantation of a fertilized egg, or both. The most effective _____ is the birth control pill, taken orally by females to block ovulation. Other methods include condoms, diaphragms, and intrauterine devices (IUDs).

episiotomy

eh peez ee OTT oh mee

12.128 To prevent tearing of the vulva and perineum during childbirth, an incision may be made through these tissues to widen the vaginal opening. The procedure is called **episiotomy.** _____ is a constructed term, written episi/o/tomy.

fetometry

fee TOM eh tree

12.129 A procedure that measures the size of a fetus is called _____. This constructed term is written fet/o/metry and means "fetal measurement." It is performed using ultrasound technology on the pregnant mother in the technique known as **obstetrical sonography** (ob STET rih kal * son OG rah fee), which is shown in Figure 12.25■.

Figure 12.25 ■
Obstetrical sonography and fetometry. (a) The procedure is performed in a clinical setting. The instrumentation includes a monitor, control panel, and ultrasound probe.
(b) Close-up view of an ultrasound probe.
(c) An ultrasound image reveals the fetus within the uterus.

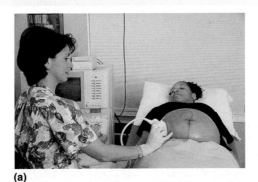
(a)

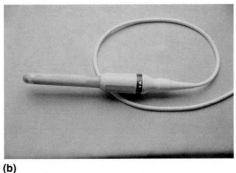
(b)

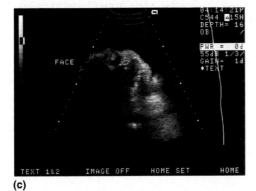
(c)

obstetrics

ob STET riks

obstetrician

12.130 The combining form obstetr/o is derived from the Latin word obstetrix, which means "midwife." The medical field of _____ is a discipline concerned with prenatal development, pregnancy, childbirth, and the postpartum period. It is abbreviated **OB**. A physician practicing in this field is called an _____ (OB steh TRISH an).

PRACTICE: Treatments, Procedures, and Devices of Obstetrics

The Right Match

Match the term on the left with the correct definition on the right.

_____ 1. cesarean section

_____ 2. miscarriage

_____ 3. abortifacient

_____ 4. therapeutic abortion

_____ 5. contraception

_____ 6. obstetrics

a. termination of pregnancy by a natural expulsion of the embryo or fetus; also called *spontaneous abortion*

b. the use of devices and drugs to prevent fertilization, implantation of a fertilized egg, or both

c. an abortion induced by surgery or drugs

d. an assisted birth procedure using a surgical incision through the abdomen and uterus

e. medical field concerned with fetal development, pregnancy, childbirth, and the postpartum period

f. a drug that induces therapeutic abortion

Linkup

Link the word parts in the list to create the terms that match the definitions. You may use word parts more than once. Remember to add combining vowels when needed—and that some terms do not use any combining vowel.

Combining Form	Suffix
amni/o	-centesis
episi/o	-metry
fet/o	-tomy

Definition   Term

1. aspiration of amniotic fluid for analysis   _____

2. an incision made through the vulva and perineum during childbirth   _____

3. procedure that measures the size of a fetus   _____

Sexually Transmitted Infections (STIs)

acquired immunodeficiency syndrome
ah KWIE erd *
ih MYOO noh deh FISH en see *
SIN drom

12.131 The disease that results from infection with the human immunodeficiency virus, or **HIV**, is called **acquired immunodeficiency syndrome**, abbreviated **AIDS**. It is acquired mainly through the exchange of body fluids during sex, such as semen, blood, and vaginal secretions. It can also be acquired by the use of contaminated instruments, such as intravenous needles. The onset of _____ _____ _____ is characterized by the development of opportunistic infections, which arise as the white blood cell count (mainly helper T cells) declines.

candidiasis
KAN dih DYE ah siss

12.132 Infection by the yeastlike fungus, *Candida albicans*, is often sexually transmitted to cause the infection known as _____. It is characterized by skin and mucuous membrane irritation and can lead to fatal systemic disease such as endocarditis and septicemia. Candidiasis may also be caused by an interference with normal flora, such as antibiotic therapy, and occurs most frequently in women.

chlamydia
klah MID ee ah

12.133 The most common bacterial STI in North America is **chlamydia**. Its symptoms include urethral or vaginal discharge and pelvic pain among women, urethritis and proctitis in men, and inflammation of the eye's conjunctiva in newborns that can lead to blindness. The term _____ is derived from the Greek word, *chlamydos*, which means "cloak."

genital herpes
JENN ih tal * HER peez

12.134 **Genital herpes** is the most common viral STI in North America. _____ _____ is caused by the herpes simplex virus Type 2, or **HSV-2**. It is characterized by periodic outbreaks of ulcerlike sores on the genital and anorectal skin and mucous membranes.

gonorrhea
gahn oh REE ah

12.135 An STI that is caused by the bacterium *Neisseria gonorrhoeae* is called _____. It produces ulcerlike lesions on the mucous membranes and skin of the genital region and is characterized by urethral discharge. The term means "a flow of seed."

hepatitis B

12.136 Hepatitis is an inflammatory disease of the liver that has many different forms that are categorized as type A through E. In _____, commonly called **hep B**, the cause is a virus that is primarily transmitted via blood exchange, often through blood transfusions or sharing IV needles. It may also be acquired through sexual exchange of body fluids. Hep B causes liver damage that can lead to liver failure and death. (Recall from Chapter 10 that hepatitis is a constructed term, hepat/itis: *hepat/o* means "liver," and *-itis* means "inflammation.")

human papillomavirus

12.137 The **human papillomavirus**, or **HPV**, is a virus that is extremely common in the human population and is transmitted during intercourse. In some people, _____ _____ forms the symptom of papillomas or genital warts, which are transient vesicles on the penis or within the vagina. There is evidence that HPV creates an increased risk of cervical cancer (Frame 12.62). A recently developed vaccine is believed to provide protection from HPV infection.

syphilis
SIFF ih liss

12.138 An STI that is caused by a bacterium called a spirochete (*Treponema pallidum*) is known as **syphilis**. It is transmitted by sexual contact and usually first appears as red, painless pustules on the skin that erode to form small ulcers known as **chancres** (SHANG kerz) (Frame 12.10). If left untreated, _____ can result in mental confusion, organ destruction, and death.

trichomoniasis
TRIK oh moh NYE ah siss

12.139 An STI caused by the protozoan *Trichomonas*, which is an amoeba-like single-celled organism, is called _____. It is spread by sexual contact and infects both women and men. In women, the sexually transmitted form is called *Trichomonas vaginalis* and causes vaginal swelling and pain. In men, the urethra and prostate gland become infected, causing inflammation and pelvic pain.

PRACTICE: Sexually Transmitted Infections (STIs)

The Right Match

Match the term on the left with the correct definition on the right.

_____ 1. chlamydia

_____ 2. genital herpes

_____ 3. acquired immunodeficiency syndrome

_____ 4. hepatitis B

_____ 5. human papillomavirus

_____ 6. syphilis

_____ 7. gonorrhea

_____ 8. trichomoniasis

_____ 9. candidiasis

a. extremely common STI that causes genital warts in some people and may also increase risk of cervical cancer

b. caused by a bacterium called a spirochete

c. the most common bacterial STI in North America; symptoms include urethritis and inflammation of the conjunctiva

d. characterized by skin and mucous membrane irritation; can lead to endocarditis and septicemia

e. a bacterial infection that produces ulcerlike lesions on the mucous membranes and skin of the genital region and urethral discharge

f. results from infection with the human immunodeficiency virus (HIV)

g. infection caused by a protozoan that causes inflammation of the urethra and prostate, and pelvic pain

h. a form of an inflammatory disease of the liver caused by a virus that is sexually transmitted

i. characterized by periodic outbreaks of ulcerlike sores on the genital and anorectal skin and mucous membranes

Abbreviations of the Reproductive System and Obstetrics

The abbreviations associated with the reproductive system and obstetrics are summarized here. Study these abbreviations, and review them in the exercise that follows.

Abbreviation	Definition
AIDS	acquired immuno-deficiency syndrome
BPH	benign prostatic hyperplasia
Bx	biopsy
CIN	cervical intraepithelial neoplasia
CIS	carcinoma in situ
C-section	cesarean section
D&C	dilation and curettage
DRE	digital rectal exam
ED	erectile dysfunction
FAS	fetal alcohol syndrome
FBD	fibrocystic breast disease
GYN	gynecology
HBV	hepatitis B virus
HIV	human immunodeficiency virus
HMD	hyaline membrane disease
HPV	human papillomavirus
HRT	hormone replacement therapy

Abbreviation	Definition
HSV-2	herpes simplex virus type 2
IDC	infiltrating ductal carcinoma
OB	obstetrics
OB/GYN	obstetrics/gynecology
Pap smear (test)	Papanicolaou smear (or test)
PID	pelvic inflammatory disease
PIH	pregnancy-induced hypertension
PMS	premenstrual syndrome
PSA	prostate-specific antigen
RDS	respiratory distress syndrome
SAB	spontaneous abortion
STI	sexually transmitted infection
TAB	therapeutic abortion
TSS	toxic shock syndrome
TURP	transurethral resection of the prostate
TVS	transvaginal sonography

PRACTICE: Abbreviations

Fill in the blanks with the abbreviation or the complete medical term.

Abbreviation	Medical Term
1. PSA	_____
2. _____	sexually transmitted infection
3. HIV	_____
4. _____	transurethral resection of the prostate
5. BPH	_____
6. _____	acquired immunodeficiency syndrome
7. HMD	_____
8. _____	hepatitis B virus
9. HSV-2	_____
10. _____	digital rectal exam
11. HPV	_____
12. _____	cervical intraepithelial neoplasia
13. D&C	_____
14. _____	carcinoma in situ
15. HRT	_____
16. _____	respiratory distress syndrome
17. PMS	_____
18. _____	therapeutic abortion
19. TSS	_____
20. _____	pelvic inflammatory disease
21. TVS	_____
22. _____	gynecology
23. Bx	_____
24. _____	Papanicolaou smear
25. ED	_____
26. _____	fibrocystic breast disease
27. OB	_____
28. _____	cesarean section
29. OB/GYN	_____
30. _____	spontaneous abortion
31. PIH	_____
32. _____	fetal alcohol syndrome
33. IDC	_____

▶▶▶▶ Chapter Review

Word Building _____

Construct medical terms from the following meanings. (Some are built from word parts, some are not.) The first question has been completed as an example.

1. absence of one or both testes   *an*orchism

2. cancer originating from a testis   testicular carcin_____

3. abnormally persistent erection   _____ism

4. constriction of the prepuce   _____mosis

5. excision of the prepuce   circum_____

6. an STI that causes liver inflammation   _____itis

7. incision into a testis   _____tomy

8. condition of an undescended testis   _____orchidism

9. condition of abnormally few sperm   _____spermia

10. inflammation of a testis   orch_____

11. herniation of veins in the spermatic cord   _____cele

12. absence of menstrual discharge   _____menorrhea

13. white or yellow discharge from the uterus   _____rrhea

14. condition of pain in the breast   _____algia

15. profuse bleeding during menstruation   meno_____

16. abnormally reduced bleeding during menstruation   _____menorrhea

17. spread of endometrial tissue into the myometrium   endometri_____

18. inflammation of the cervix   _____itis

19. closure of the uterus   _____atresia

20. condition of a sagging breast   masto_____

21. inflammation of the vulva and vagina   _____vaginitis

22. displacement of the uterus downward   _____ uterus (2 words)

23. excision of a fallopian tube and ovary   salpingo-_____ (hyphenated term)

24. suture of the perineum to correct a tear   _____tomy

25. endoscopic examination of the uterus   hystero_____

26. breast X-ray procedure   mammo_____

27. a false pregnancy   pseudo_____

28. termination of pregnancy by expulsion of the fetus   _____ (do this one on your own)

29. separation of the placenta from the uterine wall   _____ placentae (2 words)

30. abnormal discharge of amniotic fluid   amnio_____

31. surgical repair of the glans penis   _____plasty

32. surgical removal of a testis   orchid_____

33. abnormal pain during menstruation   _____menorrhea

34. severe nausea and vomiting during pregnancy   hyper_____ gravidarum (2 words)

Clinical Application Exercises

Medical Report

Read the following medical report, then answer the questions that follow.

University Hospital

5500 University Avenue
Metropolis, TX

Phone: (211) 594-4000
Fax: (211) 594-4001

Medical Consultation: Internal Medicine

Date: 7/10/2008

Patient: Marsha Williams

Patient Complaint: Dysmenorrhea accompanied by menorrhagia with possible leukorrhea between menstrual periods.

History: 45-year-old female, nulligravida, with history of occasional dysmenorrhea since puberty. No record of STI or other reproductive pathology. D&C performed on 3/1/07 but failed to correct symptoms.

Family History: Father 79-year-old with hepatic cancer in remission; mother 82-year-old with total hysterectomy at age 44 as a treatment for dysmenorrhea and menorrhagia.

Allergies: None

Evidences: Pap smear positive for anaplasia; HPV confirmed with culture; colposcopy positive for CIS and confirmed with blood test.

Treatment: Perform cervical conization to confirm CIS; if confirmed, perform cervicectomy and follow with lab tests.

Jennifer Holland, M.D.

---

1. Which patient complaints are consistent with the evidence? _____

_____

2. Why was a Pap smear performed? _____

_____

3. Why would a cervicectomy be a suitable treatment for CIS? _____

_____

Key Term	Frame	Definition	Know It?
20. breast cancer	12.60	a malignant _____ arising from breast tissue	☐
21. breech presentation	12.115	abnormal childbirth _____ in which the buttocks, feet, or knees appear through the birth canal first	☐
22. candidiasis	12.132	infection by the yeastlike _____, Candida albicans, often sexually transmitted	☐
23. carcinoma in situ	12.61	a form of cervical cancer that arises from cells of the cervix, abbreviated _____ of the cervix	☐
24. cervical cancer	12.62	a malignant tumor of the cervix; the most common form of cervical cancer is a squamous cell carcinoma, arising from the epithelial cells lining the opening into the uterus, called cervical intraepithelial _____ or CIN	☐
25. cervical conization	12.86	procedure in which a(n) _____-_____ section of precancerous or cancerous tissue of the cervix is removed	☐
26. cervicectomy	12.86	surgical removal of the _____	☐
27. cervicitis	12.63	inflammation of the _____	☐
28. cesarean section	12.126	an alternative to the nonsurgical birth of a child through the birth canal, birthing can be accomplished surgically by making an incision through the abdomen and uterus, abbreviated _____	☐
29. chancres	12.10	small _____ on the skin of the penis, a symptom of syphilis	☐
30. chlamydia	12.133	most common _____ STI in North America	☐
31. circumcision	12.34	removal of the _____, or foreskin, of the penis	☐
32. colpectomy	12.87	surgical removal of the vagina, also called _____	☐
33. colpodynia	12.49	symptom of _____ pain	☐
34. colpoplasty	12.88	surgical _____ of the vagina	☐
35. colporrhaphy	12.88	procedure involving _____ the wall of the vagina	☐
36. congenital anomaly	12.116	a(n) _____ present at birth	☐
37. contraception	12.127	use of devices and drugs to prevent fertilization, _____ of a fertilized egg, or both	☐
38. cryptorchidism	12.21	condition of an undescended testis, also called _____	☐
39. cystocele	12.64	a(n) _____ of the urinary bladder against the wall of the vagina	☐
40. digital rectal examination	12.35	a physical exam that involves the insertion of a finger into the _____ to feel the size and shape of the prostate gland through the wall of the rectum	☐
41. dilation and curettage	12.89	common procedure that is used for both diagnostic and treatment purposes, abbreviated _____	☐
42. dysmenorrhea	12.50	abnormal _____ during menstruation	☐
43. dystocia	12.108	difficult _____	☐
44. eclampsia	12.117	dangerous condition, in which the high blood pressure of pregnancy-induced _____ (PIH), or preeclampsia, worsens to cause convulsions and possibly coma and death	☐

Key Term	Frame	Definition	Know It?
45. ectopic pregnancy	12.118	a pregnancy occurring outside the _____	☐
46. endometrial ablation	12.90	procedure in which _____, electricity, or heat is used to destroy the endometrium	☐
47. endometrial cancer	12.65	a malignant tumor arising from the endometrial tissue lining the _____	☐
48. endometriosis	12.66	condition of abnormal growth of endometrial tissue throughout areas of the _____ cavity, including the external walls of the uterus, fallopian tubes, urinary bladder, and even on the peritoneum	☐
49. endometritis	12.67	inflammation of the endometrium usually caused by _____ infection	☐
50. epididymitis	12.22	inflammation of the _____	☐
51. episiotomy	12.128	an incision may be made through the vulva and _____ to widen the vaginal orifice	☐
52. erectile dysfunction	12.23	inability to achieve an erection sufficient to perform sexual intercourse, abbreviated _____, also known as impotence	☐
53. erythroblastosis fetalis	12.119	condition of neonates in which red blood cells are destroyed due to an incompatibility between the mother's blood and baby's blood, also called _____ disease of the newborn	☐
54. fetal alcohol syndrome	12.120	neonatal condition caused by excessive alcohol consumption by _____ during pregnancy	☐
55. fetometry	12.129	procedure that measures the size of a fetus using ultrasound technology on the pregnant mother in the technique known as obstetrical _____	☐
56. fibrocystic breast disease	12.68	inherited condition where one or more benign fibrous _____ develop within the breast	☐
57. fistula	12.69	an abnormal passage from one organ or cavity to another: a(n) _____ fistula occurs between the vagina and rectum, and a vesicovaginal fistula occurs between the urinary bladder and the vagina	☐
58. genital herpes	12.134	most common viral STI in North America is caused by the herpes simplex virus Type 2, or _____	☐
59. gonorrhea	12.135	_____ that is caused by the bacterium *Neisseria gonorrhoeae*	☐
60. gynecology	12.91	branch of medicine focusing on women; a physician known as an obstetrician-gynecologist combines these two areas of expertise, abbreviated _____	☐
61. gynopathology	12.91	the study of diseases that afflict _____	☐
62. hematosalpinx	12.51	condition of retained menstrual blood in a(n) _____ tube	☐
63. hepatitis B	12.136	an inflammatory disease of the _____ that has many different forms, categorized as type A through E	☐

Key Term	Frame	Definition	Know It?
64. hormone replacement therapy	12.92	therapy for hormonal management, abbreviated _____, can be very effective in correcting disrupted menstrual and ovarian cycles	☐
65. human papilloma virus	12.137	a virus that is extremely common in the human population and is transmitted during intercourse, abbreviated _____	☐
66. hyaline membrane disease	12.121	lung disorder of neonates, particularly _____ infants, in which certain cells of the lungs fail to mature at birth causing lung collapse	☐
67. hydrocele	12.24	swelling of the _____ caused by fluid accumulation, usually due to injury	☐
68. hydrocelectomy	12.36	surgical removal of a(n) _____	☐
69. hydrosalpinx	12.52	_____ accumulation within a fallopian tube	☐
70. hyperemesis gravidarum	12.109	condition of severe nausea and _____ (vomiting) during pregnancy	☐
71. hysteratresia	12.70	_____ of the uterus resulting in an abnormal obstruction within the uterine canal that may interfere with childbirth	☐
72. hysterectomy	12.93	surgical removal of the _____ and sometimes surrounding structures	☐
73. hysteropexy	12.94	surgical procedure that may be used to correct a(n) _____ uterus by strengthening its connections to the abdominal wall to correct its position	☐
74. hysteroscopy	12.95	noninvasive diagnostic technique that uses a modified endoscope, called a(n) _____, to evaluate the uterine cavity	☐
75. lactorrhea	12.110	a normal, spontaneous discharge of _____	☐
76. laparoscopy	12.95	procedure to evaluate the external appearance of the uterus and other organs of the pelvic cavity by means of a small incision through the lower abdominal wall and a(n) _____	☐
77. leiomyomas	12.71	condition of benign tumors in the muscular wall of the uterus, also known as _____ _____	☐
78. leukorrhea	12.53	white or yellow discharge from the _____, literally "white discharge"	☐
79. mammography	12.96	X-ray procedure that produces an X-ray image of a breast, called a(n) _____	☐
80. mammoplasty	12.97	surgical repair of one or both breasts, including _____ or reduction of breast size, reconstruction, or tumor removal	☐
81. mastalgia	12.54	condition of pain in the _____	☐
82. mastectomy	12.98	surgical removal of breast tissue; types include simple mastectomy, _____ mastectomy, modified radical mastectomy, and lumpectomy	☐
83. mastitis	12.72	inflammation of the breast often caused by bacterial infection of the _____ ducts within breast tissue	☐

Key Term	Frame	Definition	Know It?
84. mastoptosis	12.73	condition of a breast that is abnormally _____ or drooping	☐
85. menorrhagia	12.55	profuse _____ during menstruation	☐
86. mittelschmerz	12.56	abdominal pain occurring during _____	☐
87. obstetrician	12.130	_____ who practices obstetrics	☐
88. obstetrics	12.130	medical field concerned with prenatal development, pregnancy, childbirth, and the postpartum period, abbreviated _____	☐
89. oligomenorrhea	12.57	abnormally _____ discharge during menstruation	☐
90. oligospermia	12.11	abnormally _____ sperm count, a sign of male infertility	☐
91. oophorectomy	12.99	surgical removal of a(n) _____	☐
92. oophoropathy	12.74	general term for any disease of a(n) _____	☐
93. orchidectomy	12.37	surgical removal of a testis; removal of both testes is commonly called _____	☐
94. orchidopexy	12.38	surgical fixation of a testis is sometimes required to draw an undescended testis into the scrotum, also called _____	☐
95. orchidoplasty	12.39	surgical repair of a testis is _____, also called _____	☐
96. ovarian cancer	12.75	the most common form of reproductive _____ in women	☐
97. ovarian cyst	12.76	a cyst on an ovary that is usually _____ and asymptomatic, although in some cases it may cause pelvic pain and dysmenorrhea	☐
98. Papanicolaou smear	12.100	common diagnostic procedure that screens for precancerous cervical dysplasia and cervical cancer, also known as _____	☐
99. papillomas	12.12	wartlike lesions on the skin and _____ membranes, commonly called genital warts	☐
100. pelvic inflammatory disease	12.77	inflammation involving some or all of the female organs within the pelvic cavity, abbreviated _____	☐
101. penile implant	12.40	surgical insertion of a(n) _____, or artificial device, to correct erectile dysfunction	☐
102. Peyronie's disease	12.25	hardness, or induration, of the _____ tissue within the penis	☐
103. phimosis	12.26	congenital narrowing of the _____ opening	☐
104. placenta previa	12.122	condition in which the placenta is abnormally attached to the uterine wall in the _____ portion of the uterus	☐
105. polyhydramnios	12.111	_____ production of amniotic fluid during fetal development	☐
106. premenstrual syndrome	12.78	a collection of _____, including nervous tension, irritability, breast pain (mastalgia), edema, and headache, usually occurring during the days preceding menstruation, abbreviated PMS	☐

Key Term	Frame	Definition	Know It?
107. priapism	12.27	abnormally _____ erection of the penis, often accompanied by pain and tenderness	☐
108. prolapsed uterus	12.79	condition in which the uterus may become _____ to shift downward into the vagina	☐
109. prostate cancer	12.28	aggressive form of cancer of the prostate gland, also called _____ carcinoma	☐
110. prostatectomy	12.41	surgical _____ of the prostate gland	☐
111. prostate-specific antigen	12.42	a clinical test that measures levels of the protein, prostate-specific antigen, in the blood, commonly called _____	☐
112. prostatitis	12.13	inflammation of the _____ gland	☐
113. prostatorrhea	12.14	_____, excessive discharge from the prostate gland	☐
114. pseudocyesis	12.112	sensation of being pregnant when a true _____ does not exist	☐
115. pyosalpinx	12.58	discharge of _____ from a fallopian tube that is a sign of infection	☐
116. salpingectomy	12.101	surgical removal of a(n) _____ tube	☐
117. salpingitis	12.80	_____ of a fallopian tube	☐
118. salpingocele	12.81	a(n) _____, or herniation, of a fallopian tube wall	☐
119. salpingopexy	12.102	surgical _____ of a fallopian tube	☐
120. sonohysterography	12.103	a noninvasive diagnostic procedure that uses _____ waves to visualize the uterus within the pelvic cavity	☐
121. syphilis	12.138	STI caused by a bacterium called a(n) _____ (*Treponema pallidum*)	☐
122. testalgia	12.15	a condition of testicular pain, also known as _____ and orchidalgia	☐
123. testicular carcinoma	12.29	a cancer originating from the testis, the most common form is called _____	☐
124. testicular torsion	12.30	condition in which the _____ cord becomes twisted, causing a reduced blood flow to the testis	☐
125. toxic shock syndrome	12.82	severe bacterial infection characterized by a sudden high fever, skin rash, mental confusion, acute renal failure, and abnormal liver function, abbreviated _____	☐
126. toxoplasmosis	12.123	disease caused by the protozoan *Toxoplasma gondii* that may be contracted by exposure to animal feces, most commonly from household _____	☐
127. transurethral resection of the prostate gland	12.43	procedure involving _____ of prostate tissue to treat BPH	☐
128. transvaginal sonography	12.103	diagnostic procedure in which an ultrasound _____ is inserted through the vagina to record images of the uterine cavity and fallopian tubes	☐

Key Term	Frame	Definition	Know It?
129. trichomoniasis	12.139	STI caused by the protozoan *Trichomonas*, which is an amoebalike _____-celled organism	☐
130. tubal ligation	12.104	common form of female _____ as a contraceptive measure in which fallopian tubes are severed and closed to prevent the migration of sperm upward into the tubes	☐
131. urethritis	12.16	inflammation of the _____	☐
132. urology	12.44	department within a hospital or clinic that treats _____ tract problems (in both sexes)	☐
133. vaginal speculum	12.105	an instrument used to open the vaginal orifice wide enough to permit _____ examination of the vagina and cervix	☐
134. vaginitis	12.83	inflammation of the vagina, also called _____	☐
135. varicocele	12.31	_____ of the veins within the spermatic cord caused by failure of the valves within the veins	☐
136. vasectomy	12.45	elective sterilization procedure in which the vas deferens is severed to block the flow of _____ during ejaculation	☐
137. vasovasostomy	12.46	surgery to reverse a(n) _____	☐
138. vesiculectomy	12.47	procedure to remove the _____ vesicles	☐
139. vulvectomy	12.106	surgical removal of the _____	☐
140. vulvitis	12.84	inflammation of the external genitals, or _____	☐

Multimedia Preview ▶▶▶▶▶

Additional interactive resources and activities for this chapter can be found on the Companion Website. For videos, audio glossary, and review, access the accompanying DVD-ROM in this book.

DVD-ROM Highlights

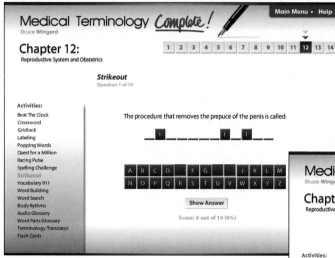

Strikeout

Click on the alphabet tiles to fill in the empty squares in the word or phrase and complete the sentence. This game quizzes your vocabulary and spelling. But choose your letters carefully because three strikes and you're out!

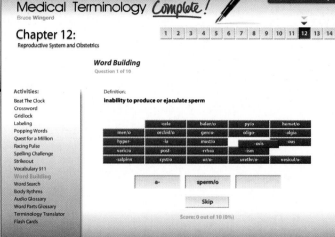

Word Building

Are you ready to master the technique of constructing terms using word parts? Put it all together by clicking and dragging the right prefixes, suffixes, roots, and combining forms together to match the definitions provided.

Website Highlights—www.prenhall.com/wingerd

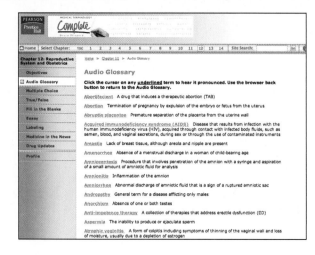

Audio Glossary

Click here and take advantage of the free-access online study guide that accompanies your textbook. You'll find an audio glossary with definitions and audio pronunciations for every term in the book. By clicking on this URL you'll also access a variety of quizzes with instant feedback, links to download mp3 audio reviews, and current news articles.

The Nervous System, Mental Health, and Special Senses ▶▶▶▶

Learning Objectives

After completing this chapter, you will be able to:

- Define and spell the word parts used to create terms for the nervous system.

- Identify the major organs of the nervous system.

- Break down and define common medical terms used for symptoms, diseases, disorders, procedures, treatments, and devices associated with the nervous system, mental health, and the special senses of vision and hearing.

- Build medical terms from the word parts associated with the nervous system, mental health, and the special senses of vision and hearing.

- Pronounce and spell common medical terms associated with the nervous system, mental health, and the special senses of vision and hearing.

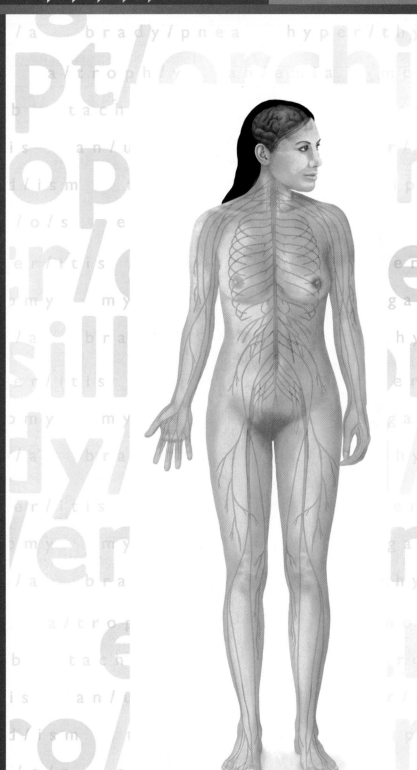

Anatomy and Physiology Terms ▶▶▶▶

The following table provides the combining forms that specifically apply to the anatomy and physiology of the nervous system, eyes, and ears. Note that the combining forms are colored red to help you identify them when you see them again later in the chapter.

Combining Form	Definition	Combining Form	Definition
blephar/o	eyelid	myel/o	spinal cord
cephal/o	head	neur/o	nerve
cerebell/o	little brain	ocul/o, opt/o, ophthalm/o	eye
cerebr/o, encephal/o	brain	ot/o	ear
conjunctiv/o	conjunctiva	phren/o, psych/o	mind
crani/o	skull, cranium	radic/o, radicul/o	nerve root
dacry/o	tear	retin/o	retina
gangli/o	swelling, knot	rhin/o	nose
ir/o	iris	scler/o	thick or hard; sclera
mast/o	breast	vag/o	vagus
mening/i, mening/o	membrane	ventricul/o	ventricle

nervous
NURR vuss

13.1 The _____ system is a complex part of the body that has been studied extensively, yet there is still much more to learn. It is composed of the brain, spinal cord, and nerves. Together, these important organs enable you to sense the world around you, integrate this information to form thoughts and memories, and control your body movements and many internal functions.

FUNCTION ▶▶▶▶

neuron

13.2 The nervous system maintains homeostasis by monitoring changes in the body and initiating responses to those changes. It is able to perform this important function by its ability to perceive changes, or stimuli, and convert this information into nerve impulses. A nerve impulse begins when a nerve cell, or **neuron**, opens its membrane channels to sodium and potassium ions, resulting in a flow of these ions across the cell membrane. The flow causes a sudden change in electrical current, which flows along the _____ and is transmitted to other adjacent neurons. The result is an impulse that can travel very quickly between the nerves in your skin and elsewhere and your spinal cord and brain.

13.3 Use the anatomy terms that appear in the left column to fill in the corresponding blanks in Figures 13.1■ through 13.4■.

1. brain
2. gray
3. ganglion
4. nerve

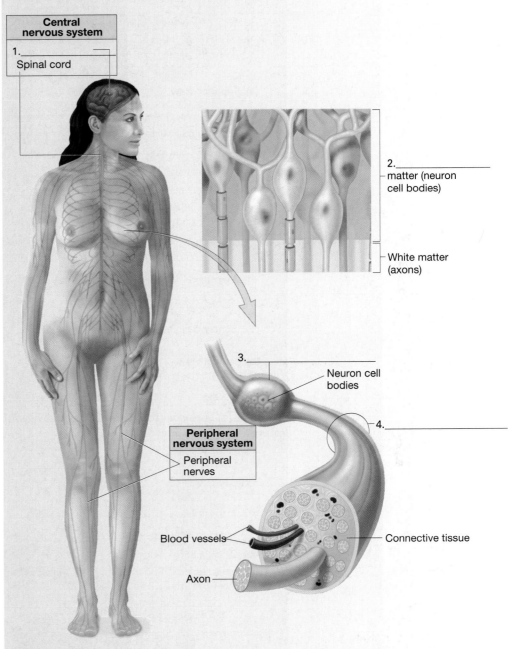

Central nervous system

1._____
Spinal cord

2._____
matter (neuron cell bodies)

White matter (axons)

3._____
Neuron cell bodies

4._____

Peripheral nervous system
Peripheral nerves

Blood vessels

Connective tissue

Axon

Figure 13.1 ■
Organization of the nervous system.

5. cerebral
6. left
7. cerebrum
8. cerebellum
9. stem

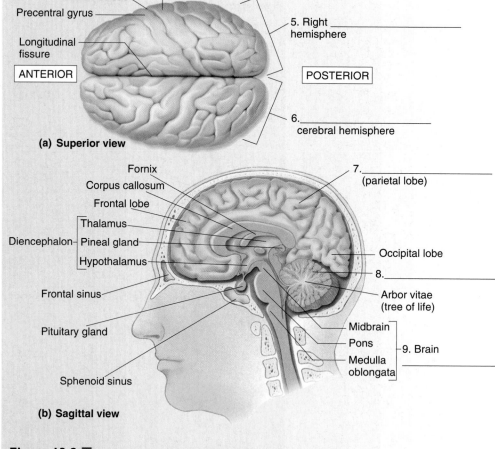

(a) Superior view

Central sulcus
Postcentral gyrus
Precentral gyrus
Longitudinal fissure
ANTERIOR
POSTERIOR
5. Right _____ hemisphere
6. _____ cerebral hemisphere

Fornix
Corpus callosum
Frontal lobe
Thalamus
Diencephalon— Pineal gland
Hypothalamus
Frontal sinus
Pituitary gland
Sphenoid sinus
7. _____ (parietal lobe)
Occipital lobe
8. _____
Arbor vitae (tree of life)
Midbrain
Pons
Medulla oblongata
9. Brain

(b) Sagittal view

Figure 13.2 ■
The brain. (a) Superior (top) view. (b) Sagittal view of a sectioned brain to reveal internal features.

10. cornea
11. lens
12. retina
13. sclera

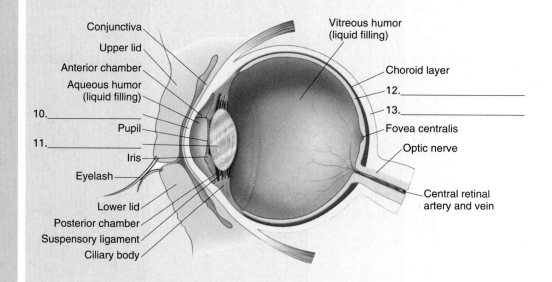

Conjunctiva
Upper lid
Anterior chamber
Aqueous humor (liquid filling)
10. _____
Pupil
11. _____
Iris
Eyelash
Lower lid
Posterior chamber
Suspensory ligament
Ciliary body

Vitreous humor (liquid filling)
Choroid layer
12. _____
13. _____
Fovea centralis
Optic nerve
Central retinal artery and vein

Figure 13.3 ■
The eye. Lateral view of a sectioned eyeball in its socket.

14. **incus**
15. **canals**
16. **cochlea**
17. **tympanic**

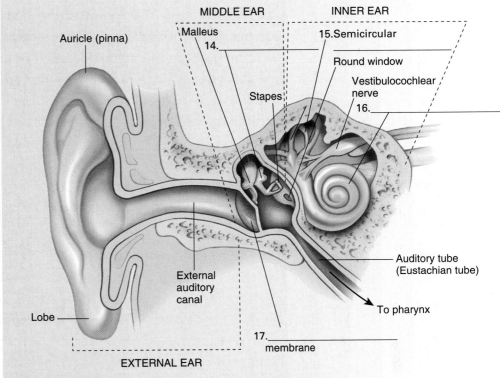

Figure 13.4 ■
The ear. Lateral view of the ear region on one side of the head.

Medical Terms for the Nervous System, Mental Health, and Special Senses ▶▶▶▶

nervous

13.4 The nervous system can experience many challenges to health. Nervous tissue is quite delicate and easily damaged. Therefore, it requires special protective features, such as bone, meninges, and cerebrospinal fluid (CSF). Protection from pathogens circulating in the bloodstream is further assisted by the blood–brain barrier, which keeps most bacteria, harmful cells, and many toxins from entering the _____ system. Usually, the unwanted substances that successfully penetrate the blood–brain barrier are eliminated by special neuroglial cells in the brain, called microglia.

brain	**13.5** Despite the measures protecting the brain and spinal cord, the nervous system may still experience infectious diseases, exposure to toxic substances, injury, and inherited conditions, any of which may lead to functional losses. For example, the most common affliction of the nervous system is stroke. Also known as cerebrovascular accident (CVA), it is a disruption of the normal flow of blood to the brain, resulting in the loss of _____ function that often proves fatal. According to the Centers for Disease Control (CDC), about 200,000 lives were lost in the United States from stroke in 2002, making it the third-most-common cause of death (behind heart disease and cancer).
study of **mind**	**13.6** The treatment of disorders affecting the nervous system is a relatively young branch of medicine known as **neurology** (noo RAHL oh jee). The combining form *neur/o* means "nerve," and the suffix *-logy* means "_____." Specialists within the broad field of neurology include **neurosurgeons** (NOO roh serj enz), whose medical practice focuses on brain or spinal cord surgery; **psychiatrists** (sye KYE ah trists), whose medical practice addresses mental illness; and **clinical psychologists** (sye KOL oh jists), who are mental health professionals trained in the treatment of behavioral disorders. The combining form *psych/o* means "_____."
	13.7 In the following sections, you will study the prefixes, combining forms, and suffixes that combine to build the medical terms of the nervous system. Complete the frames and review exercises that follow. You are on your way to mastery of the medical terms related to the nervous system, mental health, and eyes and ears!

Signs and Symptoms of the Nervous System

Following are the word parts that specifically apply to the signs and symptoms of the nervous system that are covered in the following section. Note that the word parts are color-coded to help you identify them: prefixes are blue, combining forms are red, and suffixes are purple.

Prefix	Definition
a-	without or absence of
hyper-	excessive, abnormally high, or above
hypo-	deficient, abnormally low, or below
par, para-	alongside or abnormal
poly-	excessive, over, or many

Combining Form	Definition
cephal/o	head
esthesi/o	sensation
neur/o	nerve
phasi/o	to speak

Suffix	Definition
-algesia	pain
-algia	condition of pain
-asthenia	weakness
-ia, -a	condition of

aphasia
ah FAY zee ah

a/phas/ia

13.8 The combining form *phasi/o* means "to speak," and the prefix *a-* means "without or absence of." Therefore, the inability to speak is known as _____. It is a clinical sign of a disease process causing the disability. The term is a constructed term composed of word parts. To highlight the word parts, aphasia can be written as ___/_____/_____. It literally means "without the condition of speaking."

cephalalgia
seff al AL jee ah

13.9 The clinical term for a **headache**, or a generalized pain in the region of the head, includes the combining form for head, *cephal/o*, and the suffix that means "condition of pain." The term is _____. It is a constructed term that can be written as cephal/algia, and literally means "condition of head pain." There are several forms of cephalalgia, including muscle contraction (tension) headaches resulting from sustained muscle contractions often caused by tension; cluster headaches, in which the pain is felt on one side of the head in several areas; and migraine headaches, caused by circulatory disturbances and often accompanied by nausea.

convulsion
kon VUHL shun

13.10 A **convulsion** is a series of involuntary muscular spasms caused by an uncoordinated excitation of motor neurons that triggers muscle contraction. A _____ is a sign of a neurological disorder and is also called **seizure** (SEE zhur).

hyperalgesia
HIGH per al JEE zee ah

13.11 The symptom **hyperalgesia** is an excessive sensitivity to painful stimuli. The symptom **hypoalgesia** is a deficient sensitivity to normally painful stimuli. The constructed form of _____ is written hyper/algesia, and hypoalgesia is written hypo/algesia.

hyperesthesia
HIGH per ess THEE zee ah

13.12 The combining form *esthesi/o* means "sensation." An excessive sensitivity to a stimulus, such as touch, sound, or pain, is experienced by a patient suffering from _____. This constructed term may be written as hyper/esthesi/a.

neuralgia
noo RAL jee ah

13.13 The suffix *-algia* means "condition of pain." A condition of pain in a nerve is a symptom known as _____ and can be written as neur/algia.

neurasthenia noo ras THEE nee ah	**13.14** The suffix *-asthenia* means "weakness." When the word root *neur* is included, the clinical term is spelled _____. The symptom of neurasthenia is a generalized experience of body fatigue, which is often associated with mental depression. Alternate terms sharing the same meaning include **chronic fatigue**, **fibromyalgia**, and **dysphoria**. The constructed form of *neurasthenia* is neur/asthenia.
paresthesia par ess THEE see ah	**13.15** The prefix *par-* means "alongside or abnormal." Combining it to the combining form for "sensation" forms the term _____. The symptom of paresthesia is an abnormal sensation of numbness and tingling caused by an injury to one or more nerves. It can be written as par/esthesi/a to identify its three word parts.
polyneuralgia pall ee noo RAL jee ah	**13.16** In Frame 13.13, you learned that **neuralgia** is a condition of pain in a nerve. A condition of pain in many nerves can be termed by adding the prefix that means "many," as in the clinical term _____. The term *polyneuralgia* is constructed of three word parts and can be written as poly/neur/algia.
syncope SIN ko pee	**13.17 Syncope** is a temporary loss of consciousness due to a sudden reduction of blood flow to the brain. _____ is often called "fainting." The term is a Greek word that means "a sudden loss of strength."

PRACTICE: Signs and Symptoms of the Nervous System

The Right Match

Match the term on the left with the correct definition on the right.

_____ 1. aphasia

_____ 2. cephalalgia

_____ 3. paresthesia

_____ 4. neuralgia

_____ 5. hyperesthesia

_____ 6. neurasthenia

_____ 7. convulsion

_____ 8. syncope

a. a series of involuntary muscle spasms

b. a vague condition of fatigue

c. excessive sensitivity to a stimulus

d. a headache

e. inability to speak

f. a sudden loss of consciousness

g. abnormal sensation of numbness

h. pain in a nerve

Linkup

Link the word parts in the list to create the terms that match the definitions. You may use word parts more than once. Remember to add combining vowels when needed—and that some terms do not use any combining vowel. The first one is completed as an example.

Prefix	Combining Form	Suffix
a-	algesi/o	-algia
hyper-	asthen/o	-algesia
par-	esthesi/o	-ia
poly-	neur/o	
	phasi/o	

	Definition	Term
1.	the inability to speak	*aphasia*
2.	an extreme sensitivity to painful stimuli	
3.	pain in many nerves	
4.	an excessive sensitivity to a stimulus	
5.	generalized body fatigue and weakness	
6.	pain in a nerve	
7.	abnormal sensation of numbness and tingling caused by nerve injury	

Diseases and Disorders of the Nervous System

Following are the word parts that specifically apply to the diseases and disorders of the nervous system that are covered in the following section. Note that the word parts are color-coded to help you identify them: prefixes are blue, combining forms are red, and suffixes are purple.

Prefix	Definition	Combining Form	Definition	Suffix	Definition
a-	without or absence of	ather/o	fatty substance or plaque	-al, -ar, -ic, -ion, -uss	pertaining to
epi-	upon, over, above, or on top	aut/o	self	-cele	hernia, swelling, or protrusion
		cephal/o	head		
para-	alongside or abnormal	cerebell/o	little brain, cerebellum	-ism, -osis	condition of
		cerebr/o, encephal/o	brain	-itis	inflammation
poly-	excessive, over, or many	embol/o	a plug	-lepsy	seizure
		gli/o	glue	-malacia	softening
		gnos/o	knowledge	-oma	tumor
		hydr/o	water	-pathy	disease
		later/o	side	-plegia	paralysis
		mening/i, mening/o	membrane	-rrhage	profuse bleeding or hemorrhage
		myel/o	spinal cord		
		narc/o	numbness	-troph	development
		neur/o	nerve		
		scler/o	thick, hard; sclera		
		poli/o	gray		
		thromb/o	clot		
		ventricul/o	ventricle		

cerebral palsy
seh REE bral * PAWL zee

13.27 A condition that appears at birth or shortly afterward as a partial muscle paralysis is called **cerebral palsy**. The paralysis of _____ _____ persists throughout life and is caused by a brain lesion present at birth or a brain defect that arose during development. Abbreviated **CP**, there is no treatment or cure.

cerebrovascular accident
seh REE broh VASS kyoo lar * AKS ih dent

13.28 The clinical term for a **stroke** is **cerebrovascular accident** and is abbreviated **CVA** (Figure 13.6■). A _____ _____ occurs when the blood supply to the brain is cut off, resulting in the irreversible death of brain cells followed by losses of mental function or death. A CVA may be caused by emboli (moving blood clots), a thrombus (a lodged, stationary blood clot), or a hemorrhage (perforation through a blood vessel wall).

Figure 13.6 ■
Causes of cerebrovascular accident (CVA), or stroke.

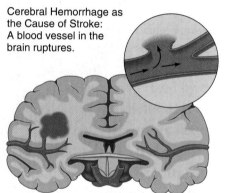

Cerebral Hemorrhage as the Cause of Stroke: A blood vessel in the brain ruptures.

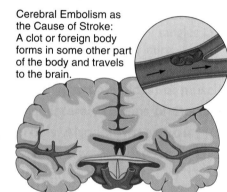

Cerebral Embolism as the Cause of Stroke: A clot or foreign body forms in some other part of the body and travels to the brain.

STROKE

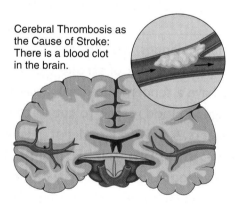

Cerebral Thrombosis as the Cause of Stroke: There is a blood clot in the brain.

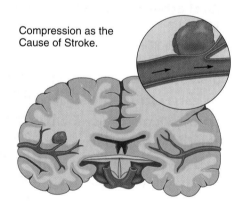

Compression as the Cause of Stroke.

coma
KOH mah

13.29 A **coma** is a general term describing several levels of abnormally decreased consciousness. The term _____ is derived from *koma*, the Greek word for "deep sleep."

concussion
kon CUSH uhn

13.30 The Latin word for "shaking" is *concussio*. This word has been used to create the medical term _____, which is an injury to soft tissue resulting from a blow or violent shaking. In a **cerebral concussion**, the cerebrum undergoes physical damage that often results in hemorrhage (bleeding) and the subsequent loss of brain cells and mental function.

encephalitis
en seff ah LYE tiss

13.31 A Greek word for brain is *encephalos*, providing us with the combining form, *encephal/o*, which is used in many medical terms associated with the brain. The term for an inflammation of the brain is _____. The condition of encephalitis is usually caused by bacterial or viral infection. The constructed term may be written as encephal/itis.

encephalomalacia
en seff ah loh mah LAY she ah
encephal/o/malacia

13.32 The suffix *-malacia* means "softening." When the combining form for brain is included, the resulting term _____ is created, which refers to a softening of brain tissue. Write the constructed form of this term: _____/___/_____. Encephalomalacia is usually caused by deficient blood flow to the brain.

epilepsy
EP ih lep see

13.33 A brain disorder characterized by recurrent seizures, including convulsions and temporary loss of consciousness, is the disease **epilepsy**. The term _____ literally means "to be seized upon."

DID YOU KNOW ?

Epilepsy

Epileptic seizures have been written about since 400 BC, when they were first described by Hippocrates in his book *Sacred Disease*. His Greek culture believed it was a punishment for offending the gods. The Greek word *epilepsia* literally means "seized upon by the gods." The misconception that epilepsy is divine punishment or a form of evil persisted until the late 19th century.

multiple sclerosis
MULL tih pull * skleh ROH siss

13.39 A disease characterized by the deterioration of the myelin sheath covering axons within the brain is known as _____ _____, abbreviated **MS** (Figure 13.9■). It is a progressive disease without a known cause, diagnosed by episodes of localized functional losses that eventually lead to paralysis and death. It is believed to be an autoimmune disease, due to evidence showing the destruction of the myelin is caused by the body's immune response. Notice the term *sclerosis* contains two word parts, scler/osis, and means "condition of thick or hard."

Figure 13.9 ■
Multiple sclerosis (MS). (a) A disease characterized by the gradual development of small areas of hardened (sclerotic) tissue in the cerebrum, it results in a gradual loss of brain function. The illustration shows a single sclerotic lesion within the right cerebral hemisphere.
(b) MRI of sclerotic lesions within the brain, which are characteristic of MS.
Source: Peter Arnold, Inc.

Multiple sclerosis lesion

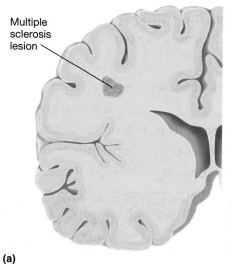
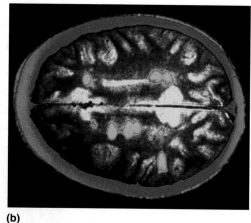

(a)

(b)

myelitis
mye eh LYE tiss

13.40 The combining form that means "spinal cord" is *myel/o*, which is derived from the Greek word meaning "marrow," *myelos*. Inflammation of the spinal cord is called _____, which can also be written as myel/itis. It is usually caused by a bacterial infection spreading from the meninges to the spinal cord and if not treated can result in muscle paralysis or sensory loss.

narcolepsy
NAR koh lep see

13.41 A sleep disorder characterized by sudden uncontrollable episodes of sleep, attacks of paralysis, and hypnagogic hallucinations (dreams intruding into the wakeful state) is called **narcolepsy.** _____ literally means "numb seizure."

neuritis
noo RYE tiss

polyneuritis
PALL ee noo RYE tiss

13.42 Inflammation of a nerve is called _____. It is usually caused by a bacterial or viral infection of the connective tissue coverings surrounding a nerve, although it may also result from physical injury to the nerve. In the condition _____, many nerves at once are inflamed. The term *polyneuritis* includes three word parts and can be written as poly/neur/itis. Polyneuritis may be an early sign of increased intracranial (*intra-* = "within"; crani/al = "pertaining to the cranium") pressure.

neuroma
noo ROH mah

13.43 A tumor originating from nerve cells is generally called a _____. This constructed term may be written as neur/oma.

neuropathy
noo ROH path ee

polyneuropathy
pall ee noo ROH path ee

13.44 A disease affecting any part of the nervous system, such as a cranial nerve or a peripheral nerve, is known as a _____. When many parts are affected by the condition, the prefix *poly-* is added to change the term to _____. The four word parts of the term *polyneuropathy* can be shown as poly/neur/o/pathy.

paraplegia
pair ah PLEE jee ah

13.45 The suffix *-plegia* means "paralysis," or the inability to contract muscles. In _____, muscles of the legs and lower body are paralyzed. Other forms of paralysis include the terms **monoplegia** (mon oh PLEE jee ah), in which one limb is paralyzed; **hemiplegia** (hem ee PLEE jee ah), paralysis on one side of the body; and **quadriplegia** (qwad rih PLEE jee ah), paralysis from the neck down including all four limbs. Note how the prefixes alter the meaning of the term: *para-* for "alongside," *mono-* for "single," *hemi-* for "half," and *quadri-* for "four."

Parkinson disease
PARK ihn son

13.46 A chronic degenerative disease of the brain characterized by tremors, rigidity, and shuffling gait is called **Parkinson disease**. The cause of _____ _____ is not yet known. It is also called **parkinsonism** and is abbreviated **PD**.

poliomyelitis
poh lee oh my eh LYE tiss

13.47 Caused by one of several viruses belonging to the family poliovirus, the disease **poliomyelitis** is characterized by inflammation of the gray matter of the spinal cord, often resulting in paralysis. _____ is commonly referred to as **polio**.

rabies
RAE beez

13.48 Rabies is an acute, often fatal, infection of the central nervous system that is caused by a virus transmitted to humans by the bite of an infected animal. _____ was formerly called **hydrophobia** (hye droh PHO bee ah), which means "fear of water," after it was observed that rabid animals avoid water. The avoidance of water is caused by the paralysis of the jaws that makes it impossible to swallow.

ventriculitis
vehn TRIK yoo LIE tiss

13.49 The condition of inflammation of the ventricles of the brain is known as _____. Its most common cause is a blockage of one of the channels that carry cerebrospinal fluid (CSF). The constructed form of this term is ventricul/itis. When it strikes an infant, it results in **hydrocephalus** (see Frame 13.35).

PRACTICE: Diseases and Disorders of the Nervous System

The Right Match

Match the term on the left with the correct definition on the right.

_____ 1. encephalitis

_____ 2. coma

_____ 3. Alzheimer disease

_____ 4. epilepsy

_____ 5. Parkinson disease

_____ 6. amyotrophic lateral sclerosis

_____ 7. Bell palsy

_____ 8. autism

_____ 9. concussion

_____ 10. stroke

_____ 11. cerebral palsy

a. recurrent seizures

b. partial muscle paralysis caused by a brain defect

c. a disease characterized by paralysis of face muscles on one side

d. an injury to the brain resulting from a blow or violent shaking

e. decreased consciousness

f. a developmental disorder that varies in severity

g. a disease characterized by brain deterioration

h. a disease characterized by tremors and rigidity

i. a cerebrovascular accident

j. a disease characterized by progressive atrophy of muscle

k. inflammation of the brain

Break the Chain

Analyze these medical terms:

   a) Separate each term into its word parts; each word part is labeled for you (**p** = prefix, **r** = root, **cf** = combining form, and **s** = suffix).

   b) For the Bonus Question, write the requested definition in the blank that follows.

The first set has been completed for you as an example.

1. a) agnosia   *a / gnos / ia*
                        p   r   s

    b) *Bonus Question:* What is the meaning of the suffix? *condition of* _____

2. a) cerebellitis   _____ / ____
                            r   s

    b) *Bonus Question:* What is the meaning of the word root? _____

3. a) encephalitis   _____ / ____
                            r   s

    b) *Bonus Question:* What is the meaning of the word root? _____

4. a) epilepsy   _____ / _____
                        p   s

    b) *Bonus Question:* What is the meaning of the suffix? _____

5. a) meningitis   _____ / _____
                          r   s

    b) *Bonus Question:* What is the meaning of the suffix? _____

6. a) paraplegia   _____ / _____
                          p   s

    b) *Bonus Question:* What is the meaning of the suffix? _____

7. a) neuroma   _____ / _____
                        r   s

    b) *Bonus Question:* What is the meaning of the suffix? _____

8. a) neuritis   _____ / _____
                        r   s

    b) *Bonus Question:* What is the definition of the word root? _____

psychiatry sigh KIGH ah tree	**13.72** The branch of medicine that addresses disorders of the brain resulting in mental and emotional disturbances is known as _____. The term may be written as psych/iatry, which means "treatment of the mind." A physician practicing in this field is a **psychiatrist**, who often uses **psychopharmacology**, or drug therapy targeting the brain, and **psychoanalysis**, or psychiatric therapy, to improve a patient's quality of life.
psychology sigh KALL oh jee **psychotherapy** SIGH koh THAIR ah pee	**13.73** In contrast to psychiatry, the field of _____ is not a medical specialty. It is the study of human behavior. The term *psychology* may be written as psych/o/logy, which means "study of the mind." However, a subdiscipline within this field, known as **clinical psychology**, uses applied psychology to treat patients suffering from behavioral disorders and emotional trauma. The technique used in treating behavioral and emotional issues is called _____.
radicotomy ray dih KOT oh mee	**13.74** Recall that the suffix *-tomy* means "surgical incision." A surgical incision into a nerve root is called _____. It is also called **rhizotomy**, since a nerve root includes two combining forms, *radic/o* and *rhiz/o*.
reflex testing	**13.75 Reflex testing** is a series of diagnostic tests performed to observe the body's response to touch stimuli. _____ _____ is useful in assessing stroke, head trauma, birth defects, and other neurological challenges. The tests include deep tendon reflexes (DTR) involving percussion at the patellar tendon and elsewhere and Babinski reflex involving stimulation of the plantar surface of the foot.
vagotomy vae GOT oh mee	**13.76** The vagus nerve is a large cranial nerve passing from the brain stem into the thoracic and abdominal cavities. During a _____, several branches of the vagus nerve are severed to reduce acid secretion into the stomach in an effort to prevent the reoccurrence of peptic ulcer. The constructed form of this term is vag/o/tomy.

PRACTICE: Treatments, Procedures, and Devices of the Nervous System

The Right Match

Match the term on the left with the correct definition on the right.

_____ 1. computed tomography

_____ 2. effectual drug therapy

_____ 3. reflex testing

_____ 4. sedative

_____ 5. analgesic

_____ 6. lumbar puncture

_____ 7. reflex testing

a. the withdrawal of CSF from the spinal cord

b. agent with a calming effect

c. treatment with medications to manage neurological disorders

d. deep tendon reflex and Babinski reflex

e. a procedure that constructs a 3-D view of the brain

f. series of tests that observe responses to touch stimuli

g. agent that relieves pain

Linkup

Link the word parts in the list to create the terms that match the definitions. You may use word parts more than once. Remember to add combining vowels when needed—and that some terms do not use any combining vowel.

Prefix	Combining Form	Suffix
an-	crani/o	-ectomy
	esthesi/o	-ia
	neur/o	-iatry
	psych/o	-logy
	vag/o	-rrhaphy
		-tomy

Definition

1. the primary type of pain management that is used during surgical procedures

2. surgical removal of part of the cranium

3. the study and medical practice of the nervous system

4. a procedure in which an incision is made through the cranium to provide surgical access to the brain

5. suture of a nerve

6. branch of medicine that addresses disorders of the brain that result in mental and emotional disturbances

7. surgical severing of several branches of the vagus nerve to reduce acid secretion in the stomach

8. the study of human behavior

Term

1. _____

2. _____

3. _____

4. _____

5. _____

6. _____

7. _____

8. _____

psychosis sy KO siss	**13.88** An individual suffering from a gross distortion or disorganization of their mental capacity, emotional response, and capacity to recognize reality and relate to others may be diagnosed with the disease known as **psychosis**. The most common form of _____ is **schizophrenia** (Frame 13.90). The term can be written as psych/osis and literally means "condition of the mind."
psychosomatic SY koh soh MAT ik	**13.89** The term **psychosomatic** literally means "pertaining to mind and body." Its word parts can be shown as psych/o/somat/ic. It refers to the influence of the mind over bodily functions, especially disease. Among some people, their mind creates symptoms that suggest an illness when physical signs are absent. In others, a _____ illness can be a real physical illness resulting from mental anxiety, such as peptic ulcer and hypertension.
schizophrenia SKIZ oh FREHN ee ah	**13.90** The most common form of psychosis is _____, which literally means "condition of split mind." It is characterized by delusions, hallucinations, and extensive withdrawal from other people and the outside world. There are many forms of schizophrenia, each type classified according to the experiences of the patient.

PRACTICE: Mental Health Diseases and Disorders

The Right Match

Match the vocabulary term on the left with the correct definition on the right.

_____ 1. anxiety disorder

_____ 2. bipolar disease

_____ 3. dementia

_____ 4. posttraumatic stress disorder

_____ 5. paranoia

_____ 6. attention deficit disorder

a. a neurological disorder characterized by short attention span and poor concentration

b. a disorder that results from severe mental strain or emotional trauma

c. alternating periods of high energy and mental confusion (mania) with low energy and mental depression

d. persistent delusions of persecution that results in mistrust and combativeness

e. impairment of mental function characterized by memory loss, disorientation, and confusion

f. a disorder in which the mental state of apprehension and fear dominates behavior

Break the Chain

Analyze these medical terms:

a) Separate each term into its word parts; each word part is labeled for you (**p** = prefix, **r** = root, **cf** = combining form, and **s** = suffix).

b) For the Bonus Question, write the requested definition in the blank that follows.

1. a) dyslexia   ___/___
                        p   s

   b) *Bonus Question:* What is the definition of the prefix? _____

2. a) neurosis   _____/___
                         r   s

   b) *Bonus Question:* What is the definition of the word root? _____

3. a) psychopathy   _____/__/____
                         cf   s

   b) *Bonus Question:* What is the definition of the suffix? _____

4. a) psychosis   _____/_____
                         r   s

   b) *Bonus Question:* What is the definition of the word root? _____

5. a) schizophrenia   _____/__/_____/_____
                         cf   r   s

   b) *Bonus Question:* What is the definition of the suffix? _____

Eye Diseases and Disorders

Following are the word parts that specifically apply to the diseases and disorders of the eye that are covered in the following section. Note that the word parts are color-coded to help you identify them: prefixes are blue, combining forms are red, and suffixes are purple.

Prefix	Definition	Combining Form	Definition	Suffix	Definition
a-	without or absence of	blephar/o	eyelid	-iasis	condition of
		conjunctiv/o	conjunctiva	-ism	condition of
dipl-	double	cyst/o	bladder or sac	-malacia	softening
hyper-	excessive, abnormally high, or above	dacry/o	tear	-opia	condition of vision
		ir/o	iris	-pathy	disease
		kerat/o	hard, cornea	-plegia	paralysis
		lith/o	stone	-ptosis	drooping
		ophthalm/o	eye	-rrhagia	condition of profuse bleeding or hemorrhage
		presby/o	old age		
		retin/o	retina		
		sinus/o	sinus cavity		
		stigmat/o	point		

blepharoptosis
BLEF ah ropp TOH siss

blephar/o/ptosis

blepharitis
BLEF ah RYE tiss

13.91 The combining form for eyelid is *blephar/o*. To describe a drooping eyelid, the suffix *-ptosis* is added to form the term _____. Write the word part construction for this term to reveal its three word parts: _____/__/_____. A common symptom of an inflammation of the eyelid is called _____. If the inflammation or a trauma damages the eyelid, it is repaired in the procedure known as **blepharoplasty** (BLEF ah roh plass tee).

cataract
KAT ah rakt

13.92 The lens of the eye is normally transparent. In the condition known as **cataract**, transparency of the lens is reduced. _____ formation is usually a normal part of the aging process.

DID YOU KNOW?

Cataract

The term *cataract* is from the Latin word that means "waterfall." It was an ancient belief that the gradual loss of vision was due to a veil that fell between the lens and the cornea, spilling over vision *like a waterfall*.

conjunctivitis
kon JUNK tih VYE tiss

13.93 The conjunctiva is a thin membrane covering the anterior, exposed part of the eye and the inner eyelid. Bacteria may infect this membrane, causing inflammation known as _____. Commonly known as "pink eye" because of the pink color of the sclera caused by the inflammation, itchy watery eyes and a crusty exudate are common signs (Figure 13.13■). The word part construction for this term can be written as conjunctiv/itis.

Figure 13.13 ■
Conjunctivitis, with the characteristic "pink eye" appearance.

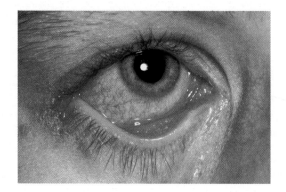

dacryolithiasis
DAK ree oh lith EYE ah siss

dacryocystitis
DAK ree oh sist EYE tiss

13.94 The lacrimal apparatus is a tear-forming gland and its associated tubes and chambers, mainly located near the medial side of each eyeball. The combining form of lacrimal is *dacry/o*. The presence of rocky particles in the apparatus is a condition known as _____. It is a painful condition that often leads to inflammation of the lacrimal apparatus, known as _____. The word part construction of dacryocystitis can be written as *dacry/o/cyst/itis*. If the inflammation should pass into the adjacent sinuses, the condition becomes **dacryosinusitis** (DAK ree oh SYE nus EYE tiss).

detached retina
dee TACHD * RET ih nah

13.95 A common cause of blindness is **detached retina**. It occurs when the retina tears away from the choroid layer of the eye. A _____ _____ can be caused by a severe blow to the head, high blood pressure, or old age.

diplopia
dih PLOH pee ah

13.96 The condition of double vision is called **diplopia**. _____ may result from weakened extrinsic eye muscles, defects in the lens, or a condition of the brain.

glaucoma
glaw KOH mah

13.97 In the disease of the eye known as **glaucoma**, a loss of vision occurs when the fluid pressure within the anterior chamber of the eyeball (called intraocular pressure) rises above normal. The rise of fluid pressure in _____ is caused by a blockage in a small opening that normally drains the fluid (Figure 13.14■).

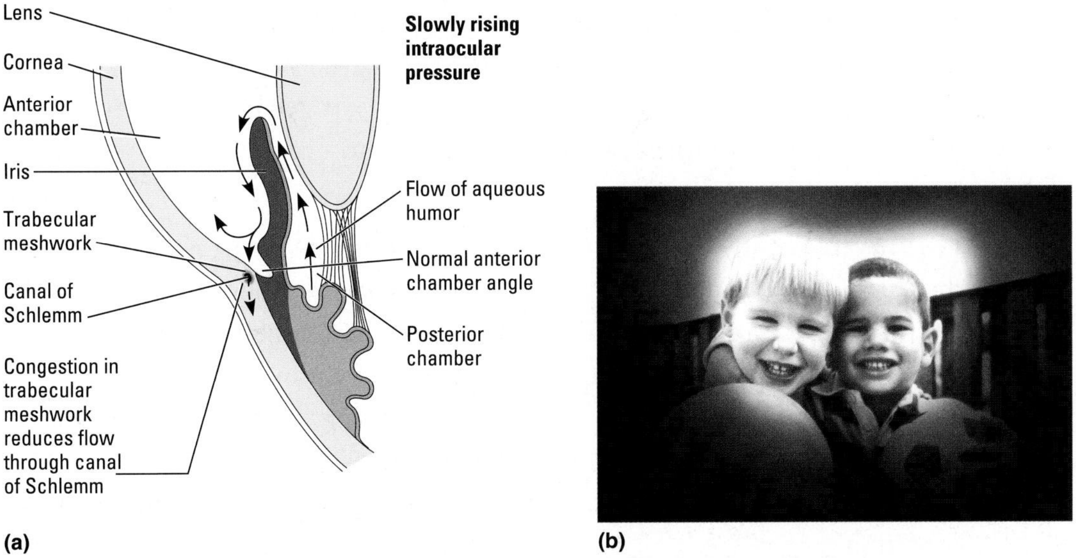

Lens
Cornea
Anterior chamber
Iris
Trabecular meshwork
Canal of Schlemm
Congestion in trabecular meshwork reduces flow through canal of Schlemm

Slowly rising intraocular pressure

Flow of aqueous humor
Normal anterior chamber angle
Posterior chamber

(a)

(b)

Figure 13.14 ■
Glaucoma. (a) A blockage of the canal of Schlemm causes rising fluid pressure in the anterior chamber.
(b) Narrowing of the optical fields is a typical symptom of untreated glaucoma.
Courtesy of the National Eye Institute: National Institutes of Health.

hordeolum
hor DEE oh lum

13.98 The meibomian gland is a small gland in the eyelid that secretes lubricating fluid onto the conjunctiva. An infection of this gland produces a local swelling of the eyelid, known as a **hordeolum**. Also called a *sty*, the term _____ is derived from the Latin word, *hordeum*, which means "barley" (Figure 13.15■). A chronic form of this infection is often called a **chalazion** (kah LAY zee on).

Figure 13.15 ■
Hordeolum (or sty).
Source: Photo Researchers, Inc.

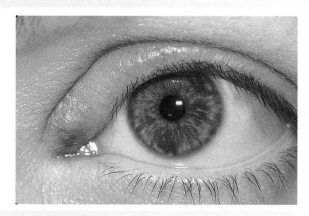

iritis
eye RYE tiss

keratitis
kair aht EYE tiss

13.99 During a bacterial infection of the eye, parts of the eye may become inflamed. When the iris is affected, the condition is known as _____, and when the cornea becomes inflamed, it is called _____. The word part construction of iritis is written as ir/itis, and keratitis is kerat/itis.

macular degeneration
MAK yoo lahr * dee jenn er AY shun

13.100 The macula lutea is a small area of the retina that contains a high density of photoreceptors, known as cone cells. Because of the high concentration of cone cells, it is the area of sharpest vision. Progressive deterioration of the macula lutea leads to a loss of visual focus, and is called **macular degeneration**. The abbreviated version of _____ _____ is **ARMD** (age-related macular degeneration), because its most common cause is age.

ophthalmomalacia
off thal moh mah LAY shee ah

ophthalmoplegia
off thal moh PLEE gee ah

ophthalmorrhagia
off thal moh RAHJ ee ah

13.101 A frequently used combining form that means "eye" is *ophthalm/o*. In the term _____, the suffix *-malacia* is included to establish the meaning "softening of the eye." The word part construction of this term is written as ophthalm/o/malacia. Similarly, paralysis of the eye is termed _____, formed by adding the suffix that means "paralysis," *-plegia*. In this eye disease, the extrinsic eye muscles are unable to move the eyeball. Also, loss of blood by hemorrhage of the eye is the condition _____. Each of these eye conditions are forms of eye disease, or **ophthalmopathy** (OFF thalm MOH path ee).

retinopathy

RETT in OPP ah thee

13.102 A general term for a disease of the retina is the term _____, which is illustrated in Figure 13.16■. The three word parts that form the term *retinopathy* can be written as retin/o/pathy.

Figure 13.16 ■
Retinopathy. Illustration of a normal retina (left) and a diseased retina (right).

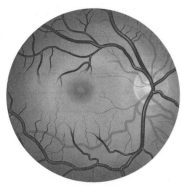
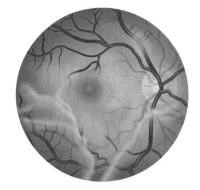

Normal retina   Diseased retina

vision disorders

13.103 Conditions of the eye that result in a reduction of vision are generally called **vision disorders**. Often caused by defects in the lens, cornea, or shape of the eyeball, _____ _____ include nearsightedness, or **myopia** (mye OH pee ah), farsightedness, or **hyperopia** (HYE per oh pee ah), and **presbyopia** (PREZ bee oh pee ah), or reduction in vision due to age. **Emmetropia** (EM eh troh pee ah) is the normal condition of the eye, abbreviated **Em**. Note that each of these terms include the suffix -*opia*, which means "condition of vision." In the condition **astigmatism** (ah STIG mah tizm), the curvature of the eye is defective to produce blurred vision. It is abbreviated **Ast**.

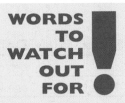

WORDS TO WATCH OUT FOR

Myopia
You may recall from Chapter 6 that *my/o* is the combining form for muscle. It is derived from the Greek word for muscle, *myos*. However, in the word *myopia*, *my* is derived from the Greek word *myein*, which means "to shut." When followed by the suffix -*opia*, the term *myopia* translates into "condition of shut vision."

PRACTICE: Eye Diseases and Disorders

The Right Match

Match the vocabulary term on the left with the correct definition on the right.

_____ 1. glaucoma

_____ 2. cataract

_____ 3. macular degeneration

_____ 4. hordeolum

_____ 5. detached retina

a. occurs when the retina tears away from the choroid layer

b. progressive deterioration of the macula lutea

c. infection of the meibomian gland; also called a *sty*

d. loss of vision as a result of increased intraocular pressure

e. a condition in which the transparency of the lens is reduced

Linkup

Link the word parts in the list to create the terms that match the definitions. You may use word parts more than once. Remember to add combining vowels when needed—and that some terms do not use any combining vowel.

Prefix	Combining Form	Suffix
a-	blephar/o	-ism
	conjunctiv/o	-itis
	dipl/o	-opia
	ophthalm/o	-pathy
	retin/o	
	stigmat/o	

Definition   Term

1.   bacterial infection of the conjunctiva   _____

2.   double vision   _____

3.   defective curvature of the eye that causes blurred vision _____

4.   inflammation of the eyelid   _____

5.   disease of the retina   _____

6.   eye disease   _____

Eye Treatments, Procedures, and Devices

Following are the word parts that specifically apply to eye treatments, procedures, and devices that are covered in the following section. Note that the word parts are color-coded to help you identify them: prefixes are blue, combining forms are red, and suffixes are purple.

Prefix	Definition	Combining Form	Definition	Suffix	Definition
intra-	within	dacry/o	tear	-ar	pertaining to
		cyst/o	bladder or sac	-logist	one who studies
		kerat/o	hard, cornea	-metrist	one who measures
		ocul/o	eye	-stomy	surgical creation of an opening
		opt/o	eye		
		rad/i	spoke of a wheel	-tomy	incision or to cut
		rhin/o	nose		

cataract extraction

13.104 During **cataract extraction**, a lens damaged by a cataract is surgically removed and replaced with a donor lens (Figure 13.17■). If a donor lens is not available for a _____ _____, an artificial **intraocular lens (IOL)** may be implanted.

Figure 13.17 ■
Cataract extraction. The procedure involves a surgical removal of a cataract lens and its replacement with an artificial lens. The artificial lens is usually an acrylic (Plexiglas) material.

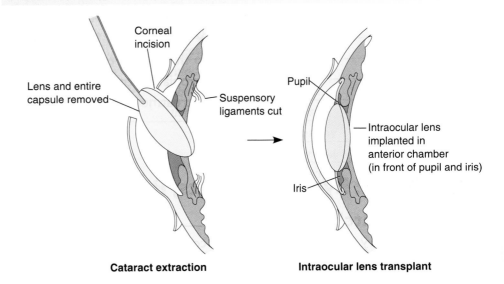

Corneal incision

Lens and entire capsule removed

Suspensory ligaments cut

Pupil

Intraocular lens implanted in anterior chamber (in front of pupil and iris)

Iris

Cataract extraction   Intraocular lens transplant

corneal grafting
KOR ne al * GRAF ting

13.105 The cornea is normally transparent, but may lose its transparency from exposure to ultraviolet light or become damaged from an injury. The most common treatment of corneal damage is **corneal grafting**. During a _____ _____, the injured cornea is removed and replaced by implantation of a donor cornea.

dacryocystorhinostomy
DAK ree o SIS toh rye NOS stoh mee

13.106 To treat dacryocystitis, antibiotic eye drops are often used to defeat the bacterial infection. In some cases, a **dacryocystorhinostomy** may be needed. During a _____, a channel is surgically created between the nasal cavity and lacrimal sac to promote drainage. This long term may be divided into its numerous word parts by writing it as dacry/o/cyst/o/rhin/o/stomy.

LASIK
LAY sik

13.107 The acronym for **laser-assisted in situ keratomileusis** is _____. It is the use of a laser to reshape the corneal tissue beneath the surface of the cornea to correct vision disorders, such as myopia, hyperopia, and astigmatism.

▶▶▶▶ Chapter Review

Word Building

Construct medical terms from the following meanings. The first question has been completed for you as an example.

1. excessive sensitivity to painful stimuli   *hyper*algesia

2. a pain in the head (headache)   _____algia

3. inflammation of the cerebellum   cerebell_____

4. a disease of blood vessels in the cerebrum   _____vascular disease

5. a tumor of neuroglial cells   gli_____

6. softening of brain tissue   encephalo_____

7. nervous system disease   neuro_____

8. excessive sensitivity to a stimulus   _____esthesia

9. inflammation of the brain   _____itis

10. protrusion of the meninges   meningo_____

11. literally a *condition of many hardened areas*   _____sclerosis

12. inflammation of the spinal cord   _____itis

13. literally *nerve weakness*   neur_____

14. a tumor arising from nervous tissue   neur_____

15. pain in a nerve   neur_____

16. abnormal sensation of numbness   par_____

17. paralysis on one side of the body   _____plegia

18. inflammation of many nerves   poly_____

19. a disease of the mind   _____pathy

20. paralysis of all four limbs   _____plegia

21. abnormally increased volume of cerebrospinal fluid (CSF)   hydro_____

22. excision of part of the skull   _____ectomy

23. incision into the skull   cranio_____

24. suture of a nerve   neuro_____

25. separating a nerve by removing adhesions   neuro_____

26. incision into a nerve   neuro_____

27. inflammation of the ventricles of the brain   ventricul_____

28. physician who specializes in neurology   _____logist

29. drug therapy that targets the brain   _____pharmacology

30. psychology technique used to treat behavioral issues   psycho_____

31. abnormally high psychomotor activity   _____ (do this one on your own!)

32. an irrational, obsessive fear   _____ (do this one on your own!)

33. inflammation of the corneum   _____itis

Clinical Application Exercises

Medical Report

Read the following medical report, then answer the questions that follow.

University Hospital

5500 University Avenue
Metropolis, TX

Phone: (211) 594-4000
Fax: (211) 594-4001

Medical Consultation: Neurology

Date: 10/11//2008

Patient: Melissa Tampico

Patient Complaint: Cephalalgia and neuralgia; polyneuritis on left upper limb and shoulder following automobile collision.

History: 19-year-old female, recently migrated from the Philippine Islands, with no prior history of medical concerns.

Family History: Father, 42-year-old, with Type 2 diabetes under dietary restrictions; Mother, 40-year-old, with no neurological history.

Allergies: None

Evidences: CT and MRI reveal subdural hemorrhage at 1.5 mm inferior to right squamosal suture.

Treatment: STAT craniotomy with insertion of shunt as needed to drain fluids; identify source of leakage and repair.

Jennifer Holland, M.D.

---

1. What patient complaint is an early indication of increasing intracranial pressure on the right side of the brain?

   _____

   _____

2. If the intracranial pressure is not relieved in time, what do you suppose might be the consequences to the patient?

   _____

   _____

Medical Report Case Study

The following Case Study provides further discussion regarding the patient in the medical report. Fill in the blanks with the correct terms. Choose your answers from the following list of terms. (Note that some terms may be used more than once.)

analgesics	craniotomy	neuralgia
cephalalgia	intracranial	paresthesia
computed tomography	magnetic resonance imaging	polyneuritis

The patient, Melissa Tampico, was examined following an automobile collision. At the time of admittance she reported

symptoms of headache, or (a) _____, generalized pain in the nerves, or (b) _____, of

the right shoulder and upper arm. Physical examination showed an inflammation of multiple nerves, or

(c) _____, of the shoulder and upper arm. Anti-inflammatory medication and pain relievers, or

(d) _____, were prescribed for treatment. Two weeks after the first exam, the patient returned with

reported abnormal sensations along the left side of the body, or (e) _____. Following a preliminary CT,

or (f) _____ _____, scan, an MRI, or (g) _____

_____ _____ was ordered for a more complete evaluation. The MRI revealed

bleeding below the dura mater (subdural hemorrhage), which was increasing the (h) _____ (within

the cranium) pressure. An incision into the cranium, or (i) _____, was performed to correct the

hemorrhage and reduce the intracranial pressure. The patient made a complete recovery.

Key Terms Double-Check

Remember that the chapter's key terms appeared alphabetically throughout this chapter. This exercise helps you to check your knowledge AND review for tests.

1. First, fill in the missing word in the definitions for the chapter's key terms.
2. Then, check your answers using Appendix F.
3. If you got the answer right, put a check mark in the right column.
4. If your answer was incorrect, go back to the frame number provided and review the content.

Use the checklist to study the terms you don't know until you're confident you know them all.

Key Term	Frame	Definition	Know It?
1. agnosia	13.18	the _____ to interpret sensory information	☐
2. Alzheimer disease	13.19	a disease characterized by gradual deterioration in _____ function	☐
3. amyotrophic lateral sclerosis	13.20	a disease characterized by progressive atrophy of _____	☐
4. analgesics	13.50	a common form of _____ management; includes aspirin, ibuprofen, and acetaminophen	☐
5. anesthesia	13.51	the primary type of pain management that is used during _____ procedures	☐
6. anxiety disorder	13.77	a mental disorder in which _____ dominates a person's behavior	☐
7. aphasia	13.8	the inability to _____	☐
8. attention deficit disorder	13.78	a neurological disorder characterized by short _____ span and poor concentration	☐
9. autism	13.21	_____ developmental disorder that varies in severity	☐
10. Bell palsy	13.22	condition characterized by _____ of the face muscles on one side	☐
11. bipolar disease	13.79	a mental disorder characterized by alternating periods of _____ energy and mental confusion with low energy and mental depression	☐
12. blepharitis	13.91	inflammation of the _____	☐
13. blepharoptosis	13.91	a _____ eyelid	☐
14. cataract	13.92	a condition in which the eye _____ transparency is reduced	☐
15. cataract extraction	13.104	the surgical removal of a cataract and replacement with a _____ lens	☐
16. cephalalgia	13.9	the clinical term for a _____, or a generalized pain in the region of the head	☐
17. cerebellitis	13.23	_____ of the cerebellum	☐
18. cerebral aneurysm	13.24	a protrusion through the _____ of a blood vessel in the brain	☐

Key Term	Frame	Definition	Know It?
19. cerebral angiography	13.52	a diagnostic procedure that reveals blood flow to the _____ by X-ray photography	☐
20. cerebral athero-sclerosis	13.25	accumulation of fatty plaques that cause arteries that supply the brain to gradually _____	☐
21. cerebral hemorrhage	13.26	_____ from cerebral blood vessels	☐
22. cerebral palsy	13.27	a condition that appears at birth or shortly afterward as a partial muscle _____	☐
23. cerebrovascular accident	13.28	irreversible death of brain cells caused by inadequate _____ supply to the brain	☐
24. coma	13.29	abnormally _____ consciousness	☐
25. computed tomography	13.53	a procedure that involves the use of a computer to interpret a series of images and construct from them a three-dimensional view of the _____	☐
26. concussion	13.30	an injury to soft tissue that results from a blow or violent _____	☐
27. conjunctivitis	13.93	_____ of the conjunctiva	☐
28. convulsion	13.10	a series of involuntary muscular _____	☐
29. corneal grafting	13.105	the surgical removal of an injured _____ and replacement with a donor cornea	☐
30. craniectomy	13.54	the surgical _____ of part of the cranium	☐
31. craniotomy	13.55	a surgical _____ through the cranium to provide access to the brain	☐
32. dacryocystitis	13.94	inflammation of the _____ apparatus	☐
33. dacryocystorhinos-tomy	13.106	a procedure in which a channel is surgically created between the _____ cavity and lacrimal sac to promote drainage	☐
34. dacryolithiasis	13.94	the presence of _____ particles in the lacrimal apparatus	☐
35. dementia	13.80	an impairment of mental function characterized by memory _____, disorientation, and confusion	☐
36. detached retina	13.95	occurs when the retina tears away from the choroid layer of the _____	☐
37. diplopia	13.96	_____ vision	☐
38. dyslexia	13.81	a reading handicap in which the brain _____ the order of some letters and numbers	☐
39. echoenceph-alography	13.56	a procedure that uses _____ technology to record brain structures	☐
40. effectual drug therapy	13.57	a general type of treatment to manage _____ disorders	☐
41. electroenceph-alography	13.58	a diagnostic procedure that records _____ impulses of the brain to measure brain activity	☐

Key Term	Frame	Definition	Know It?
42. encephalitis	13.31	inflammation of the _____	☐
43. encephalomalacia	13.32	_____ of brain tissue	☐
44. epidural	13.59	the injection of a spinal block _____ into the epidural space	☐
45. epilepsy	13.33	a brain disorder characterized by recurrent _____	☐
46. evoked potential studies	13.60	a group of diagnostic tests that measure changes in brain _____ during particular stimuli	☐
47. ganglionectomy	13.61	the surgical _____ of a ganglion	☐
48. glaucoma	13.97	a loss of vision caused by an increase in the fluid _____ within the anterior chamber of the eyeball	☐
49. glioma	13.34	a _____ of neuroglial cells	☐
50. hordeolum	13.98	an _____ of the meibomian gland that produces a local swelling of the eyelid; a sty	☐
51. hydrocephalus	13.35	a congenital disease characterized by an abnormally increased volume of cerebrospinal _____ in the brain	☐
52. hyperalgesia	13.11	an excessive sensitivity to _____ stimuli	☐
53. hyperesthesia	13.12	an _____ sensitivity to a stimulus	☐
54. iritis	13.99	_____ of the iris	☐
55. keratitis	13.99	inflammation of the _____	☐
56. lumbar puncture	13.62	the withdrawal of cerebrospinal fluid (CSF) from the _____ cord	☐
57. macular degeneration	13.100	progressive _____ of the macula lutea that leads to a loss of visual focus	☐
58. magnetic resonance imaging	13.63	a diagnostic procedure in which powerful _____ are used to observe soft tissues in the body	☐
59. mania	13.82	an emotional disorder of abnormally _____ psychomotor activity	☐
60. mastoiditis	13.109	inflammation of the _____	☐
61. Ménière disease	13.110	a chronic disease of the inner ear that causes _____ and ringing in the ears	☐
62. meningioma	13.36	a benign _____ of the meninges	☐
63. meningitis	13.37	inflammation of the _____	☐
64. meningocele	13.38	_____ of the meninges	☐
65. meningomyelocele	13.38	protrusion of the meninges and _____ _____	☐
66. multiple sclerosis	13.39	a disease characterized by the deterioration of the myelin sheath covering axons within the _____	☐
67. myelitis	13.40	inflammation of the _____ _____	☐
68. myelogram	13.64	an X-ray _____ of the spinal cord following injection of a contrast dye	☐

Key Term	Frame	Definition	Know It?
69. myelography	13.64	the diagnostic _____ in which contrast dye is injected into the spinal cord	☐
70. narcolepsy	13.41	a _____ disorder characterized by sudden uncontrollable episodes of sleep, attacks of paralysis, and hallucinations	☐
71. neuralgia	13.13	pain in a _____	☐
72. neurasthenia	13.14	generalized body _____	☐
73. neurectomy	13.65	the surgical _____ of a nerve	☐
74. neuritis	13.42	_____ of a nerve	☐
75. neurology	13.66	the study and medical practice of the _____ system	☐
76. neurolysis	13.67	the procedure of _____ a nerve by removing unwanted adhesions	☐
77. neuroma	13.43	a _____ originating from nerve cells	☐
78. neuropathy	13.44	a _____ affecting any part of the nervous system	☐
79. neuroplasty	13.68	the surgical _____ of a nerve	☐
80. neurorrhaphy	13.69	the _____ of a nerve	☐
81. neurosis	13.83	an emotional disorder that involves a counterproductive way of dealing with _____ stress	☐
82. neurotomy	13.70	incision into a _____	☐
83. ophthalmomalacia	13.101	_____ of the eye	☐
84. ophthalmoplegia	13.101	_____ of the eye	☐
85. ophthalmorrhagia	13.101	_____ of the eye	☐
86. optometrist	13.108	a health professional trained to examine _____ to correct vision problems and eye disorders	☐
87. otalgia	13.112	_____ in the ear	☐
88. otitis	13.111	inflammation of the _____	☐
89. otopathy	13.111	_____ of the ear	☐
90. otorrhea	13.112	_____ of pus into the external auditory canal	☐
91. otosclerosis	13.113	an abnormal formation of _____ within the ear	☐
92. otoscopy	13.114	a _____ examination of the ear using a handheld instrument called an otoscope	☐
93. paranoia	13.84	persistent _____ of persecution that results in mistrust and combativeness	☐
94. paraplegia	13.45	muscle _____ from the waist down	☐
95. paresthesia	13.15	abnormal sensation of _____ and tingling	☐
96. Parkinson disease	13.46	a chronic, degenerative disease of the brain characterized by _____, rigidity, and shuffling gait	☐
97. phobia	13.85	an irrational, obsessive _____	☐
98. poliomyelitis	13.47	a disease characterized by _____ of the gray matter of the spinal cord	☐
99. polyneuralgia	13.16	pain in _____ nerves	☐
100. polyneuritis	13.42	_____ of many nerves at once	☐

Key Term	Frame	Definition	Know It?
101. polyneuropathy	13.44	a disease affecting many parts of the _____ system	☐
102. positron emission tomography	13.71	a computerized procedure that involves a scan using an injected radioactive chemical to provide a map of blood _____ within the body	☐
103. posttraumatic stress disorder	13.86	a disorder caused by a severe mental strain or emotional _____ that includes sleeplessness, anxiety, and paranoia	☐
104. psychiatry	13.72	the branch of _____ that addresses disorders of the brain resulting in mental and emotional disturbances	☐
105. psychology	13.73	the study of _____ behavior	☐
106. psychopathy	13.87	a general term for a _____ or emotional disorder	☐
107. psychosis	13.88	a disease characterized by a gross _____ or disorganization of mental capacity	☐
108. psychosomatic	13.89	the influence of the _____ over bodily functions, especially disease	☐
109. psychotherapy	13.73	a technique used in treating _____ and emotional issues	☐
110. rabies	13.48	an acute, often fatal, _____ of the central nervous system	☐
111. radial keratotomy	13.108	a procedure in which _____ are made into the cornea to flatten it to correct myopia	☐
112. radicotomy	13.74	a surgical incision into a nerve _____	☐
113. reflex testing	13.75	a series of diagnostic tests performed to observe the body's response to _____ stimuli	☐
114. retinopathy	13.102	_____ of the retina	☐
115. schizophrenia	13.90	a mental condition characterized by delusions, _____, and extensive withdrawal	☐
116. syncope	13.17	temporary _____ of consciousness	☐
117. vagotomy	13.76	a procedure in which several branches of the vagus nerve are _____ to reduce acid secretion in the stomach	☐
118. ventriculitis	13.49	_____ of the ventricles of the brain	☐
119. vertigo	13.115	a _____ of whirling motion	☐
120. vision disorders	13.103	conditions of the eye that result in a _____ of vision	☐

Multimedia Preview ▶▶▶▶▶

Additional interactive resources and activities for this chapter can be found on the Companion Website. For videos, audio glossary, and review, access the accompanying DVD-ROM in this book.

DVD-ROM Highlights

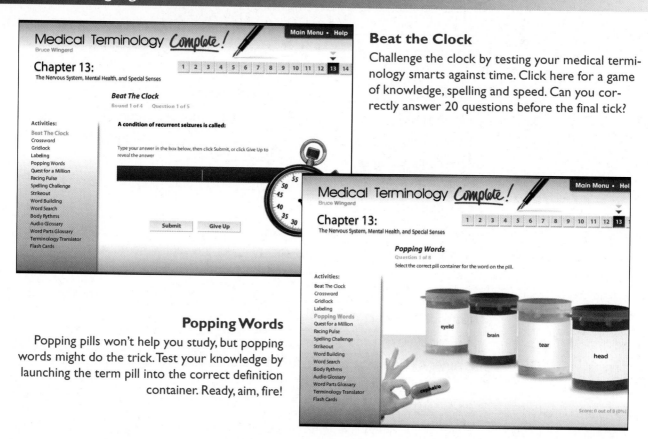

Beat the Clock

Challenge the clock by testing your medical terminology smarts against time. Click here for a game of knowledge, spelling and speed. Can you correctly answer 20 questions before the final tick?

Popping Words

Popping pills won't help you study, but popping words might do the trick. Test your knowledge by launching the term pill into the correct definition container. Ready, aim, fire!

Website Highlights—www.prenhall.com/wingerd

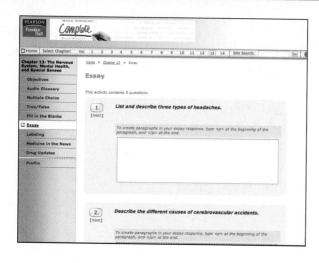

Essay Questions

Click here to take advantage of the free-access online study guide that accompanies your textbook. You'll find a series of short answer essay questions that correspond to the concepts in this chapter. By clicking on this URL you'll also access links to download mp3 audio reviews, current news articles, and an audio glossary.

The Endocrine System ▶▶▶▶▶

Learning Objectives

After completing this chapter, you will be able to:

- Define and spell the word parts used to create terms for the endocrine system.

- Identify the major organs of the endocrine system and describe their structure and function.

- Break down and define common medical terms used for symptoms, diseases, disorders, procedures, treatments, and devices associated with the endocrine system.

- Build medical terms from the word parts associated with the endocrine system.

- Pronounce and spell common medical terms associated with the endocrine system.

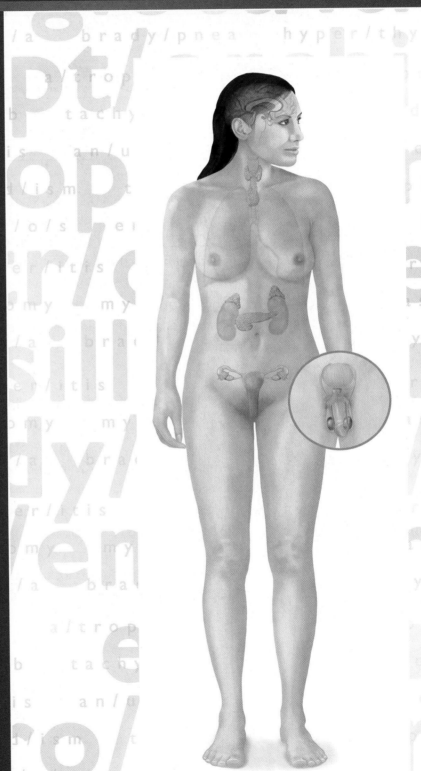

Anatomy and Physiology Terms ▶▶▶▶▶

The following table provides the combining forms that specifically apply to the anatomy and physiology of the endocrine system. Note that the combining forms are colored red to help you identify them when you see them again later in the chapter.

Combining Form	Definition
aden/o	gland
adren/o	adrenal gland
crin/o	to secrete
gonad/o	sex gland
hormon/o	to set in motion
pancreat/o	sweetbread, pancreas
ren/o	kidney
thyr/o, thyroid/o	shield, thyroid

endocrine

14.1 The **endocrine** (EN doh krin) **system** works hand in hand with the nervous system to regulate body functions. The primary organs of the _____ system include the pituitary gland attached to the hypothalamus at the base of the brain, the thyroid gland in the neck, the parathyroid glands embedded within the thyroid gland, the two adrenal glands located above each kidney, the pancreatic islets within the pancreas, and the gonads, which include the ovaries of the female and testes of the male.

FUNCTION ▶▶▶▶

hormone

14.2 Like the nervous system, the endocrine system provides a method of control to keep the body functioning despite changing conditions in the environment. Thus, the primary role of the endocrine system is to manage homeostasis, a state in which the body's equilibrium is maintained. Instead of regulating body activities with rapid nerve impulses, the endocrine organs secrete chemicals called **hormones** that are carried by the bloodstream. The result of _____ secretion is a change in cell functions, which alters body activities. When the endocrine system becomes deficient due to disease, the result is a homeostatic imbalance that often affects overall health.

14.3 Use the anatomy terms that appear in the left column to fill in the corresponding blanks in Figure 14.1■.

1. **gland**
2. **thyroid**
3. **adrenal**
4. **pancreas**
5. **testis**

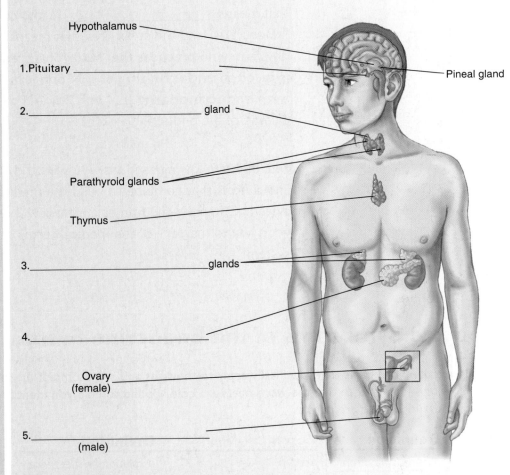

Hypothalamus

1. Pituitary _____

Pineal gland

2. _____ gland

Parathyroid glands

Thymus

3. _____ glands

4. _____

Ovary
(female)

5. _____
(male)

Figure 14.1 ■
The endocrine glands of the endocrine system are distributed throughout the body.

Medical Terms for the Endocrine System ▶▶▶▶▶

hyposecretion

14.4 An array of disorders can occur when an endocrine gland fails to deliver the quantity of hormones needed to regulate body functions. In general, endocrine disease results from either abnormally high hormone production, called **hypersecretion**, or abnormally low hormone production, called _____. Either condition upsets the homeostatic balance of the body. Hypersecretion may arise due to an inherited disease or a tumor. Often, hyposecretion occurs if an endocrine gland suffers trauma due to an injury or infection, although it also may be caused by an inherited disorder or a tumor. Sometimes, an endocrine disorder includes an array of symptoms and involves multiple organs. This type of disease is generally known as a **syndrome**.

within
study of

14.5 The treatment of endocrine diseases is a focused discipline within medicine, called **endocrinology** (EN doh krin ALL oh jee). This is a constructed term that is written endo/crin/o/logy, and includes the prefix endo- that means "_____," the combining form crin/o that means "to secrete," and the suffix -logy that means "_____ _____." A physician who practices the "study of secreting within," or endocrinology, is called an **endocrinologist** (EN doh krin ALL oh jist). In addition, the term **endocrinopathy** (EN doh krin AH path ee) is a general term for a disease of the endocrine system.

14.6 In the following sections, you will study the prefixes, combining forms, and suffixes that combine to build the medical terms of the endocrine system. Complete the frames and review exercises that follow. You are on your way to mastery of the medical terms related to the endocrine system!

Signs and Symptoms of the Endocrine System

Following are the word parts that specifically apply to the signs and symptoms of the endocrine system that are covered in the following section. Note that the word parts are color-coded to help you identify them: prefixes are blue, combining forms are red, and suffixes are purple.

Prefix	Definition
ex-	outside, away from
poly-	excessive, over, or many

Combining Form	Definition
acid/o	a solution or substance with a pH less than 7
acr/o	extremity
dips/o	thirst
ophthalm/o	eye
ket/o	ketone
hirsut/o	hairy

Suffix	Definition
-ia	condition of
-ism	condition of
-megaly	abnormally large
-osis	condition of
-s	more than one
-uria	pertaining to urine or urination

KEY TERMS A-Z

acidosis
ass ih DOH siss

14.7 Recall that the suffix -osis means "condition of." The condition of acid in the body is therefore known as _____, and the constructed form of the term is acid/osis. It occurs when carbon dioxide, the primary waste product from cellular metabolism, accumulates in tissues (including blood) to form carbonic acid. Acidosis is a symptom of diabetes mellitus (Frame 14.21) and may also be caused by respiratory or kidney disorders.

14.8 A sign that includes enlargement of bone structure is known as **acromegaly**. The enlargement causes disfigurement, especially in the hands and face, and is a sign of hypersecretion of growth hormone from the pituitary gland during adulthood (Figure 14.2■). _____ literally means "abnormally large extremity." It is a constructed term that is written acro/megaly.

acromegaly
ak roh MEG ah lee

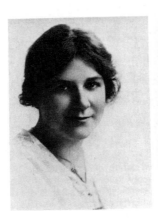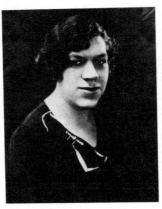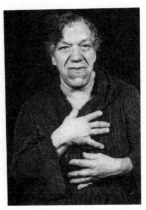

Figure 14.2 ■
Acromegaly. Acromegaly is a metabolic disorder in which excessive amounts of growth hormone are secreted during adulthood, resulting in enlarged bones.
© Dr. William H. Daughaday, University of California/Irvine. American Journal of Medicine (20) 1956. With permission of Excerpta Medica Inc.

14.9 The abnormal protrusion of the eyes is known as **exophthalmos**. It is a classic symptom of excessive activity of the thyroid gland and literally means "outside eyes" (Figure 14.3■). _____ is a constructed term that is written as ex/ophthalm/o/s.

exophthalmos
eks off THAL mos

Figure 14.3 ■
Exophthalmos. The protrusion of the eyes is a common symptom of hyperthyroidism.
Source: Custom Medical Stock Photo, Inc.

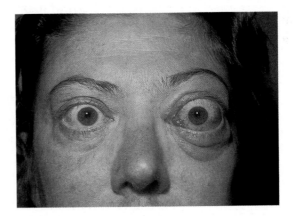

DID YOU KNOW ?

Thyroid
The shape of the thyroid gland must have reminded the Greeks of a shield because the term is derived from the Greek word for this defensive warrior gear, thyreos.

goiter
GOY ter

14.10 A common symptom of thyroid gland disease is a swelling on the anterior side of the neck in the location of the thyroid gland, known as a **goiter**. A _____ is an abnormal enlargement of the thyroid gland caused by a tumor, lack of iodine in the diet, or an infection (Figure 14.4■).

Figure 14.4 ■
Goiter. The formation of numerous nodules in the thyroid gland causes the enlargement of the neck. It is a symptom of iodine deficiency or tumors.
Source: Custom Medical Stock Photo, Inc.

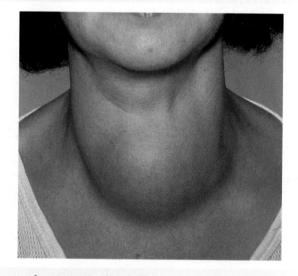

hirsutism
HER soot izm

14.11 A symptom of excessive body hair in a masculine pattern is known as **hirsutism**. The term is derived from the Latin word *hirsutus*, which means "hairy." When _____ occurs in women, it is caused by the hypersecretion of androgens by the adrenal cortex. Excessive production of androgens in women may also lead to muscle and bone growth. The resulting pattern of masculinization is known as **adrenal virilism** (add REE nal *VIHR ill izm).

ketosis
kee TOH siss

14.12 A ketone body is a waste substance produced when cells are unable to metabolize carbohydrates. The condition called _____ is an excessive amount of ketone bodies in the blood and urine and is a symptom of diabetes mellitus (Frame 14.21) and starvation. Because ketosis produces an acidic condition of the body, it is also known as **ketoacidosis** (KEE toh ass ih DOH siss). Ketoacidosis contains four word parts and is written as ket/o/acid/osis.

polydipsia
PALL ee DIP see ah

14.13 The prefix *poly-* means "excessive, over, or many." It is sometimes used to indicate an abnormally excessive amount. The combining form *dips/o* means "thirst." Thus, the symptom called _____ literally means "condition of many thirsts." An abnormal state of excessive thirst occurs during certain disorders of the pituitary gland or the pancreas.

polyuria
PALL ee YOO ree ah

14.14 As you learned in Chapter 11, the term **polyuria** includes the prefix *poly-*. It is a symptom of pituitary gland disease that arises when the hormone ADH is not produced normally. It is also a symptom of diabetes mellitus (Frame 14.21). _____ is the production of abnormally large volumes of urine.

PRACTICE: Signs and Symptoms of the Endocrine System

The Right Match

Match the term on the left with the correct definition on the right.

_____ 1. acidosis

_____ 2. ketosis

_____ 3. goiter

_____ 4. adrenal virilism

_____ 5. hirsutism

a. enlargement at the throat

b. a pattern of masculinization and hair distribution in women

c. excessive body hair

d. abnormal accumulation of waste materials that are acidic

e. excessive amount of ketone bodies in the blood and urine

Break the Chain

Analyze these medical terms:

a) Separate each term into its word parts; each word part is labeled for you (**p** = prefix, **r** = root, **cf** = combining form, and **s** = suffix).

b) For the Bonus Question, write the requested definition in the blank that follows.

The first set has been completed as an example.

1. a) *polydipsia*   poly / dips / ia
                      p   r   s

   b) *Bonus Question:* What is the definition of the suffix? condition of _____

2. a) exophthalmos   ____ / _____ / __ / ____
                           p   cf   s

   b) *Bonus Question:* What is the definition of the combining form? _____

3. a) polyuria   _____ / ____
                 p   s

   b) *Bonus Question:* What is the definition of the suffix? _____

4. a) acromegaly   ____ / __ / _____
                    cf   s

   b) *Bonus Question:* What is the definition of the combining form? _____

5. a) ketoacidosis   _____ / ____ / _____ / _____
                      cf   r   s

   b) *Bonus Question:* What is the definition of the combining form? _____

Diseases and Disorders of the Endocrine System

Following are the word parts that specifically apply to the diseases and disorders of the endocrine system that are covered in the following section. Note that the word parts are color-coded to help you identify them: prefixes are blue, combining forms are red, and suffixes are purple.

Prefix	Definition
endo-	within
hyper-	excessive, abnormally high, or above
hypo-	deficient, abnormally low, or below
para-	alongside or abnormal

Combining Form	Definition
aden/o	gland
adren/o	adrenal gland
calc/i, calc/o	calcium
carcin/o	cancer
crin/o	to secrete
glyc/o	sweet or sugar
gonad/o	sex gland
muc/o	mucus
pancreat/o	pancreas
thyr/o, thyroid/o	shield, thyroid

Suffix	Definition
-al	pertaining to
-emia	condition of blood
-ism	condition of
-itis	inflammation
-oma	tumor
-pathy	disease

KEY TERMS A–Z

adenitis
add en EYE tiss

adenopathy
add en OH path ee

aden/osis

14.15 A commonly used combining form that means "gland" is aden/o. When the suffix meaning "inflammation" is included, the term _____ is formed, which can be written in its constructed form as aden/itis. Adenitis is the general term for an inflammation of a gland. Similarly, the general term for a glandular disease is _____. Also, any disease of a gland is called an **adenosis** (add en OH siss). The constructed form of adenopathy is aden/o/pathy, and adenosis is _____/_____.

adenocarcinoma
ADD eh noh kar sih NOH mah

adenoma
ADD eh NOH mah

14.16 A malignant tumor that arises from epithelial tissue to form a glandular or glandlike pattern of cells is called an _____. As a constructed term with four word parts, it is written aden/o/carcin/oma. An adenocarcinoma is a life-threatening form of cancer. It often develops from a benign tumor of glandular cells, known as an _____. An adenoma may cause excess secretion by the affected gland.

adrenalitis
add REE nah LYE tiss

adrenomegaly
add ree noh MEG ah lee

14.17 Inflammation of the adrenal gland is a condition known as _____. It may result from tumor development or infection and is often revealed in women by the symptoms of adrenal virilism (Frame 14.11). This constructed term is written adren/al/itis. A similar disease in which one or both of the adrenal glands becomes enlarged is known as _____, which has three word parts and is written adren/o/megaly. Both adrenalitis and adrenomegaly are forms of **adrenopathy** (add ren AH path ee).

cretinism
KREE tin izm

14.18 A child suffering from the thyroid gland's inability to produce normal levels of growth hormone at birth may develop the condition called **cretinism**. A reduced mental development and physical growth occur in

_____.

Cushing syndrome
KUSH ingz * SIN drohm

14.19 A **syndrome** is a disease with an array of symptoms and involving multiple organs. A syndrome that is caused by excessive secretion of the hormone cortisol by the adrenal cortex, which affects many organs, is called **Cushing syndrome**. It is characterized by obesity, moon (round) face, hyperglycemia (Frame 14.25), and muscle weakness. A common cause of _____ _____ is a tumor of the pituitary gland.

diabetes insipidus
DYE ah BEE teez * in SIP ih duss

14.20 **Diabetes insipidus** is caused by hyposecretion of ADH by the pituitary gland. The disease _____ _____ is characterized by the symptoms of polydipsia (Frame 14.13) and polyuria (Frame 14.14).

diabetes mellitus
DYE ah BEE teez * MELL ih tuss

14.21 Although the term *diabetes* is shared by both diseases, the chronic disorder of carbohydrate metabolism known as **diabetes mellitus** has very little in common with diabetes insipidus (see the Did You Know? box to read why). Diabetes mellitus (DM) is a result of resistance of body cells to insulin, or a deficiency or complete lack of insulin production by cells of the pancreas. Two major forms of _____ _____ strike human health. Type 1, which is less common, usually requires hormone replacement therapy with insulin and appears during childhood or adolescence. The more common Type 2 usually appears during adulthood and is often associated with obesity. Unlike Type 1, Type 2 can usually be managed with dietary restrictions and regular exercise, and it can be controlled with oral antidiabetic drugs. Common symptoms of both types include polydipsia (Frame 14.13), polyuria (Frame 14.14), and the presence of sugar in the urine (glycosuria). If unmanaged, diabetes mellitus causes large fluctuations in blood sugar levels, leading to circulatory deficiencies that result in kidney damage called **diabetic nephropathy** (DYE ah BET ik * nef ROHP ah thee), peripheral nerve damage known as **diabetic neuropathy** (DYE ah BET ik * noo ROH path ee), and a form of potentially sight-threatening damage to the eye called _____ _____ .

diabetic retinopathy
DYE ah BET ik * ret in NOP ah thee

Diabetes

The term *diabetes* is a Greek word that means "to pass through" or "to pass over." Another meaning is "siphon." The term was first used during the Middle Ages when a siphon was used by physicians to withdraw a sample of urine from a patient to test for an excess of sugar, which was often done by taste. The siphon "passed urine through" to a collection device. A sweet taste indicated sugar excess and a crude diagnosis of diabetes mellitus. The term *mellitus* is a Latin word that means "sweetened with honey." If the "taste test" did not indicate sweetness, but the patient still complained of excessive urination, the diagnosis was diabetes insipidus. As you might guess, the term *insipidus* is a Latin word that means "lacking flavor."

endocrinopathy
en doh krin OPP ah thee

14.22 The general term for a disease of the endocrine system is _____. It is a constructed term with four word parts, written as endo/crin/o/pathy. In most cases, endocrinopathy is the result of either an excessive production of one or more hormones by an endocrine gland or deficient production of one or more hormones. To identify which, the prefixes *hyper-* (excessive, abnormally high, or above) and *hypo-* (deficient, abnormally low, or below) are frequently used with the endocrine gland that is diseased.

hyperadrenalism
HIGH per add REN al izm

hypoadrenalism
HIGH poh add REN al izm

14.23 Excessive activity of one or more adrenal glands is the disease called _____. It is a constructed term written hyper/adren/al/ism. In time, hyperadrenalism produces the symptoms that characterize **Cushing syndrome** (Frame 14.19). The opposite disorder occurs when the adrenal gland activity becomes abnormally reduced. Called _____, it may lead to a chronic form called **Addison disease** if left untreated. The constructed form of this term is written hypo/adren/al/ism.

Addison Disease

In 1855, a series of signs and symptoms were connected for the first time into a disease. They included "feeble heart action, anemia, irritability of the stomach, and a peculiar change in the color of the skin." The syndrome was named to recognize its discoverer, the English physician Thomas Addison, who correlated the symptoms and signs to a failure of the adrenal cortex.

hypercalcemia
HIGH per kal SEE mee ah

hypocalcemia
HIGH poh kal SEE mee ah

14.24 The suffix -*emia* means "condition of blood." When calcium levels in the blood become abnormally high, the disease is known as _____. The constructed form of this term is hyper/calc/emia. The disease is a result of the abnormal release of calcium from bones, which leads to softening of the bones if left untreated. It is caused by excessive activity of the parathyroid glands. The condition of abnormally low levels of calcium in the blood is called _____ and is also called **calcipenia** (KAL sih PEE nee ah). It is caused by the abnormally low activity of the parathyroid glands to produce insufficient parathyroid hormone (PTH). *Calcipenia* is a constructed term, written as calc/i/penia.

hypoglycemia
HIGH poh glye SEE mee ah

14.25 Another use of the suffix -*emia* is in the term **hyperglycemia**, which literally means "condition of blood excessive sugar." The constructed form of this term is hyper/glyc/emia. The chronic form of the disease often indicates the body may not be producing enough insulin or insulin receptor sites are resistant and may lead to Type 2 diabetes mellitus (Frame 14.21). In the opposite condition, _____, blood sugar levels fall to abnormally low levels. It is caused by excessive insulin administration or excessive production by the pancreas and is often accompanied by headache, malaise (weakness), tremors, hunger, and anxiety. If left untreated, it can lead to coma and death.

hypoparathyroidism
HIGH poh pair ah THIGH royd izm
hypo/para/thyroid/ism

14.26 The excessive production of PTH by the parathyroid glands is a disorder known as **hyperparathyroidism**. This lengthy term contains four word parts: hyper/para/thyroid/ism. Usually caused by a tumor, it results in excessive calcium levels in the blood, or hypercalcemia (Frame 14.24). In the opposite condition called _____, PTH levels are reduced and the condition of hypocalcemia (Frame 14.24) occurs. The constructed form of this term is written ____/____/_____/____.

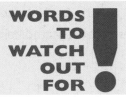
WORDS TO WATCH OUT FOR

para-
Note that the prefix *para-* doesn't always appear at the beginning of a term. In the term *hypoparathyroid*, it appears in the middle of the term. But don't let that confuse you: it is still a prefix, and it still means "alongside or abnormal."

hyperthyroidism
HIGH per THIGH royd izm

14.27 Excessive activity of the thyroid gland produces abnormally high levels of thyroid hormone in the disease _____. The constructed form of this term is hyper/thyroid/ism. Symptoms include exophthalmos (Frame 14.9), goiter (Frame 14.10), rapid heart rate, and weight loss. One form of chronic hyperthyroidism, called **Graves disease**, is believed to be an autoimmune disease. Another form known as **thyrotoxicosis** (THIGH roh toks ih KOH siss) is an acute event that is triggered by infection or trauma and can become life threatening.

hypothyroidism
HIGH poh THIGH royd izm

14.28 When thyroid gland activity becomes deficient, thyroid hormone blood levels drop below normal in the disease called _____. The constructed form is written hypo/thyroid/ism. The symptoms of hypothyroidism include a slow heart rate, dry skin, low energy, and weight gain. In the chronic form of hypothyroidism known as **myxedema** (miks eh DEE mah), the subcutaneous layer beneath the skin becomes thick and hard and the body retains water, aging the skin prematurely while puffing the face and thickening the tongue and hands. Myxedema literally means "swollen mucus."

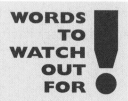
WORDS TO WATCH OUT FOR !

hyper- or *hypo-*?
The spelling of these two prefixes is very similar, but the difference in meaning is great. *Hyper-* means "excessive, abnormally high, or above"; whereas *hypo-* means "deficient, abnormally low, or below." An easy way to remember the difference is to think of the "low" sound of the word "low," which matches the sound of the vowel in *hypo-*.

hypogonadism
HIGH poh GOH nad izm

hypo/gonad/ism

14.29 In the disease **hypogonadism**, abnormally low amounts of follicle-stimulating hormone (FSH) and luteinizing hormone (LH) are produced by the pituitary gland, which reduces the production of the sex hormones testosterone (produced by the male testes) and estrogen/progesterone (produced by the female ovaries). Also known as pituitary _____, it results in reduced sexual interest and reproductive capacity. If it occurs prior to puberty, the gonads (male testes and female ovaries) fail to develop. Hypogonadism is a constructed term, which is written as _____/_____/_____.

pancreatitis
PAN kree ah TYE tiss

14.30 Inflammation of the pancreas is a disorder known as
_____. It often results in a deficient production of insulin,
which leads to hyperglycemia (Frame 14.25). Pancreatitis is an acute reaction to infection or trauma and can become life threatening. The term includes only two word parts, pancreat/itis.

pituitary gigantism
pih TOO ih tair ee * JYE gant izm

14.31 Because the pituitary gland produces numerous hormones, a tumor
or congenital defect of the pituitary can affect many body functions. In
pituitary dwarfism (pih TOO ih tair ee * DWARF izm), the pituitary
growth hormone is deficient at birth, resulting in short stature. An abnormally high production of pituitary growth hormone before adolescence results in _____ _____, and if it occurs
after adolescence, it results in acromegaly (Frame 14.8). Dwarfism and
gigantism are illustrated in Figure 14.5■.

Figure 14.5 ■
Growth hormone disorders.
Photograph of a pituitary giant and a
pituitary dwarf, both adults of about
the same age.
Source: Ewing Galloway, Inc.

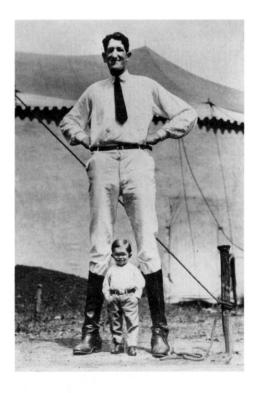

thyroiditis
THYE royd EYE tiss

14.32 Inflammation of the thyroid gland is called _____.
The constructed form is thyroid/itis. Acute thyroiditis is usually caused by a
local infection, while there are many forms of chronic thyroiditis that often
lead to hyperthyroidism (Frame 14.27).

PRACTICE: Diseases and Disorders of the Endocrine System

The Right Match _____

Match the term on the left with the correct definition on the right.

_____ 1. Addison disease

_____ 2. diabetic nephropathy

_____ 3. diabetes insipidus

_____ 4. pituitary gigantism

_____ 5. Cushing syndrome

_____ 6. Graves' disease

_____ 7. diabetic retinopathy

_____ 8. diabetes mellitus

_____ 9. pituitary dwarfism

_____ 10. cretinism

a. caused by excessive secretion of adrenal cortex

b. a form of chronic hyperthyroidism; may be an autoimmune disease

c. chronic disorder of carbohydrate metabolism

d. kidney damage caused by diabetes mellitus

e. potentially vision-threatening damage to the eye in diabetics

f. caused by hyposecretion of adrenal cortex

g. short stature resulting from a deficiency in pituitary growth hormone

h. caused by hyposecretion of ADH by the pituitary

i. reduced mental development and physical growth that results from a lack of thyroid hormone at birth

j. results from an abnormally high production of pituitary growth hormone before adolescence

Linkup _____

Link the word parts in the list to create the terms that match the definitions. You may use word parts more than once. Remember to add combining vowels when needed—and that some terms do not use any combining vowel. The first one is completed as an example.

Prefix	Combining Form	Suffix
hyper-	aden/o	-al
hypo-	adrenal/o	-emia
para-	calc/o	-ism
	carcin/o	-itis
	glyc/o	-oma
	pancreat/o	-pathy
	thyr/o	
	thyroid/o	

Definition

1. inflammation of a gland

2. glandular disease

3. malignant tumor that arises from epithelial tissue to form a glandular or glandlike pattern of cells

4. excessive activity of one or more adrenal glands

Term

1. *adenitis*

2. _____

3. _____

4. _____

5.   a disease that results from abnormally high levels of calcium in the blood   _____

6.   abnormally low blood sugar level   _____

7.   excessive production of parathyroid hormone by the parathyroid glands   _____

8.   a disease that results from abnormally low blood levels of thyroid hormone   _____

9.   inflammation of the pancreas   _____

10.   inflammation of the thyroid   _____

Treatments, Procedures, and Devices of the Endocrine System

Following are the word parts that specifically apply to the treatments, procedures, and devices of the endocrine system that are covered in the following section. Note that the word parts are color-coded to help you identify them: prefixes are blue, combining forms are red, and suffixes are purple.

Prefix	Definition	Combining Form	Definition	Suffix	Definition
endo-	within	adren/o	adrenal gland	-al	pertaining to
para-	alongside or abnormal	crin/o	to secrete	-ectomy	surgical excision or removal
		thyr/o, thyroid/o	shield, thyroid	-logy	study of
				-oma	tumor
				-tomy	incision or to cut

KEY TERMS A-Z

adrenalectomy
add REE nal EK toh mee

14.33 A procedure involving the surgical excision, or removal, of one or both of the adrenal glands is known as **adrenalectomy**. The constructed form of this term is adren/al/ectomy. An _____ may become necessary if hormone therapy fails to correct hyperadrenalism (Frame 14.23).

endocrinology
en doh krin ALL oh jee

14.34 The term *endocrine* literally means "to secrete within." The field of medicine focusing on the study and treatment of endocrine disorders is called _____. It is a constructed term that is written endo/crin/o/logy. A physician specializing in this field is known as an **endocrinologist** (en doh krin ALL oh jist). In general, any disease affecting the endocrine system is called an **endocrinopathy** (Frame 14.22).

thyroidectomy
THIGH royd EK toh mee

thyroidotomy
THIGH royd OTT oh mee

14.42 Recall the meaning of the suffix *-ectomy* is "surgical excision or removal." The surgical removal of the thyroid gland is therefore called _____. The constructed form is written thyroid/ectomy, and the procedure is illustrated in Figure 14.8■. Because the suffix *-tomy* means "incision or to cut," a _____ is a procedure in which the thyroid gland is surgically entered. This constructed term is written thyroid/o/tomy.

Figure 14.8 ■
Thyroidectomy. In this procedure, the thyroid gland is accessed by a vertical incision through the neck and removed.

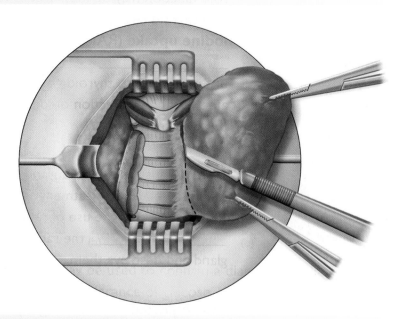

thyroparathyroidectomy
THIGH roh pair ah THIGH royd
EK toh mee
thyr/o/**para**/thyroid/ectomy

14.43 In some cases, the parathyroid glands must be surgically removed with the thyroid gland. This procedure is called _____. Write the constructed form of this term:
_____/___/_____/_____/_____.

thyroxine test
THIGH rox een

14.44 Thyroxine is one of several hormones produced by the thyroid gland. It regulates glucose metabolism and cell division in most cells of the body. A diagnostic test measuring thyroxine levels in the blood is simply called a _____ _____. It is often used as a diagnostic test for hyperthyroidism (Frame 14.27) or hypothyroidism (Frame 14.28).

PRACTICE: Treatments, Procedures, and Devices of the Endocrine System

The Right Match

Match the term on the left with the correct definition on the right.

_____ 1. fasting blood sugar

_____ 2. glucose tolerance test

_____ 3. hormone replacement therapy

_____ 4. radioactive iodine uptake

_____ 5. thyroid scan

_____ 6. thyroxine test

_____ 7. radioiodine therapy

a. synthetic or extracted hormones used to counteract hyposecretion

b. a procedure used to determine amount of iodine taken into thyroid cells

c. a test that examines a patient's tolerance of glucose

d. a procedure in which blood sugar levels are measured after a 12-hour fast

e. a diagnostic test that measures thyroxine levels in the blood

f. treatment for a thyroid tumor that targets cells within the thyroid gland and destroys them

g. a procedure that obtains an image of the thyroid to measure thyroid function

Break the Chain

Analyze these medical terms:

a) Separate each term into its word parts; each word part is labeled for you (**p** = prefix, **r** = root, **cf** = combining form, and **s** = suffix).

b) For the Bonus Question, write the requested definition in the blank that follows.

1. a) adrenalectomy _____/__/_____
                                r   s   s

   b) *Bonus Question:* What is the definition of the **first** suffix? _____

2. a) endocrinology ___/_____/__/____
                            p   cf   s

   b) *Bonus Question:* What is the definition of the combining form? _____

3. a) thyroidoma _____/____
                          r   s

   b) *Bonus Question:* What is the definition of the suffix? _____

4. a) thyroidotomy _____/__/_____
                            cf   s

   b) *Bonus Question:* What is the definition of the suffix? _____

5. a) thyroparathyroidectomy _____/__/_____/____/__/_____
                          cf   p   r   s   s

   b) *Bonus Question:* What is the definition of the **second** (last) suffix? _____

Abbreviations of the Endocrine System

The abbreviations that are associated with the endocrine system are summarized here. Study these abbreviations, and review them in the exercise that follows.

Abbreviation	Definition
ADH	antidiuretic hormone
DI	diabetes insipidus
DM	diabetes mellitus
FBS	fasting blood sugar
FSH	follicle-stimulating hormone
GH	growth hormone

Abbreviation	Definition
GTT	glucose tolerance test
HRT	hormone replacement therapy
LH	luteinizing hormone
PH	parathyroid hormone
PPBS	postprandial blood sugar
RAIU	radioactive iodine uptake

PRACTICE: Abbreviations

Fill in the blanks with the abbreviation or the complete medical term.

Abbreviation

1. GTT

2. _____

3. PPBS

4. _____

5. FBS

6. _____

7. DM

Medical Term

_____

radioactive iodine uptake

_____

diabetes insipidus

_____

hormone replacement therapy

_____

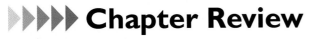 # Chapter Review

Word Building

Construct medical terms from the following meanings. The first question has been completed as an example.

1. inflammation of a gland   aden*itis*_____

2. excessive production of thyroid hormones   _____thyroidism

3. peripheral nerve damage during diabetes mellitus   diabetic neuro_____

4. inflammation of the adrenal gland   adrenal_____

5. disease of the endocrine system   _____pathy

6. excessive calcium levels in the blood   hyper_____

7. a tumor of the parathyroid gland   parathyroid_____

8. caused by too much GH in adulthood   pituitary gigant_____

9. abnormally reduced adrenal activity   _____adrenalism

10. excessive body hair   _____ism

11. deficient production of PTH   hypo_____

12. abnormally low blood sugar levels   hypo_____

13. acute form of hyperthyroidism triggered by infection or trauma   thyro_____

14. form of hypothyroidism that involves water retention and swelling   myx_____

15. caused by deficient FSH and LH that results in reduced reproductive capacity   _____gonadism

Clinical Application Exercises

Medical Report

Read the following medical report, then answer the questions that follow.

University Hospital

5500 University Avenue
Metropolis, TX

Phone: (211) 594-4000
Fax: (211) 594-4001

Medical Consultation: Endocrinology

Date: 12/15/2008

Patient: Anita Del Rio

Patient Complaint: Malaise between meals, polydipsia, polyuria, cephalalgia, difficulty sleeping.

History: 12-year-old Hispanic female, 15 pounds underweight at 75 lbs. No blood tests recorded in file prior to visit.

Family History: Father 54-year-old with Type 1 DM, Mother 44-year-old with no medical file.

Allergies: None

Evidences: Blood test positive for ketone bodies and slight acidosis; FBS 220 confirmed with GTT; urinalysis high in glucose but otherwise clear.

Treatment: Treat as Type 1 DM with regular insulin injection and follow with FBS and GTT. Place on insulin regimen and enroll in DM management class with parent.

Jonathon McClary, M.D.

---

1. What patient complaints are consistent with the signs? _____

   _____

2. Is the diagnosis temporary and capable of a cure with the prescribed treatment? _____

   _____

3. Why does the treatment plan include enrollment in a DM management class along with a parent?

   _____

   _____

Medical Report Case Study

The following Case Study provides further discussion regarding the patient in the medical report. Fill in the blanks with the correct terms. Choose your answers from the following list of terms. (Note that some terms may be used more than once.)

acidosis	glucose	ketosis
endocrinology	hyperglycemia	polydipsia
fasting blood sugar	insulin	Type 1 diabetes

A 12-year-old patient, Anita Del Rio, was referred by her personal physician for an endocrinological evaluation in the

(a) _____ department, following a four-week history of symptoms of energy loss between meals, exces-

sive thirst, or (b) _____, headache, polyuria (excessive urination), and sleeplessness. A routine blood

test had also been recorded by the physician and had shown ketone bodies in the blood, or (c) _____,

combined with a lowered blood pH, or (d) _____. Endocrinological evaluation included an FBS, or

(e) _____ _____ _____ test, followed by a

(f) _____ tolerance test, and a urinalysis. The tests indicated the patient suffered from excessive sugar

levels in the blood, or (g) _____, that was due to a failure of islet beta cells to produce proper levels of

the hormone (h) _____. A diagnosis of (i) _____ _____

_____ was recorded. The patient was treated with regular insulin, trained in self-glucose testing and

insulin administration, and referred to a local educational program in diabetes management to include her parents'

participation.

▶▶▶▶▶ Key Terms Double-Check

Remember that the chapter's key terms appeared alphabetically throughout this chapter. This exercise helps you to check your knowledge AND review for tests.

   1. First, fill in the missing word in the definitions for the chapter's key terms.

   2. Then, check your answers using Appendix F.

   3. If you got the answer right, put a check mark in the right column.

   4. If your answer was incorrect, go back to the frame number provided and review the content.

Use the checklist to study the terms you don't know until you're confident you know them all.

Key Term	Frame	Definition	Know It?
1. acidosis	14.7	the condition of _____ in the body	☐
2. acromegaly	14.8	_____ of bone structure	☐
3. adenitis	14.15	inflammation of a(n) _____	☐
4. adenocarcinoma	14.16	a malignant _____ with a glandular or glandlike pattern of cells	☐
5. adenoma	14.16	a(n) _____ tumor of glandular cells	☐
6. adenopathy	14.15	the general term for a glandular _____	☐
7. adrenalectomy	14.33	the surgical _____ of one or both of the adrenal glands	☐
8. adrenalitis	14.17	_____ of the adrenal gland	☐
9. adrenomegaly	14.17	_____ of one or both of the adrenal glands	☐
10. cretinism	14.18	a condition in which the thyroid gland is unable to produce normal levels of _____ hormone	☐
11. Cushing syndrome	14.19	a disease characterized by excessive secretion of _____ that affects many organs	☐
12. diabetes insipidus	14.20	a disease characterized by polydipsia and _____	☐
13. diabetes mellitus	14.21	a chronic disorder of _____ metabolism	☐
14. diabetic retinopathy	14.21	a form of _____ that can occur in diabetes mellitus	☐
15. endocrinology	14.34	the field of _____ that focuses on the study and treatment of endocrine disorders	☐
16. endocrinopathy	14.22	a general term for disease of the _____ system	☐
17. exophthalmos	14.9	abnormal protrusion of the _____	☐
18. fasting blood sugar	14.35	a procedure that measures blood sugar levels after a 12-hour _____	☐
19. glucose tolerance test	14.36	a test in which glucose is given orally or intravenously and blood _____ levels are measured at timed intervals	☐
20. goiter	14.10	a swelling on the anterior side of the _____ in the area of the thyroid gland	☐
21. hirsutism	14.11	excessive body _____	☐
22. hormone replacement therapy	14.37	a common therapy to counteract _____ of hormones	☐

Key Term	Frame	Definition	Know It?
23. hyperadrenalism	14.23	_____ activity of one or more adrenal glands	☐
24. hypercalcemia	14.24	abnormally high levels of _____ in the blood	☐
25. hyperglycemia	14.25	excessive sugar in the _____	☐
26. hyperparathyroidism	14.26	a disease characterized by the excessive production of parathyroid hormone (PTH) by the _____ glands	☐
27. hyperthyroidism	14.27	a disease characterized by abnormally high levels of _____ hormone	☐
28. hypoadrenalism	14.23	abnormally _____ activity of the adrenal glands	☐
29. hypocalcemia	14.24	abnormally _____ levels of calcium in the blood	☐
30. hypoglycemia	14.25	abnormally low levels of _____ in the blood	☐
31. hypogonadism	14.29	a disease characterized by abnormally low amounts of _____-stimulating hormone (FSH) and luteinizing hormone (LH)	☐
32. hypoparathyroidism	14.26	a disease characterized by the abnormally _____ production of PTH by the parathyroid glands	☐
33. hypothyroidism	14.28	a disease characterized by abnormally low levels of _____ hormone	☐
34. ketosis	14.12	a(n) _____ amount of ketone bodies in the blood and urine	☐
35. pancreatitis	14.30	inflammation of the _____	☐
36. parathyroidectomy	14.38	the _____ _____ of a parathyroid gland	☐
37. pituitary gigantism	14.31	acromegaly due to a(n) abnormally _____ amount of pituitary growth hormone	☐
38. polydipsia	14.13	excessive _____	☐
39. polyuria	14.14	the production of abnormally large volumes of _____	☐
40. radioactive iodine	14.39	a substance used in a radioactive iodine uptake test, a diagnostic procedure in which radioactive iodine is used to track and measure its entry into _____ _____ cells	☐
41. radioiodine therapy	14.40	a treatment for a thyroid tumor that involves the use of radioactive _____	☐
42. thyroid scan	14.41	a procedure in which a(n) _____ of the thyroid gland is obtained	☐
43. thyroidectomy	14.42	the surgical _____ of the thyroid gland	☐
44. thyroiditis	14.32	_____ of the thyroid gland	☐
45. thyroidoma	14.41	a thyroid _____	☐
46. thyroidotomy	14.42	a(n) _____ into the thyroid gland	☐
47. thyroparathyroid-ectomy	14.43	the surgical removal of the _____ glands as well as the thyroid gland	☐
48. thyroxine test	14.44	a diagnostic test that measures _____ levels in the blood	☐

Combining Form	Definition	Chapter
hepat/o	liver	1
hidr/o	sweat	5
hirsut/o	hairy	14
hom/o	same	4
home/o	same	4
hormon/o	to set in motion	14
hydr/o	water	11
hyster/o	uterus	1
iatr/o	physician	7
idi/o	individual	7
ile/o	ileum, to roll	10
ili/o	flank, hip, groin, ilium of the pelvis	4
immun/o	exempt, immunity	7
infer/o	below	4
inguin/o	groin	4
ir/o	iris	13
ischem/o	hold back, blockage	8
ischi/o	haunch, hip joint, ischium	6
jejun/o	empty, jejunum	10
kerat/o	horny tissue	5
ket/o	ketone	11
keton/o	ketone	11
kinesi/o	motion	6
kyph/o	hump	6
lact/o	milk	12
lamin/o	thin, lamina	6
lapar/o	abdomen	10
laryng/o	larynx, voice box	1
later/o	side	13
lei/o	smooth	12
leuk/o	white	1
lingu/o	tongue	10
lip/o	fat	10
lith/o	stone	1
lob/o	a rounded part, lobe	9
lord/o	bent forward	6
lumb/o	loin, lower back	4
lymph/o	clear water or fluid	7
mamm/o	breast	1
man/o	gas	8
mast/o	breast	1
maxim/o	biggest, highest	1
meat/o	opening, passage	11
med/o	middle	13

Combining Form	Definition	Chapter
medi/o	middle	4
melan/o	dark, black	5
men/o	month, menstruation	12
mening/o	membrane	13
menisci/o	meniscus	6
menstru/o	month, menstruation	12
ment/o	mind	1
metr/o	uterus	12
muc/o	mucus	9
muscul/o	muscle	6
my/o	muscle	6
myc/o	fungus	5
myel/o	bone marrow; spinal cord; medulla; myelin	6
myos/o	muscle	6
narc/o	numbness	13
nas/o	nose	9
nat/o	birth	1
necr/o	death	7
nephr/o	kidney	11
neur/o	nerve	1
noct/o	night	11
nosocom/o	hospital	7
nucle/o	kernel, nucleus	7
obstetr/o	midwife, prenatal development	12
ocul/o	eye	13
olig/o	few in number	11
onych/o	nail	5
oophor/o	ovary	12
ophthalm/o	eye, vision	13
opt/o	eye	13
or/o	mouth	10
orch/o	testis or testicle	12
orchi/o	testis or testicle	12
orchid/o	testis or testicle	12
orex/o	appetite	10
organ/o	tool	4
orth/o	straight	6
ost/o	bone	6
oste/o	bone	6
ot/o	ear	13
ovar/o	ovary	12
ox/o	oxygen	9
palat/o	roof of mouth, palate	10

Appendix D

Combining Forms for Terms Describing Color

Combining Form	Meaning
albin/o	white
chlor/o	green
chrom/o	color
cirrh/o	orange
cyan/o	blue
erythr/o	red
jaund/o	yellow
leuk/o	white
melan/o	black
xanth/o	yellow

5b. motion
6a. dys/troph/y
6b. process of
7a. hyper/troph/y
7b. excessive
8a. my/algia
8b. muscle
9a. ten/o/dynia
9b. condition of pain

Practice: Diseases and Disorders of the Skeletal and Muscular Systems

The Right Match
1. i
2. e
3. a
4. b
5. c
6. h
7. j
8. f
9. g
10. d

Linkup
1. (provided in chapter)
2. polymyositis
3. lordosis
4. epicondylitis
5. arthritis
6. osteomalacia
7. bursitis
8. osteitis
9. bursolith
10. meniscitis
11. tenosynovitis

Practice: Treatments, Procedures, and Devices of the Skeletal and Muscular Systems

The Right Match
1. e
2. c
3. d
4. a
5. b
6. h
7. i
8. j
9. g
10. f

Break the Chain
1a. arthr/o/desis
1b. surgical fixation
2a. chondr/ectomy
2b. cartilage
3a. crani/o/tomy
3b. no
4a. lamin/ectomy
4b. excision
5a. electr/o/my/o/graphy
5b. muscle
6a. orth/o/tic/s

6b. straight
7a. oste/o/clasis
7b. break apart
8a. ten/o/my/o/plasty
8b. surgical repair
9a. oste/o/plasty
9b. bone

Practice: Abbreviations
1. SCI
2. total knee arthroplasty
3. RA
4. Duchenne's muscular dystrophy
5. HNP
6. electromyogram
7. ACL
8. total hip replacement
9. L1 through L5
10. carpal tunnel syndrome
11. ROM
12. osteoarthritis
13. TKR
14. the twelve thoracic vertebrae
15. DJD
16. temporomandibular joint disease
17. MG

Chapter Review

Word Building
1. osteomalacia
2. osteoporosis
3. paraplegia
4. scoliosis
5. tenosynovitis
6. arthrogram
7. meniscitis
8. arthrotomy
9. myasthenia
10. myocele
11. carpal tunnel syndrome
12. arthrolysis
13. Paget's disease
14. herniated disk
15. arthroplasty
16. tenodynia
17. bursolith
18. ankylosis
19. bradykinesia
20. decalcification
21. arthrodesis
22. degenerative joint disease
23. external fixation
24. fibromyalgia
25. myeloma
26. atrophy

Medical Report
1. Broken skin at right ankle and X-rays
2. To confirm the diagnosis
3. Family history of diabetes indicates a chance of slow

healing, requiring follow-up evaluations.

Medical Report Case Study
a. compound; b. tendonitis;
c. myalgia; d. myositis;
e. polymyositis; f. Pott's;
g. tendonitis

Key Terms Double-Check
1. cartilage
2. joint
3. pain
4. inflammation
5. joints
6. puncture
7. broken
8. fixation
9. recording
10. loosened
11. repair
12. joint
13. incision
14. movement
15. development
16. slow
17. toe
18. bursa
19. inflammation
20. stone
21. wrist
22. hand
23. vertebral
24. removal
25. cartilage
26. rib
27. muscular
28. cranium
29. incision
30. calcium
31. DJD
32. disk
33. weakness
34. movement
35. development
36. electrical
37. inflammation
38. fascia
39. pain
40. bone
41. normal
42. acid
43. rupture
44. growth
45. posterior
46. anterior
47. growth
48. meniscus
49. muscle
50. serious
51. tumor
52. protrusion
53. repair
54. sutures

55. inflammation
56. pharmacological
57. orthopedic
58. excision
59. bone
60. Paget's
61. cancer
62. breaking
63. growth
64. softening
65. marrow
66. musculoskeletal
67. surgical
68. density
69. bone
70. paralysis
71. foot
72. many
73. four
74. calcium
75. shoulder
76. lateral
77. column
78. inflammation
79. tear
80. stretching
81. temporomandibular
82. tendon
83. pain
84. tendon
85. sutures
86. synovial
87. incisions
88. vertebrae

Chapter 7

Practice: Signs and Symptoms of the Blood and the Lymphatic System

The Right Match
1. d
2. a
3. i
4. g
5. b
6. c
7. f
8. e
9. h

Break the Chain
1a. & 1b. (provided in the chapter)
2a. thromb/o/penia
2b. clot
3a. leuk/o/penia
3b. abnormal reduction in
4a. hem/o/lysis
4b. loosen, dissolve
5a. leuk/o/cyt/o/penia
5b. white

Practice: Diseases and Disorders of the Blood and the Lymphatic System

The Right Match
1. b
2. c
3. h
4. g
5. a
6. d
7. f
8. e
9. j
10. i

Linkup
1. (provided in chapter)
2. thymoma
3. anemia
4. botulism
5. hematoma
6. iatrogenic
7. hemophilia
8. hemoglobinopathy
9. lymphadenitis
10. mononucleosis
11. hydrophobia

Practice: Treatments and Procedures of the Blood and the Lymphatic System

The Right Match
1. c
2. f
3. j
4. b
5. a
6. e
7. d
8. g
9. h
10. i

Break the Chain
1a. immun/o/therapy
1b. treatment
2a. splen/ectomy
2b. spleen
3a. lymph/aden/ectomy
3b. gland
4a. immun/o/logy
4b. exempt
5a. hom/o/logous
5b. same
6a. hemat/o/logy
6b. study of
7a. aut/o/logous
7b. self
8a. anti/coagulant
8b. against
9a. hem/o/stasis
9b. standing still
10a. thromb/o/lysis
10b. loosen, dissolve

Practice: Abbreviations
1. AIDS
2. complete blood count
3. PLT
4. red blood cell or red blood count
5. HGB, Hgb
6. prothrombin time
7. PTT
8. white blood cell or white blood count
9. HCT, Hct
10. human immunodeficiency virus

Chapter Review

Word Building
1. (provided in chapter)
2. anisocytosis
3. dyscrasia
4. malaria
5. erythropenia
6. hemophilia
7. leukemia
8. macrocytosis
9. staphylococcemia
10. autoimmune disease
11. polycythemia
12. poikilocytosis
13. septicemia
14. anticoagulant
15. homologous transfusion
16. hematocrit
17. hemostasis
18. platelet count
19. Hodgkin's disease
20. lymphadenitis
21. diphtheria

Medical Report
1. Persistent mild fever and body aches, tenderness of the armpit and groin lymph nodes.
2. Antibiotics may fail if the bacterial strain is resistant to its effects.
3. No.

Medical Report Case Study
a. lymphadenitis; b. lymphoma; c. Hodgkin's disease; d. spleno-megaly; e. differential count; f. infection; g. septicemia; h. staphylococcemia; i. antibiotic; j. immunodeficiency; k. immunotherapy

Key Terms Double-Check
1. immune
2. allergens
3. life threatening
4. oxygen
5. red
6. bioterrorism

7. bacterial
8. clotting
9. viruses
10. vaccine
11. healthy
12. blood
13. bacteria
14. plasma
15. infection
16. volume
17. botulinum
18. clot
19. another
20. diagnostic
21. white
22. throat
23. abnormal
24. fluid
25. reduced
26. fungal
27. bloodstream
28. red
29. blood
30. blood
31. hemoglobin
32. hemoglobin
33. rupture
34. bleeding
35. blood
36. bleeding
37. stoppage
38. lymph
39. donated
40. medical
41. cause
42. immunity
43. immune
44. study
45. reduction
46. infectious
47. destruction
48. disease
49. swelling
50. respiratory
51. cancer
52. white
53. surgical
54. lymph
55. tumor
56. large
57. liver
58. enlarged
59. death
60. hospital
61. infectious
62. platelets
63. cells
64. increase
65. treatment
66. animal
67. number
68. bacteria

69. viral
70. removal
71. spleen
72. blood
73. bacterium
74. neurotoxin
75. clot
76. platelets
77. tumor
78. toxins
79. inoculation
80. response

Chapter 8

Practice: Signs and Symptoms of the Cardiovascular System

The Right Match
1. f
2. e
3. g
4. a
5. d
6. h
7. c
8. b

Break the Chain
1a. & 1b. (provided in the chapter)
2a. brady/card/ia
2b. heart
3a. cardi/o/dynia
3b. condition of pain
4a. cardi/o/genic
4b. pertaining to producing
5a. cyan/osis
5b. blue
6a. angi/o/spasm
6b. sudden, involuntary muscle spasm

Practice: Diseases and Disorders of the Cardiovascular System

The Right Match
1. e
2. k
3. i
4. f
5. g
6. a
7. d
8. b
9. j
10. c
11. h

Linkup
1. (provided in chapter)
2. cardiomyopathy
3. atherosclerosis
4. angioma
5. pericarditis

6. angiocarditis
7. varicosis
8. thrombosis
9. hypertension

Practice: Treatments, Procedures, and Devices of the Cardiovascular System

The Right Match
1. d
2. g
3. e
4. f
5. a
6. h
7. c
8. b
9. j
10. i

Break the Chain
1a. arteri/o/gram
1b. a record or image
2a. ech/o/cardi/o/graphy
2b. sound
3a. embol/ectomy
3b. a plug
4a. sphygm/o/man/o/metry
4b. process of measuring
5a. phleb/o/tom/ist
5b. vein
6a. electr/o/cardi/o/graphy
6b. recording process
7a. cardi/o/pulmon/ary resuscitat/ion
7b. lung
8a. end/arter/ectomy
8b. within
9a. valvul/o/plasty
9b. surgical repair

Practice: Abbreviations
1. CHF
2. atrial septal defect
3. CABG
4. myocardial infarction
5. PET
6. cardiopulmonary resuscitation
7. ASHD
8. atrioventricular
9. ECG, EKG
10. coronary artery disease

Chapter Review

Word Building
1. (provided in chapter)
2. angiocarditis
3. angiostenosis
4. angioma
5. arteriosclerosis
6. bradycardia
7. cardiodynia
8. endarterectomy
9. cardiomegaly
10. endocarditis

11. dysrhythmia
12. hypertension
13. myocardial infarction
14. myocarditis
15. electrocardiography
16. phlebitis
17. angiogram
18. angioplasty
19. angioscopy
20. arteriotomy
21. auscultation
22. echocardiography

Medical Report
1. Mild chest pain that is not characteristic of angina pectoris.
2. The mild chest pain combined with the dental extractions suggests a bacterial infection that originated from the mouth.
3. Reporting the allergy to penicillin informs the team to treat with a different antibiotic to avoid complications associated with the allergy.

Medical Report Case Study
a. angina pectoris; b. cardiology; c. cardiologist; d. electrocardiography; e. stress ECHO; f. block; g. myocardial infarction; h. angiostenosis; i. atherosclerosis; j. pericarditis; k. endocarditis

Key Terms Double-Check
1. bulging
2. oxygen
3. heart
4. CAT scan
5. hemangioma
6. balloon
7. endoscope
8. muscular
9. vessel
10. catheter
11. incision
12. diastole
13. aorta
14. inflammation
15. aortogram
16. dysrhythmia
17. arteriogram
18. artery
19. elasticity
20. artery
21. plaques
22. atria
23. ventricles
24. atrioventricular
25. stethoscope
26. slow
27. cessation
28. catheter

29. SA node
30. fluid
31. cardialgia
32. originates
33. enlarged
34. myocardium
35. paralyzed
36. respiration
37. heart murmur
38. stenosis
39. CHF
40. pulmonary
41. CABG
42. coronary
43. blockage
44. graft
45. deficiency
46. momentarily
47. ultrasound
48. echocardiogram
49. ECG
50. embolus
51. clot
52. fatty
53. endocardium
54. uncoordinated
55. electrical
56. auscultation
57. varicose
58. electrocardiograph
59. essential
60. low
61. blood
62. death
63. myocardium
64. vasodilator
65. heartbeat
66. opening
67. surrounding
68. surgical
69. vein
70. phlebotomist
71. many
72. PET scan
73. bloodstream
74. sphygmomanometer
75. rapid
76. birth
77. dissolve
78. blood clots
79. exercise
80. valve
81. pool
82. birth

Chapter 9

Practice: Signs and Symptoms of the Respiratory System

The Right Match
1. i
2. f
3. d

4. e
5. a
6. b
7. c
8. j
9. g
10. h
11. k

Break the Chain
1a. & 1b. (provided in the chapter)
2a. dys/phonia
2b. condition of sound or voice
3a. dys/pnea
3b. difficult
4a. epi/staxis
4b. dripping
5a. hyper/pnea
5b. breath
6a. laryng/o/spasm
6b. larynx

Practice: Diseases and Disorders of the Respiratory System

The Right Match
1. h
2. e
3. g
4. a
5. i
6. d
7. c
8. j
9. f
10. b

Linkup
1. (provided in chapter)
2. sinusitis
3. bronchiectasis
4. tracheostenosis
5. asphyxia
6. tonsillitis
7. bronchogenic carcinoma
8. pneumoconiosis
9. tuberculosis
10. legionellosis
11. pulmonary embolism

Practice: Treatments, Procedures, and Devices of the Respiratory System

The Right Match
1. j
2. f
3. g
4. c
5. b
6. e
7. i
8. d
9. h
10. a

Break the Chain

1a. trache/o/tomy
1b. incision or to cut
2a. thora/centesis
2b. chest, thorax
3a. pneumon/ectomy
3b. lung, air
4a. bronch/o/scopy
4b. process of viewing
5a. aden/oid/ectomy
5b. resembling
6a. bronch/o/dilat/ion
6b. process
7a. lob/ectomy
7b. round part, lobe
8a. rhin/o/plasty
8b. nose
9a. sept/o/plasty
9b. surgical repair

Practice: Abbreviations

1. LTB
2. hyaline membrane disease
3. TB
4. adult (or acute) respiratory distress syndrome
5. CXR
6. cardiopulmonary resuscitation
7. CF
8. upper respiratory infection

Chapter Review

Word Building

1. (provided in chapter)
2. anoxia
3. bronchitis
4. respiratory distress syndrome (or ARDS, HMD, or NRDS)
5. auscultation
6. hypoxia
7. dyspnea
8. hypercapnia
9. bronchiectasis
10. pneumoconiosis
11. bronchogenic carcinoma
12. cystic fibrosis
13. tracheitis
14. asphyxia
15. bronchogram
16. pleurocentesis (or thoracentesis)
17. oximetry

Medical Report

1. Dyspnea, thoracalgia, and malaise support the diagnosis of TB infection.
2. It is likely that the TB infection originated from exposure brought home by either of his parents.
3. The greatest threat to full recovery is the resistivity of the TB strain to antibiotics.

Medical Report Case Study

a. coryza (or acute rhinitis);
b. laryngotracheobronchitis;
c. bronchodilating; d. tuberculosis (TB); e. acid-fast; f. tuberculosis; g. chest X-rays

Key Terms Double-Check

1. absence
2. TB (or tuberculosis)
3. adenoid
4. oxygen
5. histamines
6. voice
7. inability
8. carbon dioxide
9. absence
10. suction
11. narrowing
12. alveoli
13. sounds
14. slowing
15. dilation
16. inflammation
17. inhaler
18. cancer
19. X-ray
20. lobar
21. viewing
22. contraction
23. computed tomography
24. radiograph
25. breathing
26. obstruction
27. fungal
28. infection
29. cough
30. mucus
31. voice
32. breathing
33. respiratory
34. chronic
35. trachea
36. inflammation
37. nose
38. expel
39. blood
40. pleural
41. excessive
42. breathing
43. rapid
44. shallow
45. gas
46. low
47. expansion
48. removal
49. inflammation
50. laryngoscope
51. contractions
52. incision
53. pneumonia
54. lobe
55. adenocarcinoma
56. respiratory

57. nose
58. mist
59. breathe
60. oxygen
61. convulsion
62. coughing
63. pharynx
64. fluid
65. inflammation
66. puncture
67. dust
68. lung
69. viral
70. cause
71. air
72. circulation
73. injury
74. clot
75. capacity
76. respiratory
77. pus
78. adults
79. breathing
80. nasal
81. repair
82. viral
83. inflammation
84. lungs
85. rapid
86. tuberculosis
87. pain
88. fluid
89. puncture
90. incision
91. inflammation
92. trachea
93. repair
94. narrowing
95. opening
96. surgical
97. infection
98. nasal
99. nuclear

Chapter 10

Practice: Signs and Symptoms of the Digestive System

The Right Match

1. c
2. a
3. b
4. f
5. i
6. e
7. h
8. d
9. g

Break the Chain

1a. & 1b. (provided in the chapter)
2a. dys/peps/ia

2b. digestion
3a. gastr/o/dynia
3b. stomach
4a. hemat/emesis
4b. vomiting
5a. steat/o/rrhea
5b. fat
6a. hepat/o/megal/y
6b. liver

Practice: Diseases and Disorders of the Digestive System

The Right Match

1. i
2. j
3. n
4. c
5. k
6. l
7. e
8. a
9. h
10. b
11. g
12. f
13. o
14. r
15. p
16. m
17. d
18. q

Linkup

1. (provided in chapter)
2. glossitis
3. cholelithiasis
4. proctoptosis
5. hepatoma
6. gastromalacia
7. esophagitis
8. gastroenteritis
9. pancreatitis
10. dysentery
11. anorexia nervosa
12. polyposis

Practice: Treatments, Procedures, and Devices of the Digestive System

The Right Match

1. f
2. c
3. h
4. g
5. e
6. d
7. i
8. a
9. j
10. b

Break the Chain

1a. anti/emetic
1b. vomiting
2a. gloss/o/rrhaphy

2b. tongue
3a. sigmoid/o/scopy
3b. the letter S (sigmoid)
4a. hemorrhoid/ectomy
4b. surgical removal
5a. lapar/o/tomy
5b. abdomen, abdominal cavity
6a. pylor/o/plasty
6b. surgical repair
7a. anti/diarrhe/al
7b. against
8a. gingiv/ectomy
8b. gums
9a. vag/o/tomy
9b. incision

Practice: Abbreviations
1. barium enema
2. IBD
3. upper GI series
4. GERD
5. nausea and vomiting
6. UGI
7. irritable bowel syndrome
8. LGI
9. stool culture and sensitivity
10. GI
11. fecal occult blood test
12. EGD

Chapter Review
Word Building
1. (provided in chapter)
2. hepatomegaly
3. dysphagia
4. cheilitis
5. cholecystitis
6. cholelithiasis
7. colitis
8. colorectal cancer
9. enteritis
10. gastromalacia
11. diverticulosis
12. hepatoma
13. sialoadenitis
14. hemorrhoidectomy
15. colostomy
16. proctoscopy
17. laparoscopy
18. glossorrhaphy
19. polypectomy

Medical Report
1. Crohn's disease
2. Progressive intestinal pain with diarrhea and cramping, inflammation of the ileum
3. A laparoscopy would observe the external features of the ileum, and a SCS would determine if infection is a possible cause.

Medical Report Case Study
a. diarrhea; b. flatus; c. constipation; d. lactose intolerance;
e. irritable bowel syndrome;
f. Crohn's disease; g. inflammatory bowel; h. barium enema;
i. laparoscopy; j. diverticulitis;
k. intussusception; l. colectomy

Key Terms Double-Check
1. paracentesis
2. eating disorder
3. acidity
4. vomiting
5. peristalsis
6. eating
7. removal
8. appendix
9. abdomen
10. gorging
11. waves
12. inflammation
13. suturing
14. removal
15. gallstones
16. cholecystogram
17. common bile duct
18. gallstones
19. gallbladder
20. connective
21. space
22. colon
23. ulcerative colitis
24. polyp
25. anus
26. infrequent
27. regional ileitis
28. watery
29. diverticula
30. duodenum
31. GI
32. indigestion
33. swallowing
34. small
35. reflux
36. FOBT
37. gas
38. botulism
39. stretching
40. entire
41. stomach
42. irrigated
43. ulcer
44. stomach
45. gastralgia
46. small
47. GERD
48. softening
49. nose
50. infection
51. endoscope
52. shake
53. gums
54. gingiva
55. tongue
56. repair
57. breath
58. blood
59. hemorrhoids
60. swollen
61. viral-induced
62. hepatocellular
63. enlargement
64. hiatus
65. opening
66. IBD
67. infolding
68. chronic
69. liver
70. enzyme
71. incision
72. absorbing
73. N&V
74. pancreas
75. mumps
76. tract
77. membrane
78. polyps
79. cancer
80. anus
81. prolapse
82. valve
83. regurgitation
84. feces
85. SCS
86. vagus
87. twisting

Chapter 11

Practice: Signs and Symptoms of the Urinary System
The Right Match
1. g
2. c
3. i
4. f
5. b
6. e
7. a
8. h
9. d

Break the Chain
1a. & 1b. (provided in chapter)
2a. azot/emia
2b. urea, nitrogen
3a. dys/uria
3b. pertaining to urine or urination
4a. an/uresis
4b. without or absence of
5a. py/uria
5b. pus

Practice: Diseases and Disorders of the Urinary System
The Right Match
1. b
2. c
3. e
4. f
5. a
6. d
7. j
8. g
9. i
10. k
11. h
12. m
13. l

Linkup
1. (provided in chapter)
2. glomerulonephritis
3. pyelonephritis
4. nephrolithiasis
5. hydronephrosis
6. nephroma
7. pyelitis

Practice: Treatments, Procedures, and Devices of the Urinary System
The Right Match
1. d
2. e
3. a
4. b
5. c
6. h
7. k
8. i
9. l
10. f
11. g
12. j

Break the Chain
1a. cyst/o/graphy
1b. recording process
2a. cyst/o/lith/o/tomy
2b. incision or to cut
3a. lith/o/tripsy
3b. stone
4a. hem/o/dia/lysis
4b. through
5a. cyst/o/rrhaphy
5b. no
6a. nephr/o/lysis
6b. loosen or dissolve
7a. nephr/o/gram
7b. a record or image
8a. nephr/o/tom/o/graphy
8b. kidney
9a. ureter/o/stomy
9b. surgical creation of an opening

Practice: Abbreviations
1. urinalysis
2. RP
3. catheter, catheterization
4. VCUG
5. intravenous pyelogram
6. UTI
7. hemodialysis

Chapter Review

Word Building

1. (provided in chapter)
2. anuria
3. bacteriuria
4. cystolith
5. nephritis
6. hematuria
7. ureterocele
8. enuresis
9. nephrolithiasis
10. nephropexy
11. pyelostomy
12. urethroplasty
13. ureterotomy
14. cystogram
15. nephrography
16. intravenous pyelogram
17. nephroscope
18. blood urea nitrogen (BUN)
19. urinometer
20. urinalysis

Medical Report

1. Lumbar pain, malaise, hematuria, loss of appetite, generalized body aches
2. Yes; mother lost a kidney at 72 years old due to polycystic disease.
3. Dialysis is ordered prior to surgery to stabilize the patient's condition, which will reduce the surgical risk of death.

Medical Report Case Study

a. urinalysis; b. albuminuria; c. hematuria; d. nephroto-mography; e. nephroscopy; f. nephromegaly; g. polycystic kidney disease; h. pyelonephritis; i. hemodialysis; j. renal transplant

Key Terms Double-Check

1. urine
2. inability
3. day
4. blood
5. bacteria
6. kidney
7. protein
8. removal
9. bladder
10. herniation
11. cystography
12. stone
13. incision
14. repair
15. suturing
16. bladder
17. opening
18. incision
19. image

20. urine
21. pain
22. involuntary
23. congenital
24. electric
25. inflammation
26. glucose
27. blood
28. remove
29. blockage
30. ventrally
31. urination
32. abnormal
33. crush (or dissolve)
34. removal
35. kidney
36. tumor
37. image
38. stones
39. medical
40. loosens
41. kidney
42. enlargement
43. fixation
44. downward
45. nephroscope
46. ultrasound
47. kidney
48. structure
49. night
50. reduced
51. cleanse (or filter)
52. numerous (or many)
53. excessive
54. urine
55. renal
56. cystoscope
57. removal
58. nephrons
59. repair
60. pus
61. donor
62. kidney
63. density
64. abnormal
65. blood
66. surgical removal
67. ureter
68. herniated
69. stones
70. opening
71. fixation
72. surgical repair
73. urethra
74. incision
75. urine
76. bladder
77. observe (or view)
78. accumulation (or retention)
79. kidneys
80. urethra
81. instrument

82. urology
83. stabilizes

Chapter 12

Practice: Signs and Symptoms of the Male Reproductive System

The Right Match
1. d
2. a
3. b
4. e
5. c

Break the Chain
1a. & 1b. (provided in chapter)
2a. oligo/sperm/ia
2b. little
3a. test/algia
3b. testis
4a. urethr/itis
4b. inflammation
5a. a/sperm/ia
5b. without or absence of

Practice: Diseases and Disorders of the Male Reproductive System

The Right Match
1. d
2. a
3. e
4. b
5. f
6. c

Linkup
1. (provided in chapter)
2. balanitis
3. epididymitis
4. hydrocele
5. varicocele

Practice: Treatments, Procedures, and Devices of the Male Reproductive System

The Right Match
1. c
2. a
3. e
4. b
5. d

Break the Chain
1a. vas/ectomy
1b. vas deferens
2a. hydr/o/cel/ectomy
2b. hernia, swelling, or protrusion
3a. orchid/o/pexy
3b. testis
4a. prostat/ectomy
4b. surgical removal
5a. vas/o/vas/o/stomy
5b. surgical creation of an opening

Practice: Signs and Symptoms of the Female Reproductive System

Linkup
1. amenorrhea
2. colpodynia
3. mastalgia
4. menorrhagia
5. hematosalpinx
6. oligomenorrhea

Practice: Diseases and Disorders of the Female Reproductive System

The Right Match
1. b
2. c
3. a
4. e
5. f
6. d
7. i
8. g
9. j
10. k
11. h

Break the Chain
1a. vulv/itis
1b. vulva
2a. salping/o/cele
2b. fallopian tube
3a. a/mast/ia
3b. breast
4a. endo/metr/i/osis
4b. within
5a. lei/o/my/oma
5b. smooth

Practice: Treatments, Procedures, and Devices of the Female Reproductive System

The Right Match
1. i
2. e
3. a
4. h
5. c
6. g
7. d
8. b
9. f

Linkup
1. vulvectomy
2. colpoplasty
3. gynecology
4. hysterectomy
5. colporrhaphy
6. hysteropexy
7. mammogram
8. oophorectomy
9. salpingectomy

Practice: Signs and Symptoms of Obstetrics

Break the Chain
1a. dys/toc/ia
1b. condition of
2a. hyper/emesis
2b. excessive
3a. pseud/o/cyesis
3b. false
4a. poly/hydr/amni/o/s
4b. amnion

Practice: Diseases and Disorders of Obstetrics

The Right Match
1. c
2. f
3. a
4. h
5. g
6. b
7. e
8. d

Practice: Treatments, Procedures, and Devices of Obstetrics

The Right Match
1. d
2. a
3. f
4. c
5. b
6. e

Linkup
1. amniocentesis
2. episiotomy
3. fetometry

Practice: Sexually Transmitted Infections (STIs)

The Right Match
1. c
2. i
3. f
4. h
5. a
6. b
7. e
8. g
9. d

Practice: Abbreviations
1. prostate-specific antigen
2. STI
3. human immunodeficiency virus
4. TURP
5. benign prostatic hyperplasia
6. AIDS
7. hyaline membrane disease
8. HBV
9. herpes simplex virus type 2
10. DRE

11. human papilloma virus
12. CIN
13. dilation and curettage
14. CIS
15. hormone replacement therapy
16. RDS
17. premenstrual syndrome
18. TAB
19. toxic shock syndrome
20. PID
21. transvaginal sonography
22. GYN
23. biopsy
24. Pap smear
25. erectile dysfunction
26. FBD
27. obstetrics
28. C-section
29. obstetrics/gynecology
30. SAB
31. pregnancy-induced hypertension
32. FAS
33. infiltrating ductal carcinoma

Chapter Review

Word Building
1. (provided in chapter)
2. testicular carcinoma
3. priapism
4. phimosis
5. circumcision
6. hepatitis
7. orchidotomy
8. cryptorchidism
9. oligospermia
10. orchitis
11. varicocele
12. amenorrhea
13. leukorrhea
14. mastalgia
15. menorrhagia
16. oligomenorrhea
17. endometriosis
18. cervicitis
19. hysteratresia
20. mastoptosis
21. vulvovaginitis
22. prolapsed uterus
23. salpingo-oophorectomy
24. episiotomy
25. hysteroscopy
26. mammography
27. pseudocyesis
28. abortion
29. abruptio placentae
30. amniorrhea
31. balanoplasty
32. orchidectomy
33. dysmenorrhea
34. hyperemesis gravidarum

Medical Report
1. Dysmenorrhea, menorrhagia are both consistent with evidences that point to CIS.
2. A Pap smear was performed to evaluate stages of cervical cell changes as an examination for CIS, which is characterized by cell changes.
3. A cervicectomy is a suitable treatment for CIS because in this condition the cancer cells are localized to the cervix and have not yet metastasized.

Medical Report Case Study
a. dysmenorrhea; b. menorrhagia; c. leukorrhea; d. dilation and curettage; e. Papanicolaou (Pap) smear; f. HPV (human papillomavirus); g. colposcopy; h. carcinoma in situ of the cervix; i. cervical conization

Key Terms Double-Check
1. therapeutic
2. pregnancy
3. placenta
4. immunodeficiency
5. lack
6. absence
7. fluid
8. amnion
9. ruptured
10. males
11. testes
12. dysfunction
13. sperm
14. semen
15. glans
16. penis
17. discharge
18. BPH
19. analysis
20. tumor
21. presentation
22. fungi
23. CIS
24. neoplasia
25. cone-shaped
26. cervix
27. cervix
28. C-section
29. ulcers
30. bacterial
31. prepuce
32. vaginectomy
33. vaginal
34. repair
35. suturing
36. abnormality

37. implantation
38. cryptorchism
39. protrusion
40. rectum
41. D&C
42. pain
43. labor
44. hypertension
45. uterus
46. lasers
47. uterus
48. pelvic
49. bacterial
50. epididymis
51. perineum
52. ED
53. hemolytic
54. mother
55. sonography
56. cysts
57. rectovaginal
58. HSV-2
59. STI
60. OB/GYN
61. women
62. fallopian
63. liver
64. HRT
65. HPV
66. premature
67. scrotum
68. hydrocele
69. fluid
70. emesis
71. closure
72. uterus
73. prolapsed
74. hysteroscope
75. milk
76. laparoscope
77. fibroid tumors
78. vagina
79. mammogram
80. enlargement
81. breast
82. radical
83. lactiferous
84. pendulous
85. bleeding
86. ovulation
87. physician
88. OB
89. reduced
90. low
91. ovary
92. ovary
93. castration
94. orchiopexy
95. orchidoplasty, orchioplasty
96. cancer
97. benign
98. Pap smear

99. mucous
100. PID
101. prosthesis
102. erectile
103. prepuce
104. lower
105. excessive
106. symptoms
107. persistent
108. displaced
109. prostatic
110. removal
111. PSA
112. prostate
113. abnormal
114. pregnancy
115. pus
116. fallopian
117. inflammation
118. protrusion
119. fixation
120. ultrasound
121. spirochete
122. orchialgia
123. seminoma
124. spermatic
125. TSS
126. cats
127. removal
128. probe
129. single
130. sterilization
131. urethra
132. urinary
133. visual
134. colpitis
135. herniation
136. sperm
137. vasectomy
138. seminal
139. vulva
140. vulva

Chapter 13

Practice: Signs and Symptoms of the Nervous System

The Right Match
1. e
2. d
3. g
4. h
5. c
6. b
7. a
8. f

Linkup
1. (provided in chapter)
2. hyperalgesia
3. polyneuralgia
4. hyperesthesia
5. neurasthenia

6. neuralgia
7. paresthesia

Practice: Diseases and Disorders of the Nervous System

The Right Match
1. k
2. e
3. g
4. a
5. h
6. j
7. c
8. f
9. d
10. i
11. b

Break the Chain
1a. & 1b. (provided in chapter)
2a. cerebell/itis
2b. little brain or cerebellum
3a. encephal/itis
3b. brain
4a. epi/lepsy
4b. seizure
5a. mening/itis
5b. inflammation
6a. para/plegia
6b. paralysis
7a. neur/oma
7b. tumor
8a. neur/itis
8b. nerve

Practice: Treatments, Procedures, and Devices of the Nervous System

The Right Match
1. e
2. c
3. d
4. b
5. g
6. a
7. f

Linkup
1. anesthesia
2. craniectomy
3. neurology
4. craniotomy
5. neurorrhaphy
6. psychiatry
7. vagotomy
8. psychology

Practice: Mental Health Diseases and Disorders

The Right Match
1. f
2. c
3. e
4. b
5. d
6. a

Break the Chain
1a. dys/lexia
1b. bad, abnormal, painful, or difficult
2a. neur/osis
2b. nerve
3a. psych/o/pathy
3b. disease
4a. psych/osis
4b. mind
5a. schiz/o/phren/ia
5b. condition of

Practice: Eye Diseases and Disorders

The Right Match
1. d
2. e
3. b
4. c
5. a

Linkup
1. conjunctivitis
2. diplopia
3. astigmatism
4. blepharitis
5. retinopathy
6. ophthalmopathy

Practice: Eye Treatments, Procedures, and Devices

The Right Match
1. c
2. d
3. b
4. a

Break the Chain
1a. opt/o/metrist
1b. eye
2a. dacry/o/cyst/o/rhin/o/stomy
2b. surgical creation of an opening
3a. ophthalm/o/logist
3b. eye

Practice: Medical Terms of the Ear and Hearing

The Right Match
1. c
2. d
3. b
4. a

Linkup
1. otitis
2. otosclerosis
3. otalgia
4. mastoiditis

Practice: Abbreviations
1. EP
2. positron emission tomography
3. OM
4. electroencephalogram
5. CAT scan
6. magnetic resonance imaging

7. PD
8. cerebral palsy
9. EchoEG
10. deep tendon reflexes
11. MS
12. cerebrovascular accident
13. AD
14. amyotrophic lateral sclerosis
15. ADD
16. attention deficit hyperactivity disorder
17. Ast
18. emmetropia
19. LASIK
20. intraocular lens

Chapter Review

Word Building
1. hyperalgesia
2. cephalalgia
3. cerebellitis
4. cerebrovascular disease
5. glioma
6. encephalomalacia
7. neuropathy
8. hyperesthesia
9. encephalitis
10. meningocele
11. multiple sclerosis
12. myelitis
13. neurasthenia
14. neuroma
15. neuralgia
16. paresthesia
17. hemiplegia
18. polyneuritis
19. psychopathy
20. quadriplegia
21. hydrocephalus
22. craniectomy
23. craniotomy
24. neurorrhaphy
25. neurolysis
26. neurotomy
27. ventriculitis
28. neurologist
29. psychopharmacology
30. psychotherapy
31. mania
32. phobia
33. keratitis

Medical Report
1. The early sign is the polyneuritis reported on the left limb and shoulder, which indicates possible brain damage to the right side.
2. The primary possible consequence to the patient is brain damage to the right temporal lobe.

Medical Report Case Study
a. cephalalgia; b. neuralgia;
c. polyneuritis; d. analgesics;
e. paresthesia; f. computed
tomography; g. magnetic
resonance imaging;
h. intracranial; i. craniotomy

Key Terms Double-Check
1. inability
2. brain
3. muscle
4. pain
5. surgical
6. anxiety
7. speak
8. attention
9. congenital
10. paralysis
11. high
12. eyelid
13. drooping
14. lens
15. donor
16. headache
17. inflammation
18. wall
19. brain
20. close
21. bleeding
22. paralysis
23. blood
24. decreased
25. brain
26. shaking
27. inflammation
28. spasms
29. cornea
30. removal
31. incision
32. lacrimal
33. nasal (or nose)
34. rocky (or rocklike)
35. loss
36. eye
37. double
38. reverses
39. ultrasound
40. neurological
41. electrical
42. brain
43. softening
44. anesthetic
45. seizures
46. waves
47. removal
48. pressure
49. tumor
50. infection
51. fluid
52. painful
53. excessive
54. inflammation

55. corneum
56. spinal
57. deterioration
58. magnets
59. high
60. mastoid (or part that
    resembles a breast)
61. dizziness
62. tumor
63. meninges
64. protrusion
65. spinal cord
66. brain
67. spinal cord
68. photograph
69. procedure
70. sleep
71. nerve
72. fatigue
73. removal
74. inflammation
75. nervous
76. separating
77. tumor
78. disease
79. repair
80. suture
81. mental
82. nerve
83. softening
84. paralysis
85. hemorrhage
86. eyes
87. pain
88. ear
89. disease
90. discharge
91. bone
92. visual
93. delusions
94. paralysis
95. numbness
96. tremors
97. fear
98. inflammation
99. many
100. inflammation
101. nervous
102. flow
103. trauma
104. medicine
105. human (or mind, mental)
106. mental
107. distortion
108. mind
109. behavioral
110. infection
111. incisions
112. root
113. touch
114. disease
115. hallucinations

116. loss
117. severed (with an incision)
118. inflammation
119. sensation
120. reduction

Chapter 14

Practice: Signs and Symptoms of the Endocrine System

The Right Match
1. d
2. e
3. a
4. b
5. c

Break the Chain
1a. & 1b. (provided in chapter)
2a. ex/ophthalm/o/s
2b. eye
3a. poly/uria
3b. pertaining to urine
    or urination
4a. acr/o/megaly
4b. extremity
5a. ket/o/acid/osis
5b. ketone

Practice: Diseases and Disorders of the Endocrine System

The Right Match
1. f
2. d
3. h
4. j
5. a
6. b
7. e
8. c
9. g
10. i

Linkup
1. (provided in chapter)
2. adenopathy
3. adenocarcinoma
4. hyperadrenalism
5. hypercalcemia
6. hypoglycemia
7. hyperparathyroidism
8. hypothyroidism
9. pancreatitis
10. thyroiditis

Practice: Treatments, Procedures, and Devices of the Endocrine System

The Right Match
1. d
2. c
3. a
4. b
5. g

6. e
7. f

Break the Chain
1a. adren/al/ectomy
1b. pertaining to
2a. endo/crin/o/logy
2b. to secrete
3a. thyroid/oma
3b. tumor
4a. thyroid/o/tomy
4b. incision or to cut
5a. thyr/o/para/thyr/oid/ectomy
5b. surgical excision or removal

Practice: Abbreviations
1. glucose tolerance test
2. RAIU
3. postprandial blood sugar
4. DI
5. fasting blood sugar
6. HRT
7. diabetes mellitus

Chapter Review

Word Building
1. (provided in chapter)
2. hyperthyroidism
3. diabetic neuropathy
4. adrenalitis
5. endocrinopathy
6. hypercalcemia
7. parathyroidoma
8. pituitary gigantism
9. hypoadrenalism
10. hirsutism
11. hypoparathyroidism
12. hypoglycemia
13. thyrotoxicosis
14. myxedema
15. hypogonadism

Medical Report
1. Malaise between meals,
   polydipsia, polyuria,
   cephalalgia
2. No, the diagnosis is lifelong
   and not presently curable.
3. The patient is a minor,
   which demands parental
   participation.

Case Study
a. endocrinology; b. polydipsia;
c. ketosis; d. acidosis; e. fasting
blood sugar; f. glucose; g. hyperglycemia; h. insulin; i. type I
diabetes

Key Terms Double-Check
1. acid
2. enlargement
3. gland
4. tumor
5. benign
6. disease

7. removal
8. inflammation
9. enlargement
10. growth
11. cortisol
12. polyuria
13. carbohydrate
14. blindness
15. medicine
16. endocrine
17. eyes

18. fast
19. sugar
20. neck
21. hair
22. hyposecretion
23. excessive
24. calcium
25. blood
26. parathyroid
27. thyroid
28. low

29. low
30. sugar
31. follicle
32. low
33. thyroid
34. excessive (or high)
35. pancreas
36. surgical removal
37. high
38. thirst
39. urine

40. thyroid gland
41. iodine
42. image
43. removal
44. inflammation
45. tumor
46. incision
47. parathyroid
48. thyroxine

Glossary-Index ▶▶▶▶

Terms that appear in boldface are Key Terms from the chapters. Definitions are provided here for these terms.

Body (*cont.*)
   organization of, 60–80
   planes, 69*f*
   regions of, 69–71, 70*t*
   systems in, 63–66
Bone grafting, a procedure that stimulates the healing process of a fracture, 145
Bones, 118
   of skeleton, 120*f*
   parts of, 119*f*
Botulism, life-threatening food-borne illness caused by *Clostridium botulinum,* 170, 292
Bowman's capsule, a hollow, ball-shaped structure located at one end of a nephron that includes an internal membrane that filters fluid passing out of the glomerulus; named for its 18th-century discoverer, Sir William Bowman, abbreviated BC, 324*f*
BPH. *See* **Benign prostatic hyperplasia**
Bradycardia, an abnormally slow heart rate, 52, 203
Bradykinesia, abnormally slow movements, 52, 123
Bradypnea, abnormal slowing of the breathing rhythm, 240
Brain, 425, 426*f*, 428
Breast cancer, a malignant tumor arising from breast tissue, 381, 381*f*
Breech, abnormal childbirth presentation in which the buttocks, feet, or knees appear through the birth canal first, 399
Bronchiectasis, abnormal dilation of the bronchi, 247
Bronchiole, 237
Bronchitis, inflammation of the bronchi, 247
Bronchodilation, procedure that uses a bronchodilating agent in an inhaler to reduce bronchial constriction, 257
Bronchogenic carcinoma, aggressive form of cancer in cells of the bronchi, 247, 247*f*
Bronchogram, X-ray image of the bronchi, 258
Bronchography, the X-ray imaging of the bronchi using a contrast medium to highlight the bronchial tree, 258
Bronchopneumonia, acute inflammatory disease that involves the bronchioles and alveoli; also called lobar pneumonia, 248
Bronchoscope, a modified endoscope that is a flexible fiber-optic tube with a small lens and eyepiece for viewing the bronchi on a computer monitor, 258
Bronchoscopy, evaluation of the trachea and bronchi using a bronchoscope, which is inserted through the nose, 258*f*
Bronchospasm, a narrowing of the airway caused by contraction of smooth muscles in the bronchioles, 29, 240
Bulimia, eating disorder involving repeated gorging with food followed by induced vomiting or laxative abuse, 289
BUN. *See* **Blood urea nitrogen**
Bunion, abnormal enlargement of the joint at the base of the big toe, 128
Burn, caused by excessive exposure to fire, chemicals, or sunlight and measured by total body surface area (TBSA) and depth of the damage, 94
   classification, 95*f*
Bursectomy, a surgery involving the removal of a bursa from a joint, 143
Bursitis, inflammation of a bursa, 129
Bursolith, a calcium deposit or stone within a bursa, 129
Bx. *See* **Biopsy**

C
CABG. *See* **Coronary artery bypass graft**
CAD. *See* **Coronary artery disease**
Calcipenia. *See* **Hypocalcemia**
Cancer, 239
Candida albicans, 407
Candidiasis, infection by the yeastlike fungi, *Candida albicans,* often sexually transmitted, 407
Carbon dioxide, 237
Carbuncle, a skin infection composed of a cluster of boils, 95, 95*f*

Carcinoma, skin cancer; varieties include basal cell carcinoma and squamous cell carcinoma, 95
Carcinoma in situ, a form of cervical cancer that arises from cells of the cervix; abbreviated CIS of the cervix, 382
Cardiac arrest, the cessation of heart activity, 209
Cardiac catheterization, insertion of a narrow flexible tube, called a catheter, through a blood vessel leading into the heart, 218
Cardiac or coronary angiography, a diagnostic procedure that includes X-ray photography, MRI, or CAT scan images of the heart after injection of a contrast medium; a form of angiography, 216
Cardiac pacemaker, a battery-powered device that is implanted under the skin and wired to the SA node in the heart to produce timed electric pulses that replace the function of the SA node, 218, 218*f*
Cardiac tamponade, acute compression of the heart due to the accumulation of fluid within the pericardial cavity, 209
Cardiac ultrasonography, another term for echocardiography, an ultrasound procedure that directs sound waves through the heart to evaluate heart function; recorded data is typically called an echocardiogram, 221
Cardialgia, heart pain, more frequently called cardiodynia, 203
Cardiodynia, heart pain, less frequently called cardialgia, 203
Cardiogenic, a symptom or sign that originates from a condition of the heart, 203
Cardiologist, 201
Cardiology, the study of the heart; a clinical ward specializing in the treatment of heart disease, 10, 12, 23
Cardiomegaly, an enlarged heart, which occurs when the heart must work harder than normal to meet the oxygen demands of body cells, 209
Cardiomyopathy, the general term for a disease of the myocardium of the heart, 210
Cardioplasty, 12
Cardioplegia, a sign in which the heart has become paralyzed, 203
Cardiopulmonary, pertaining to the heart and lungs, 12
Cardiopulmonary resuscitation, artificial respiration that is used to restore breathing by applying a combination of chest compression and artificial ventilation at intervals, 219, 263
Cardiovalvulitis, inflammation of the valves of the heart that is usually diagnosed from the presence of a heart murmur, which is a gurgling sound detected during auscultation, 210
Cardiovascular, 198, 201
Cardiovascular system, 63, 197–234, 199*f*
   abbreviations of, 226
   anatomy and physiology, 198–200
   clinical application exercises for, 228–29
   diseases and disorders of, 205–15
   medical terms of, 201
   signs and symptoms of, 201–4
   treatments, procedures, devices of, 216–24
Carpal tunnel syndrome, a repetitive stress injury of the wrist, 129, 141*f*
Carpoptosis, weakness of the wrist that results in difficulty supporting the hand, 129
Castration, 374
CAT scan, acronym for computed axial tomography scanning, it is a diagnostic imaging procedure that uses X-ray technology with computer enhancement and analysis to observe internal body structures, 77, 78, 78*f*, 283
Cataract, a condition in which the eye lens transparency is reduced, 454
Cataract extraction, the surgical removal of a cataract and replacement with a donor lens, 459, 459*f*
Cathartic, an agent that stimulates strong waves of peristalsis of the colon, 304
Catheter, 218, 348
Cavities, internal spaces of the body that are lined with a membrane and house one or more organs, 71, 72*f*

CBC. *See* **Complete blood count**

Cecum, 281

Cell, the most basic unit of life, 61

Cellulite, a local uneven surface of the skin caused by fat deposition, 86

Cellulitis, inflammation of the connective tissue in the dermis caused by an infection, 96, 96*f*

Cephalalgia, the clinical term for a headache, or a generalized pain in the region of the head, 429

Cerebellitis, inflammation of the cerebellum, 433

Cerebellum, 426

Cerebral aneurysm, a protruding wall of a blood vessel in the brain, 433, 433*f*

Cerebral angiography, a diagnostic procedure that reveals blood flow to the brain by X-ray photography, 443, 443*f*

Cerebral atherosclerosis, accumulation of fatty plaques that cause arteries supplying the brain to gradually close, 433

Cerebral concussion, physical damage to the cerebrum that often results in hemorrhage (bleeding) and the subsequent loss of brain cells and mental function, 435

Cerebral embolism, a moving blood clot in an artery of the brain, 433

Cerebral hemorrhage, bleeding from cerebral blood vessels, 433

Cerebral palsy, a condition that appears at birth or shortly afterward as a partial muscle paralysis, 434

Cerebral thrombosis, condition of a stationary blood clot in an artery of the brain, 433

Cerebrovascular accident, irreversible death of brain cells caused by inadequate blood supply to the brain, 434
causes of, 434*f*

Cervical cancer, a malignant tumor of the cervix; the most common form of cervical cancer is a squamous cell carcinoma, arising from the epithelial cells lining the opening into the uterus, called cervical intraepithelial neoplasia or CIN, 382

Cervical conization, procedure in which a cone-shaped section of precancerous or cancerous tissue of the cervix is removed, 389

Cervical intraepithelial neoplasia, the abnormal development of cells within the cervix resulting in tumor formation, which has the potential of becoming cancerous; abbreviated CIN, 382

Cervicectomy, surgical removal of the cervix, 389

Cervicitis, inflammation of the cervix, 382

Cervix, 372

Cesarean section, an alternative to the nonsurgical birth of a child through the birth canal, birthing can be accomplished surgically by making an incision through the abdomen and uterus, abbreviated C-section, 404

CF. *See* **Cystic fibrosis**

Chalazion, an infection of an eyelid, 456

Chancres, small ulcers on the skin of the penis, a symptom of syphilis, 365, 408

Cheilitis, inflammation of the lip, 289

Cheilorrhaphy, procedure of suturing a lip, 304

Cheilosis, condition of the lip, including splitting of the lips and angles of the mouth, 289

Chemical peel, a procedure in which a chemical agent is used to remove the outer epidermal layers to treat acne, wrinkles, and sun-damaged skin, 105

Chest CT scan, diagnostic imaging of the chest by computed tomography (CT), 258, 258*f*

Chest radiograph, another term for chest X-ray, an X-ray image of the thoracic cavity used to diagnose TB, tumors, and other lung conditions, 259

Chest X-ray, X-ray image of the thoracic cavity used to diagnose TB, tumors, and other lung conditions; also called chest radiograph, 259, 259*f*

Cheyne-Stokes respiration, a sign characterized by a repeated pattern of distressed breathing with a gradual increase of deep breathing, then shallow breathing, and apnea, 241

CHF. *See* **Congestive heart failure**

Chiropractic, the field of therapy that is centered on manipulation of bones and joints, most commonly the vertebral column, 33, 143

Chiropractor, a practitioner of the field of therapy centered on manipulation of bones and joints, most commonly the vertebral column, 143

Chlamydia, the most common bacterial STI in North America, 407

Cholecystectomy, surgical removal of the gallbladder, 304

Cholecystitis, inflammation of the gallbladder, usually caused by gallstones lodged within it, 289

Cholecystogram, 305

Cholecystography, procedure of producing an X-ray image, or cholecystogram, of the gallbladder, 305

Choledochitis, inflammation of the common bile duct, 289

Choledocholithiasis, presence of stones within the common bile duct, 289

Choledocholithotomy, surgery that involves the removal of one or more obstructive gallstones from the common bile duct, 305

Cholelithiasis, generalized condition of stones lodged within the gallbladder or bile ducts, 17, 290, 290*f*

Chondrectomy, surgical removal, or excision, of the cartilage associated with a joint, 34, 143

Chondroplasty, surgical repair of cartilage, 144

Chorioamnionitis, inflammation of the amnion and the chorion, 399

Chronic, a disease of long duration, 76

Chronic fatigue, 430

Chronic obstructive pulmonary disease, general term for several different forms of pulmonary obstruction, including chronic bronchitis, bronchospasm, cystic fibrosis, and emphysema, 248

Cicatrices, 86

Cicatrix, clinical term for scar tissue, 86

CIN. *See* **Cervical intraepithelial neoplasia**

Circumcision, removal of the prepuce, or foreskin, of the penis, 52, 373, 373*f*

Cirrhosis, chronic, progressive liver disease characterized by the gradual loss of liver cells and their replacement by fat and other forms of connective tissue, 290, 290*f*

Clavicle, 120

Cleft lip, 305

Cleft palate, a congenital defect in which the bones supporting the roof of the mouth, or hard palate, fail to fuse during fetal development, leaving a space between the oral cavity and nasal cavity, 305, 400

Clinical application exercises
for blood and lymphatic system, 191–92
for cardiovascular system, 228–29
for digestive system, 314–15
for endocrine system, 496–97
for integumentary system, 110–11
for muscular and skeletal system, 151–52
for nervous system, mental health, eye, ear, 467–68
for respiratory system, 270–71
reproductive system and obstetrics, 413–14
urinary system, 353–54

Clinical psychologists, mental health professionals trained in the treatment of behavioral disorders, 428

Clinical psychology, 448

Closed fracture, 145

Clostridium botulinum, 170, 292

Clostridium tetani, 179

Coagulation time, blood test that determines the time required for a blood clot to form, 184

Coarctation of the aorta, a congenital defect characterized by aortic stenosis that is present at birth; it causes reduced systemic circulation of blood and accumulation of fluid in the lungs, 210